NEW DEVELOPMENTS IN

MYOCARDIAL IMAGING

TECHNETIUM ^{99m}Tc SESTAMIBI

NEW DEVELOPMENTS IN

MYOCARDIAL IMAGING

TECHNETIUM ^{99m}Tc SESTAMIBI

M-P Larock S H Braat H Sochor
M Maisey P Rigo

MARTIN DUNITZ

First published in 1993 by
Martin Dunitz Ltd, The Livery House, 7–9
Pratt Street, London NW1 0AE

Reprinted, with corrections, 1993
Reprinted 1994.

A CIP catalogue record for this title is available from the British Library.

ISBN 1-85317-112-3

Publisher's Note
The views expressed are those of the authors and are not necessarily those of the publisher. Clinical judgement must guide each physician in the assessment of benefits of treatment versus risk of toxicity. Certain chapters and references therein may indicate uses of drugs at dosages and for periods of time and in combinations not included in current prescribing information.

Composition by Scribe Design,
Gillingham, Kent
Origination by Adroit Photolitho Ltd,
Birmingham
Printed in Singapore for
Imago Productions (F.E.) Pte. Ltd.

CONTENTS

CONTRIBUTORS

Simon H Braat MD
Department of Cardiology, Academic Hospital Maastricht, University of Limburg, P Debyelaan 25, 6202 AZ Maastricht, The Netherlands

Marie-Paule Larock MD
Division of Nuclear Medicine, Centre Hospitalier Universitaire de Liège, Domaine Universitaire du Sart Tilman, B 35-4000 Liège 1, Belgium

Michael N. Maisey BSc MD FRCP FRCR
Professor of Radiological Sciences, United Medical and Dental Schools of Guy's and St Thomas's Hospitals, London SE1 9RT, UK

Pierre Rigo MD
Chief, Division of Nuclear Medicine, Centre Hospitalier Universitaire de Liège, Domaine Universitaire du Sart Tilman, B 35-4000 Liège 1, Belgium

Heinz Sochor MD
Associate Professor of Medicine (Cardiology), Director, Cardiovascular Nuclear Imaging, Department of Cardiology, University of Vienna Medical Centre - AKH, Währinger Gürtel 18-20, A-1090 Vienna, Austria

with a contribution to Chapter 1 from

Petra J. Jeffery MBBS
Department of Nuclear Medicine, United Medical and Dental Schools of Guy's and St Thomas's Hospitals, London SE1 9RT, UK

ACKNOWLEDGEMENT

The Authors would like to thank their colleagues and collaborators for their help in the selection of cases and in the preparation of the illustrations and of the manuscript.

FOREWORD

Nuclear cardiology has undergone continuous growth since the mid seventies. Myocardial imaging is responsible for most of this growth as it not only provides information on perfusion, but can also be used to assess myocardial function and, possibly, myocardial viability. The advance of new Tc-labelled myocardial tracers has significantly increased the potential impact of these studies as a result of improved physical properties, different biological characteristics and increased availability.

The aim of this book is to illustrate the potential applications of ^{99m}Tc sestamibi in the management of patients with a wide variety of daily occurring cardiological problems. We hope that this practical rather than theoretical approach will be of special interest both to those performing and those requesting nuclear cardiology studies.

THE EDITORS

1 INTRODUCTION TO THE BASIS OF NUCLEAR CARDIOLOGY

Nuclear Medicine in Cardiology

Cardiology was one of the earliest clinical disciplines to benefit from the application of radionuclide tracer technology. The first application of a tracer technique to the measurement of human physiological functions was in 1943 when Blumgart used the timing of a tracer injected into a peripheral vein to measure circulation times in health and disease. Subsequently this was developed by Norman Veall and others as a method of measuring cardiac output and pulmonary transit times. This has evolved into a wide variety of highly sophisticated functional imaging and measurement techniques, all of which contribute to the understanding of cardiac physiology and the management of patients with cardiac disease.

Characteristics of nuclear medicine techniques

Nuclear medicine techniques are of particular importance in cardiology, as they provide a non-invasive means of assessing functional information which complements anatomical investigations.

Non-invasive

Most nuclear medicine studies involve no more than an intravenous injection of a radiotracer – either by a rapid bolus injection for first-pass ventricular function measurements, or by an injection of a radiotracer at peak exercise for the assessment of myocardial perfusion. Consequently the morbidity and mortality of nuclear medicine studies are very low compared to more traditional anatomical investigations such as angiography.

Functional

Most of the investigational methods used in cardiology provide anatomical information about cardiac structure and vascular anatomy, whereas nuclear medicine techniques provide functional information. Nuclear medicine techniques can measure right and left ventricular contractile as well as the diastolic function, and also can directly assess myocardial perfusion. With the introduction of positron emission tomography (PET) myocardial metabolism may also be evaluated.

Scope of nuclear cardiology

Nuclear cardiology includes an extensive range of investigations for the assessment of cardiac disease but the most important areas are the measurement of ventricular function, the assessment of myocardial perfusion, the identification of myocardial infarction and the measurement of myocardial metabolism. In most clinical situations, knowledge of both normal and abnormal anatomy and physiology is crucial to the complete assessment of any clinical problem.

Ventricular function

Global and regional myocardial function may be measured by radiotracers utilizing two different methodologies. The first-pass method for measuring ventricular function requires the rapid intravenous injection of a bolus of a radiotracer ($^{99m}TcO_4$ or ^{99m}Tc-labelled red blood cells). As the bolus travels through the cardiac chambers, rapid sequence image acquisition with a gamma camera is used to measure the global ejection fractions of the right and left ventricles (Fig. 1.1). The use of cine

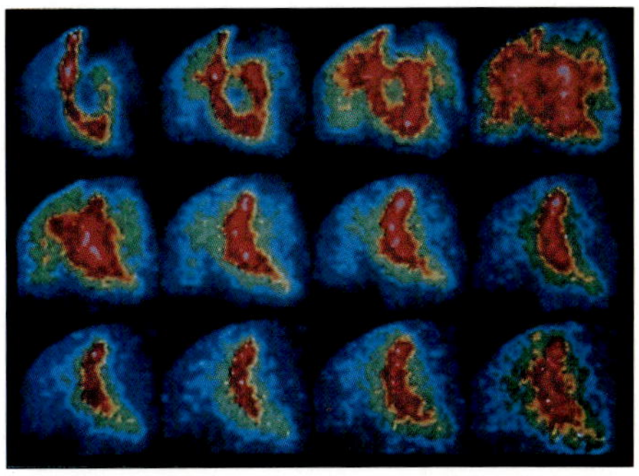

Figure 1.1
The initial images show the tracer bolus entering the right ventricle via the superior vena cava following which the lung fields and then the left ventricle are visualized.

display of the accumulated data together with computer-generated iso-count contour provides the necessary information concerning regional wall motion abnormalities (Figs. 1.2a,b,c).

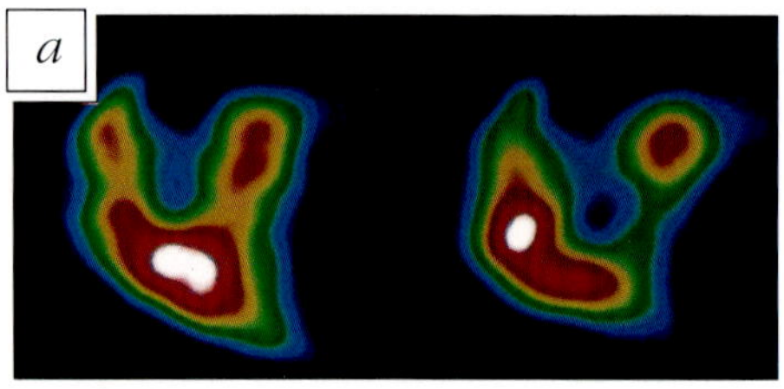

Figure 1.2a
These images show right ventricular phase of a first-pass study, left in diastole, right in systole.

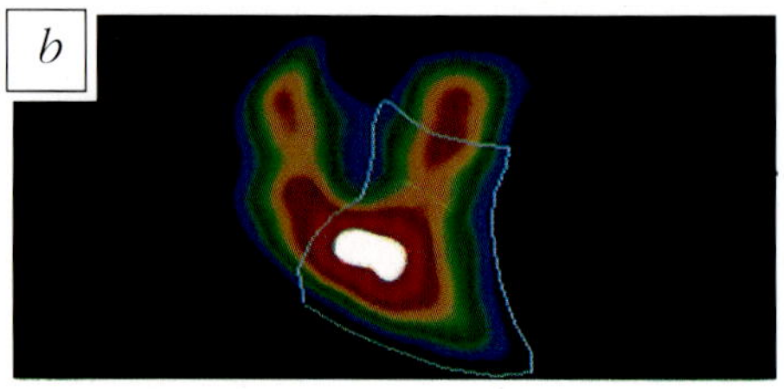

Figure 1.2b
From these images a region of interest representing the right ventricular cavity can be drawn to generate a right ventricular time–activity curve.

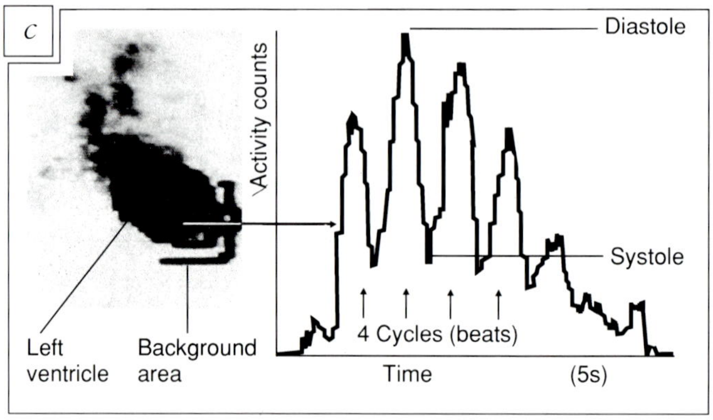

Figure 1.2c
Beat-to-beat changes in left ventricular counts are used to measure left ventricular ejection fraction (LVEF).

The alternative method of measuring ventricular function is the gated equilibrium ventriculography method. In this method a radiotracer that remains in the vascular space (usually ^{99m}Tc-labelled red blood cells) is injected intravenously and allowed to reach equilibrium. Imaging with a gamma camera displays the labelled blood-filled cardiac chambers and if the collection of data is linked ('gated') to the ECG signal of the patient (Figs. 1.3a,b,c) data can be acquired in multiple small time sections, each corresponding to a set period of the cardiac cycle. Over several hundred cardiac cycles, a dynamic image of ventricular contraction is built up. From this, measurements of ventricular contractile function, ejection fraction and diastolic function, with filling times and rates, are derived. Computer-generated cine displays allow the assessment of global and regional wall motion. By the use of Fourier transform calculations, single images (parametric images) incorporating time-related displays of atrial and ventricular volume variations (amplitude images) and the timing of wall motion contraction (phase images) can be produced (Fig. 1.4).

Myocardial perfusion

Coronary artery disease (CAD) is the single most important cardiac pathology in the adult population of the Western World. The consequence of CAD is abnormal myocardial perfusion that may result in angina, impaired myocardial function and/or myocardial infarction. Although angiography is capable of demonstrating the physical abnormalities of the coronary artery system, nuclear cardiology is the only technique able to demonstrate the consequences of coronary artery stenosis, that is, abnormalities of regional and global myocardial perfusion. This is probably the single most important measurement of the effect of CAD and will be the subject of this volume.

Myocardial infarction

Nuclear medicine techniques can be used to demonstrate both recent and old myocardial infarction. Recent

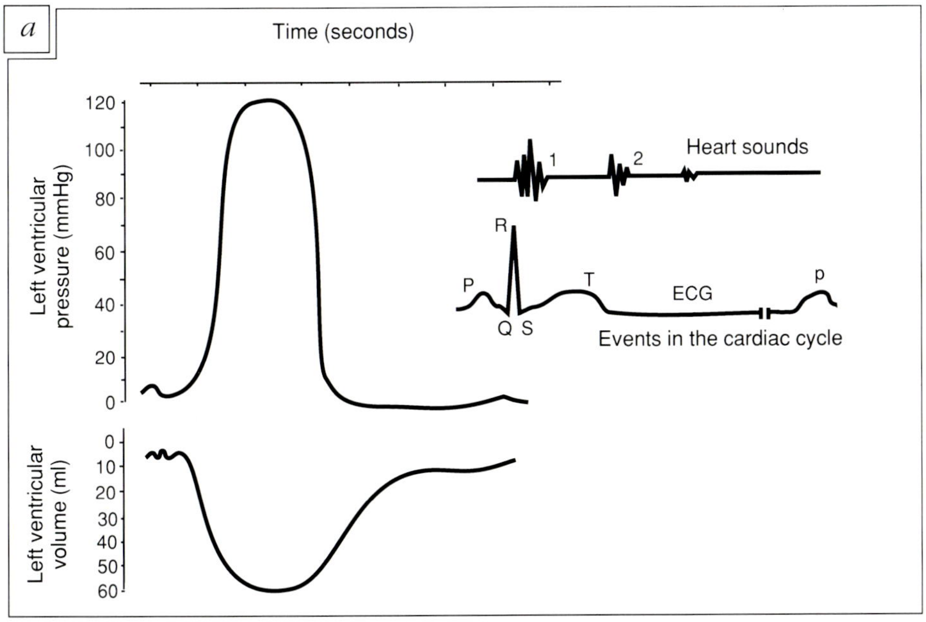

Figure 1.3a
The constant physiological relationship between electrical and mechanical phases of the heart permits the gamma camera–computer system to be linked to the ECG signal. Images from each phase of the cycle are stored until the necessary data are available to produce a statistically valid image of ventricular contraction (typically in 3–10 min).

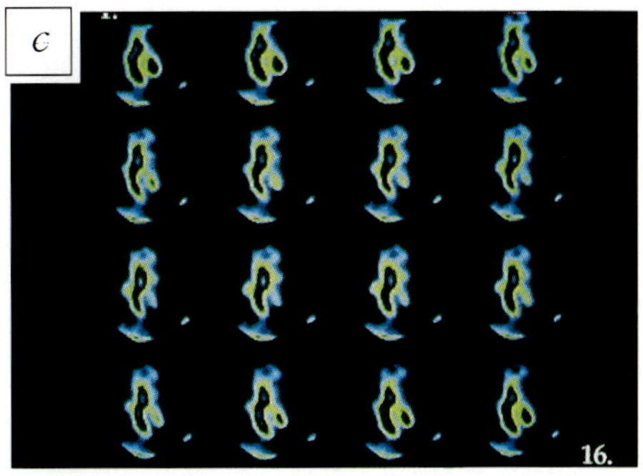

Figure 1.3c
A series of images from the left anterior oblique (LAO) view showing the volume changes during a cardiac cycle.

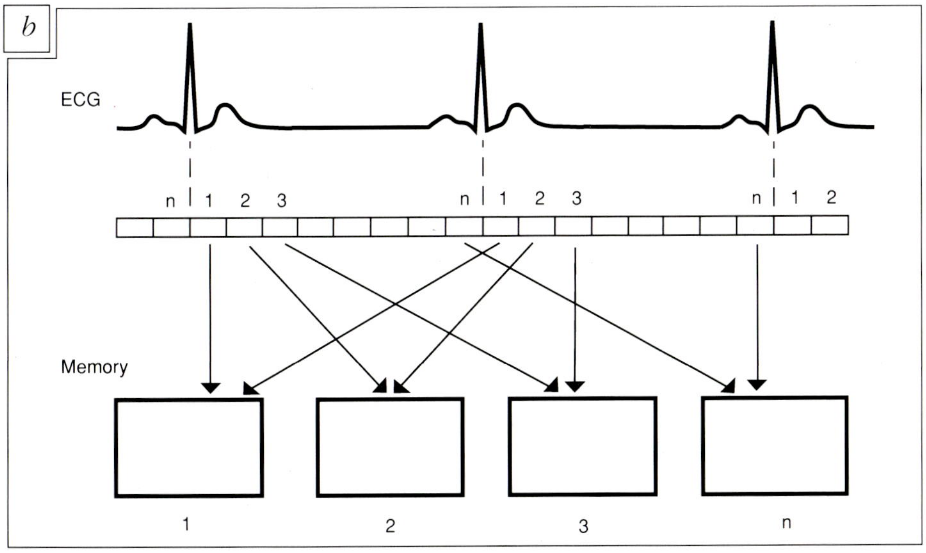

Figure 1.3b
With modern gamma cameras and computers, up to 64 intervals from each cardiac cycle can be stored until an adequate total number of counts can be collected.

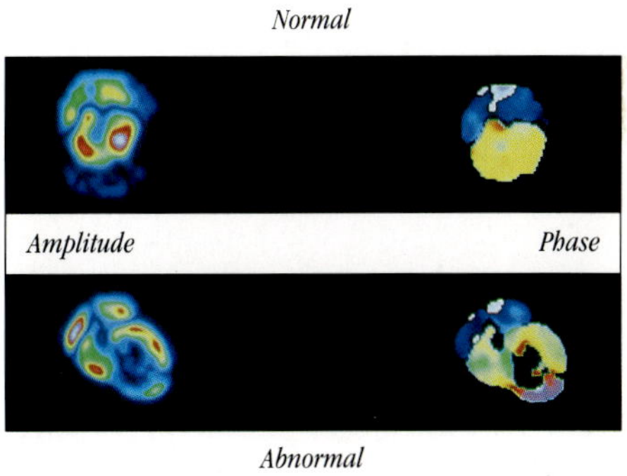

Figure 1.4
Parametric images. An aneurysm is indicated by a localized area of dyskinesis and there is often a well-defined junction between the aneurysmal zone and the more normally contracting ventricle. Usually a number of views are needed to demonstrate the aneurysm's full extent. As in this case, aneurysms are often best demonstrated using amplitude and phase images.

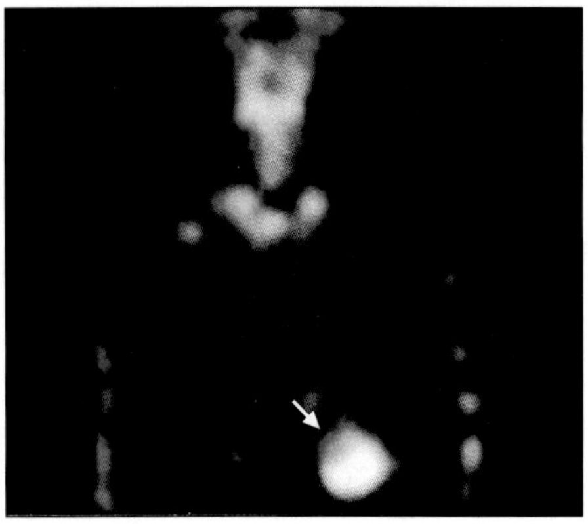

Figure 1.5
Recently infarcted myocardium that has accumulated ^{99m}Tc pyrophosphate visualized on one coronal slice after tomography (arrow).

infarcted myocardium accumulates ^{99m}Tc pyrophosphate and other bone imaging agents (Fig. 1.5). The development of superior instrumentation producing tomographic images has improved the separation of the heart from the overlying bony rib cage, which also accumulates pyrophosphate. More recently monoclonal antibodies, in particular antimyosin antibodies labelled with indium-111, have been used to demonstrate myocardial infarction of recent origin.

Both acute and chronic myocardial infarction result in loss of perfusion to part of the myocardium. Thallium-201 (^{201}Tl) or ^{99m}Tc sestamibi are both capable of identifying the site and extent of the myocardial infarct. This may be important in the diagnosis of myocardial infarction and also in the monitoring of treatment with thrombolytic and other agents (see Chapter 11).

Myocardial metabolism

The close link between myocardial perfusion and myocardial metabolism has been well known for many years. It is only with the recent extension of PET into clinical practice that the potential importance of changes in myocardial metabolism has been recognized. PET studies with ^{18}F-FDG (fluorine-18 fluorodeoxyglucose – a glucose analogue) are able to demonstrate regions of viable myocardium which would have been classified as infarcted using conventional criteria such as hypokinesis or akinesis or ECG Q-waves. This is improving the management of patients with severe CAD by identifying those who should benefit from revascularization procedures.

Cardiac Physiology

An understanding of the anatomy and physiology of the coronary circulation together with the haemodynamic effects of coronary stenosis is required to fully understand and interpret any cardiac imaging studies.

Coronary blood flow and basic anatomy

The myocardium is perfused via the coronary circulation, which consists of the right and left coronary arteries, the latter dividing into the left anterior descending and the circumflex artery (Fig. 1.6). There is a considerable amount of inter-individual variation in the relative contributions of the right and left coronary arteries. Although in man the left coronary artery predominates, three types of coronary circulation are described depending on the origin of the posterior descending branch. In 84% of cases, the posterior descending branch originates from the right coronary artery (right dominant coronary distribution), in 12% of cases, it originates from the left circumflex (left dominant coronary distribution), while in the remaining 4%, two posterior descending branches are present (balanced circulation). Collateral channels are present, which in the normal individual are potential rather than actual vessels of blood flow. These become critically important when there are significant coronary artery lesions.

Coronary flow reserve

Nuclear medicine myocardial perfusion studies are based on the concept of coronary blood flow reserve. The resting myocardial blood flow is close to 1 ml/g per min. Under conditions of stress, particularly dynamic exercise, the oxygen demand of the myocardium increases in response to the increased cardiac output. This in turn produces coronary vasodilatation. The difference between the resting myocardial blood flow and the myocardial blood flow when the coronary vasculature is maximally dilated is known as the coronary flow reserve. Regional coronary flow reserve is the first parameter to be compromised

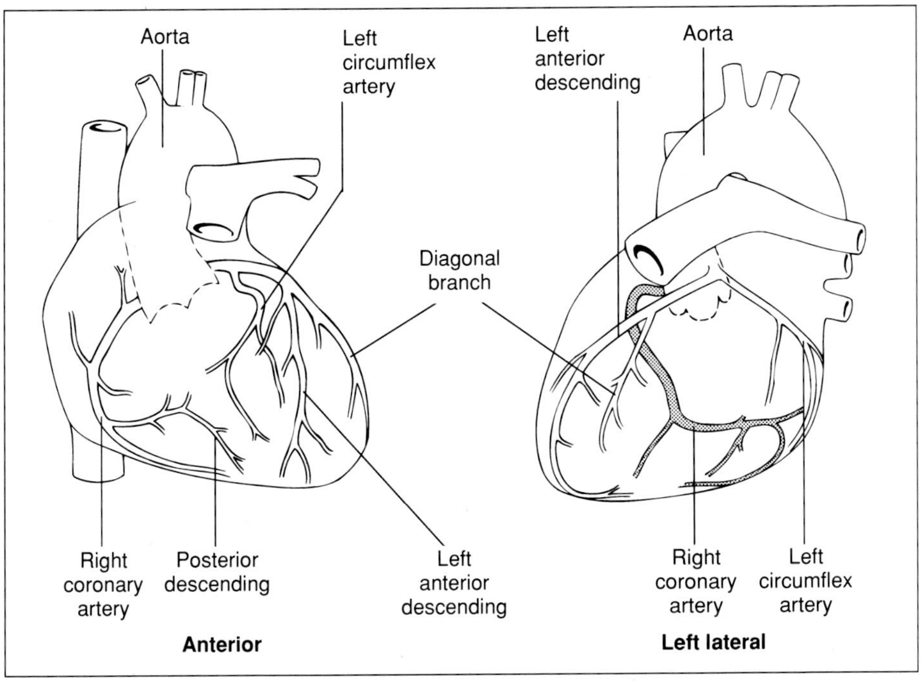

Figure 1.6
Diagram of the normal coronary arteries.

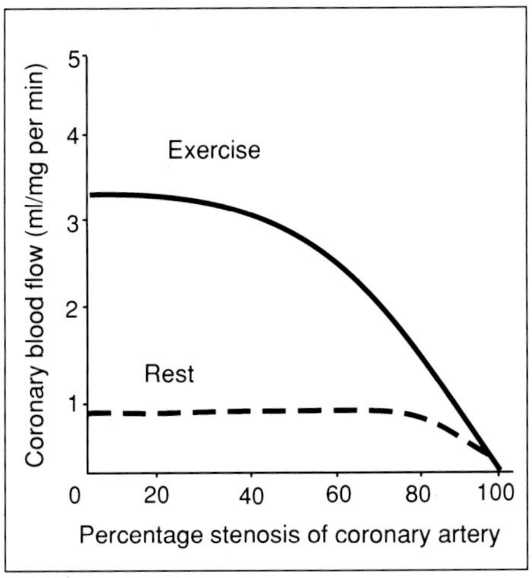

Figure 1.7
The effect of coronary narrowing on the coronary blood flow at rest (bottom) and during maximal contrast-induced hyperaemia (top).

when there is a stenotic lesion of a coronary artery (Fig. 1.7). A coronary lesion needs to affect approximately 90% of the luminal area before it reduces myocardial perfusion at rest. However, a 40–50% stenosis will decrease the measured coronary reserve. Consequently most protocols which aim to demonstrate early coronary artery lesions by perfusion imaging utilize techniques that increase coronary blood flow and thus unmask focally diminished flow reserve.

Effect of exercise on coronary blood flow

Dynamic physical exercise can potentially increase resting coronary blood flow by a factor of 2–3. Whether this flow increase will be achieved depends on many factors including the individual patient's ability to exercise maximally. Often exercise tolerance is restricted by factors such as dyspnoea, fatigue, claudication and arthritis as well as chest pain. Isometric exercise also increases blood flow, but to a lesser extent. When a stenotic coronary lesion is present the blood flow distal to the lesion cannot increase to the same degree as that in areas supplied by normal coronary arteries. This produces an apparent 'defect' – really an area of diminished coronary reserve. Myocardial ischaemia, whether exercise-induced or spontaneous, can also result from an absolute reduction in regional myocardial blood flow.

Effect of drugs on coronary blood flow

It is also possible to increase coronary blood flow using drugs. The drugs used to do this include dipyridamole (Persantin), dobutamine and adenosine.

Dipyridamole Dipyridamole given intravenously in a dose of 0.56 mg/kg is capable of increasing the coronary blood flow five-fold. The mechanism of action of dipyridamole is not fully elucidated, but probably involves an increase in local adenosine levels (see later). When combined with light exercise (isometric or gentle dynamic exercise such as walking on the spot) it is capable of increasing the coronary blood flow still further.

Adenosine Adenosine is produced naturally by myocardial cells in response to hypoxia or increased oxygen demand. It is a potent vasodilator, acting on specific adenosine receptors. This produces a rise in intracellular cAMP levels which in turn leads to vascular smooth muscle relaxation. Exogenously administered adenosine produces the same but more marked effect by the same mechanism.

Dobutamine Dobutamine given intravenously has predominately β_1 agonist activity. It produces a dose-related increase in myocardial oxygen demand, mainly through increases in pulse rate and blood pressure and increases coronary blood flow approximately two-fold.

Myocardial metabolism

The primary energy source of the normal myocardium is fatty acids and, to a lesser extent, carbohydrates; lactate, pyruvate, ketone bodies and amino acids are also utilized in small amounts. The exact relationship between these energy sources in the normal myocardium depends upon such factors as dietary state and insulin level, with increasing glycolysis in the post-prandial, hyperinsulinaemic state. With increasing myocardial ischaemia, there is a shift in metabolism from an emphasis on fatty acid metabolism to an increasing dependence on glucose metabolism. As the severity of the ischaemia increases, anaerobic glycolytic metabolism will be enhanced. It has been shown that severely ischaemic myocardium may still receive sufficient perfusion to permit anaerobic or even aerobic glycolysis to take place. However, with the most severe ischaemia, accumulation of lactate and other by-products will finally inhibit glycolysis.

Relationship of flow, metabolism and function

Normal ventricular contraction depends on normal tissue perfusion, enabling the delivery of essential substrates and the removal of waste products of metabolism. With severe ischaemia this balance may be disturbed, resulting in decreased or absent contractility shown by the usual investigative criteria (for example, gated isotope angiograms, ultrasound) and even the presence of Q-waves on the ECG. The residual blood flow and substrate delivery may be sufficient to maintain some myocardial cell viability due to the reduction in oxygen demand.

Hibernating and stunned myocardium

Two important situations are often referred to as hibernating myocardium and stunned myocardium. Hibernating myocardium occurs when coronary artery disease has chronically caused such a severe reduction in myocardial perfusion that contraction ceases through insufficient energy production even though the tissue remains viable. Under these circumstances cell integrity is maintained by an almost complete switch from fatty acid metabolism to glycolytic metabolism – largely anaerobic. With reversal of the perfusion abnormality by a revascularizing procedure, flow and hence delivery of substrates returns, resulting in normal or improved ventricular contraction. In clinical practice this means it is critically important to identify myocardium which appears infarcted but is in fact viable. Failure to do this may deny a patient a revascularization procedure which may significantly improve ventricular function.

'Stunned myocardium' is the term applied to non-infarcted myocardium that fails to regain contractility following reversal of an acute ischaemic event (either spontaneous or following medical thrombolysis or angioplasty). Under these circumstances the perfusion may be normal but the acute ischaemic damage has caused temporary but reversible functional changes resulting in loss of contractility. With time the functions may return to normal and contractility may return. As with hibernating myocardium some of the conventional diagnostic procedures may suggest myocardial infarction. Table 1.1 demonstrates the perfusion, metabolic and contractility findings in normal, hibernating and stunned myocardium. If hibernating myocardium is clinically suspected, even in the presence of an apparent

Myocardial condition	Flow	Metabolism	Contraction
Normal	Normal	Fatty acid > aerobic glycolytic	Normal
Hibernating	Very low/apparent absence	Predominantly glycolytic aerobic/anaerobic	Severe hypo-/akinesis
Stunned	Normal/decreased	Oxidative metabolism is usually depressed	Severe hypo-/akinesis

Table 1.1
Perfusion, metabolism and contraction in hibernating and stunned myocardium.

myocardial infarction, evaluation can be performed using either thallium rest injection or re-injection techniques or PET. Thallium re-injection techniques may show uptake of thallium in regions seen to have low or absent perfusion on redistribution images. Reversible perfusion abnormalities are also seen on sestamibi studies. PET is more sensitive, however, and uptake of ^{18}F-FDG confirms the viability of the underlying tissue in spite of absent flow and contractility.

Myocardial Perfusion Agents

Historical development of nuclear medicine techniques for the assessment of myocardial perfusion

Early studies into myocardial perfusion in the 1960s involved the injection of radiolabelled microspheres into the left ventricle or preferably the left atrium, or into the coronary arteries at the time of invasive catheterization. Labelled microspheres are completely cleared from the blood during their first passage through the first capillary bed of the coronary artery circulation (100% extraction fraction). By using different radioactive labels – one for microspheres injected into the right coronary artery and one for microspheres injected into the left coronary artery – differential regional perfusion can be assessed with great accuracy. Fractionation of cardiac output into the different vascular beds can also be assessed by this technique. This technology remains the gold standard for the assessment of myocardial perfusion. However, it is invasive and consequently cannot be used in the routine clinical assessment of patients with CAD.

Next, radiotracers that are taken up by the myocardium in proportion to local blood flow were evaluated. These have largely been based on analogues of potassium and have included caesium-131, rubidium-82, as well as potassium-43. By far the most successful has been thallium-201, which was introduced in 1975 and until recently has been the standard clinical method for investigating myocardial perfusion.

Mechanisms of myocardial radiotracer uptake

Radiotracers are generally distributed in the myocardium in proportion to local myocardial blood flow. This may occur via several mechanisms, dependent upon the radiopharmaceutical involved.

1 Complete first pass uptake/clearance from the coronary blood during its passage through the myocardium, for example, radiolabelled microspheres trapped in the coronary microcirculation.
2 A proportion of the tracer may be extracted from the coronary blood on each pass through the coronary circulation and may remain in the myocardium with no significant subsequent wash-out; examples are sestamibi and ammonia.

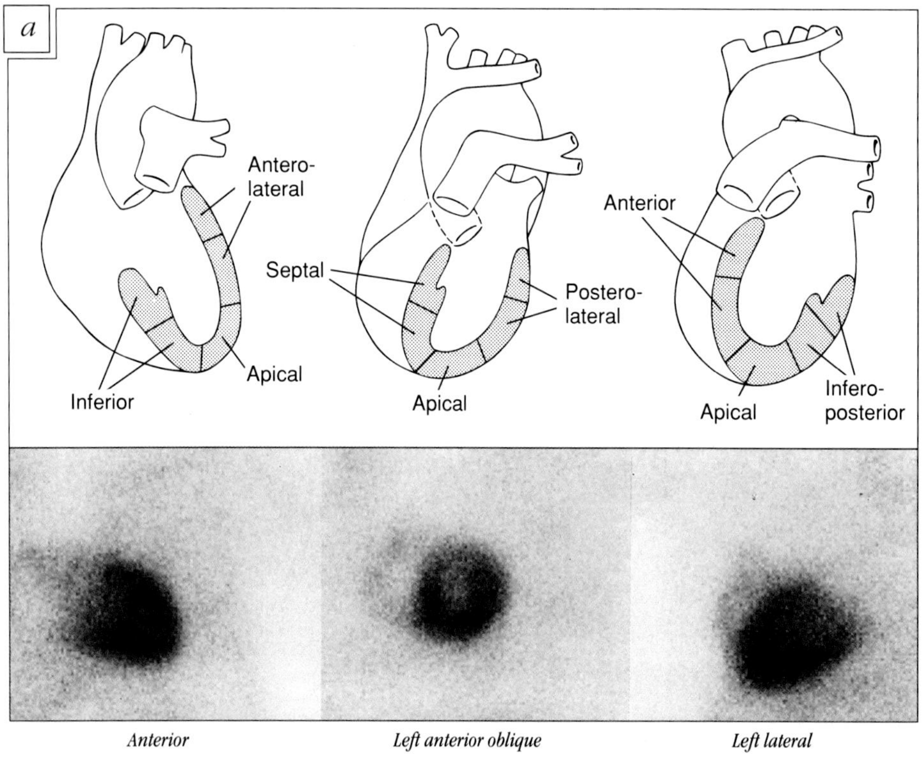

Figure 1.8a
Segmentation of the myocardial planar views. With planar imaging, the most useful views are the anterior, a 45° left anterior oblique, and a 70° left anterior oblique, or a left lateral.

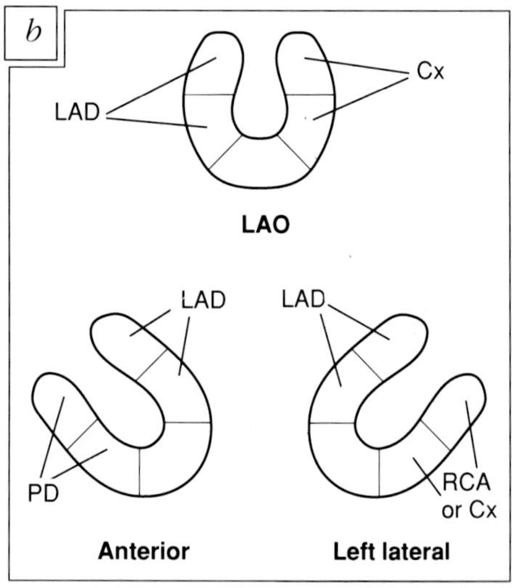

Figure 1.8b
The relationship of the myocardium to the normal coronary supply.

3 A proportion of the radiotracer may be extracted by the myocardium from the coronary blood taken up into the myocardial cell and then released in dynamic equilibrium with the tracer in the blood. An example of this is ^{201}Tl which is shown together with the relationship of the myocardium to the normal coronary supply in Figs. 1.8a,b.

Extraction fraction

The extraction fraction of any radiopharmaceutical is the fraction of the radiopharmaceutical extracted from the coronary blood flow during one passage through the myocardium. Table 1.2 shows the extraction fractions of commonly used radiopharmaceuticals. The extraction fraction is not the same as the percentage uptake in the myocardium. A radiopharmaceutical that is taken up and fixed in the myocardium will gradually 'build up'. Therefore the percentage of injected dose taken up by the heart may be much greater with these perfusion tracers than with those that are extracted but re-equilibrate.

Relationship of uptake to coronary blood flow

The ideal radiopharmaceutical to measure regional coronary blood flow

Radiopharmaceutical	Extraction fraction (%)	Significant decrease in extraction fraction at high flow rates?
Radiolabelled microspheres	100	No
Thallium	85–88	Yes
Sestamibi	50–65	Yes
$H_2{}^{15}O$ (water)	95	No
Ammonia	70	Yes
Rubidium	50–60	Yes

Table 1.2
Extraction fractions of commonly used pharmaceuticals.

will be taken up in direct linear proportion to myocardial perfusion over a wide range of flow values, unaffected by changes in cellular metabolism. This is not the case with most radiopharmaceuticals which have extraction fractions <100%. Usually there is a reasonably linear relationship between flow and uptake over the physiological range of coronary blood flow, but with increased flow, for example, with stress, the extraction fraction decreases as shown in Fig. 1.9.

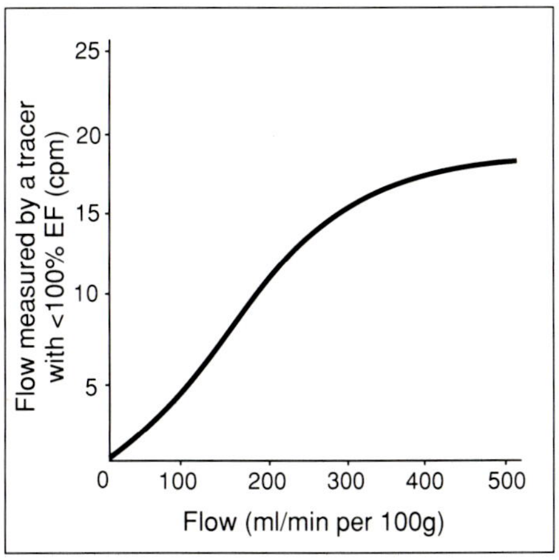

Figure 1.9
The relationship between flow and uptake over the physiological range of coronary blood flow. The extraction fraction (EF) decreases as the flow increases, hence uptake will underestimate flow at high flow rates.

The ideal myocardial perfusion agent

The properties of an ideal radiopharmaceutical for myocardial perfusion are shown in Table 1.3. ^{201}Tl falls short of these ideal properties in several respects, including extraction fraction of less than 100%, a relatively low energy resulting in unnecessary scatter and attenuation, and a half-life that significantly exceeds the measurement time. For this and other reasons a more suitable agent, particularly one that is labelled with the most widely used radiotracer technetium-99m (^{99m}Tc), has been sought.

Toxicity/dosimetry
Non-toxic pharmaceutical in doses administered
Isotope with half-life approximately equal to the study duration
Isotope with pure low–medium energy gamma emission
Significant proportion of injected dose taken up into myocardium
Low uptake into organs with carcinogenic/teratogenic potential, e.g. gonads
No known interaction with cardiac medications/dipyridamole

Perfusion agent ideals
Extraction fraction = 100%
Uptake directly proportional to myocardial blood flow over physiological and supra-physiological range

Imaging
Isotope emitting gamma rays of optimal energy for detection with standard gamma camera (i.e. *c.* 140 keV)
High heart/background ratio
No redistribution from heart during the period of imaging

Economic
Capable of simple in-house preparation
Cheap

Table 1.3
Properties of the 'ideal' myocardial perfusion agent.

^{99m}Tc sestamibi is a technetium-labelled myocardial perfusion agent that is taken up by the myocardial cell in proportion to myocardial regional blood flow and remains fixed in the myocardial cell over a long period of time. It has many logistical and imaging advantages over ^{201}Tl that will be discussed more fully in subsequent sections. Although thallium and sestamibi remain agents that can be used widely because of available instrumentation, PET techniques are important for the assessment of myocardial perfusion in specific circumstances. One of the advantages of PET perfusion imaging is its ability to produce high resolution quantitative flow images that can be matched exactly with metabolic abnormalities.

Relationship of myocardial perfusion imaging to other cardiac diagnostic methods

Often clinical assessment of patients from their history, and to a lesser extent physical examination, will be sufficient to make a diagnosis of CAD causing myocardial ischaemia. This is based largely on a history of chest pain typical of angina with known risk factors, which together may provide a diagnostic accuracy of >95%. In these instances further investigation will be directed at the extent and the severity of disease, the prognostic stratification and the choice of therapy. In other patients with less clear or ambiguous histories and/or examinations, imaging is required for diagnosis.

Exercise testing

By far the most widely used method to investigate myocardial ischaemia is the ECG in association with exercise stress testing. The advantages of this method are its wide availability and relatively low cost. It suffers from poor sensitivity and specificity and provides only limited information regarding the localization and extent of disease. The exercise test may be combined with myocardial perfusion studies using either ^{201}Tl or sestamibi, which considerably improves the diagnostic accuracy.

Ultrasound

Modern cardiac ultrasound techniques increasingly provide information on myocardial ischaemia by detecting regions of hypo- or akinesis with the patient either at rest or under stress, for example, when receiving dobutamine.

Angiography

The gold standard for the diagnosis of coronary artery disease remains coronary angiography. Coronary angiography indicates the site and extent of coronary artery disease but only provides limited information on the effects of vascular stenoses on the myocardium, and the ability of collateral blood flow to compensate. The determination of coronary artery lesions by angiography remains largely subjective, although newer techniques employing digitization improve objectivity. Techniques to measure the shape and length of coronary lesions – factors that have a significant effect on the distal blood flow – are only at early stages of development.

Radionuclide angiography

Decreased myocardial perfusion results in impairment of myocardial contractility. Non-invasive methods of assessing left ventricular function such as stressed first-pass and gated equilibrium blood pool scans may therefore be used to diagnose and assess the consequences of coronary artery lesions. The first-pass technique in particular may become increasingly important as it can be combined with myocardial perfusion studies when a technetium-labelled radiopharmaceutical such as sestamibi is used. These methods depend critically on the ability of the individual patient to achieve maximum workloads with exercise. Furthermore, although the presence of exercise-induced wall motion abnormalities has been shown to be a sensitive predictor of the presence of CAD, it is not specific and can result from many other cardiac pathological conditions.

Positron emission tomography

PET techniques using ^{18}F-FDG for metabolism and rubidium-82 or $^{13}NH_3$ (ammonia) for perfusion can be regarded as potential competitors with single photon myocardial perfusion methods. Ammonia and rubidium are both accurate quantitative methods for measuring myocardial perfusion. PET scans using FDG will demonstrate the effect of perfusion abnormalities on the balance between fatty acid and glucose uptake. It is unlikely that PET will have a major role in diagnosing and assessing perfusion abnormalities in clinical practice due to the limited availability and expense of the technique. It should therefore be restricted to well-defined clinical problems that cannot be answered by conventional imaging methods.

Sestamibi

Pharmacology of sestamibi

Structure and chemistry

Sestamibi belongs to a family of hexakisisonitrile compounds which have been investigated for their ability to be taken up and fixed into the myocardial tissue in proportion to regional myocardial blood flow. The structure of ^{99m}Tc sestamibi is shown in Fig. 1.10. Once it has entered the myocardium, it remains trapped, probably in the mitochondria as a result of the transmembrane potential gradient.

The effective dose equivalent for an injected total of 1480 MBq cardiac stress and rest study is 12.2 mSv. Sestamibi can be prepared simply and quickly in any radiopharmacy from pyrogen-free vials and ^{99m}Tc pertechnetate, as compared to ^{201}Tl which must be obtained to order.

Whole body distribution

The whole body distribution of sestamibi following intravenous injection is shown in Fig. 1.11. If the radiotracer is injected immediately following exercise there is increased myocardial uptake. Table 1.4 shows the percentage uptake at exercise and rest following intravenous sestamibi injection. Myocardial imaging is usually optimal 1–2 h after injection following the clearance from liver and lung.

Sestamibi is excreted via the hepatobiliary system and the kidneys. The emptying of radiotracer from the gallbladder may be accelerated by eating after injection.

Comparison of sestamibi with other agents

Due to the most favourable dosimetry characteristics of ^{99m}Tc over ^{201}Tl, a much higher dose can be administered. This higher photon flux

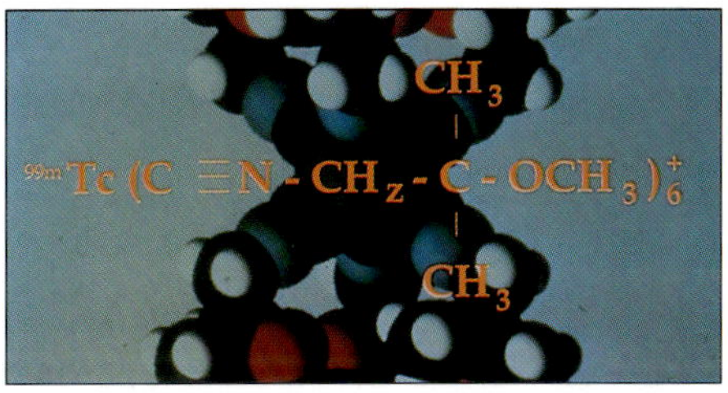

Figure 1.10
The structure of ^{99m}Tc sestamibi.

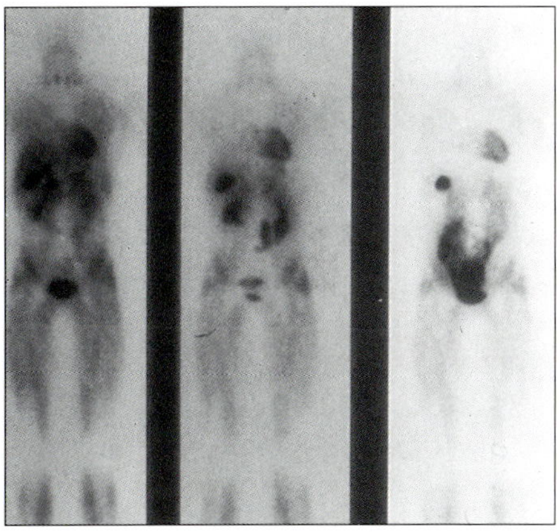

Figure 1.11
Whole body distribution of sestamibi: initial injection (left panel); 1 h after injection (middle panel); 4 h after injection (right panel).

Table 1.4
*Whole body distribution of sestamibi at rest and after exercise given as the mean percentage of the injected dose. (Adapted from Wackers et al, J Nucl Med (1989) **30**: 301–311.)*

Organ	Rest			Exercise		
	5 min	60 min	240 min	5 min	60 min	240 min
Heart	1.2	1.0	0.8	1.5	1.4	1.0
Lung	2.6	0.9	0.4	2.7	1.4	0.3
Liver	19.6	5.6	0.7	5.9	2.4	0.3
Gallbladder	1.2	3.5	2.7	0.6	2.5	2.6
Kidney	13.6	6.7	3.9	10.6	6.7	3.3
Thyroid	0.2	0.2	0.1	0.06	0.2	0.1
Leg muscles	10.1	11.1	10.9	21.2	22.2	22.5
Bladder	5.6	8.7	2.6	2.5	2.6	0.9
Spleen	2.5	1.0	0.1	1.0	0.4	0.1

along with the better imaging characteristics (from 140 keV photons as opposed to 68–82 keV for ^{201}Tl) significantly improves image quality and enables first-pass studies to be performed if required. Table 1.5 compares the characteristics of an ideal radiopharmaceutical with those of sestamibi and thallium.

Imaging methodology with sestamibi

Cardiac nuclear medicine is the most complex of all nuclear medicine techniques and careful attention to detail in all aspects of the methodology is essential to achieve optimum results.

Patient preparation

Patient preparation is very important in cardiac studies. Preparation includes:

Drug withdrawal If clinically appropriate beta-blockers should ideally be withdrawn for 48 h prior to the study. Failure to do so may jeopardise the exercise test by decreasing exercise capacity and maximum heart rate achievable, and hence the increased oxygen demand which produces the vasodilatation. Other drugs that need to be withdrawn are the methylxanthine-based drugs, for example, theophylline, and also food and drink containing caffeine and caffeine-like compounds (Table 1.6). This is particularly true if a dipyridamole-stimulated myocardial perfusion study is known to be scheduled. Unfortunately this may not always be known in advance and patients who

Property	'Ideal'	Thallium	Sestamibi
Toxicity	None	None	None
Effective dose equivalent (EDE) for standard study	Lowest EDE/ dose ratio	25 mSv per 80 MBq	12.2 mSv per 1480 MBq
Half-life	4–6 h	73.5 h	6.02 h
Mode of decay	All gamma	>99% gamma	>99% gamma
Energy of gamma emission	120–169 keV	68–80 keV	140 keV
Extraction fraction (EF)	100%	85–88%	50–65%
Linearity of uptake	Over all flow rates	↓EF at high flow	↓EF at high flow
Myocardial uptake	High	3.5–4.5%	1–1.5%
Organ to background ratio	High stress and rest	Moderate stress, poor at rest	Moderate stress and rest
Redistribution	None	Significant	None
Mode production	In-house	Cyclotron	In-house
Cost	Cheap	Moderate	Moderate

Table 1.5
Comparison between sestamibi, thallium and an ideal myocardial perfusion pharmaceutical.

Methylxanthine drugs	Caffeine-containing foods	Non-prescription drugs containing caffeine
Aminophylline	Coffee	Anacin
Choline theophyllinate	Tea	Midol
Enpropyllin	Chocolate	Excedrin
Oxpentifylline	Bananas	Vanquish
Theophylline preparations:	Cola drinks	No-Doz
Theo-Dur		Pro Plus
Slo-phyllin		Cold remedies
Elixophyllin		
Nuelin		
Uniphyllin		
Franol		

Table 1.6
Medications that counteract dipyridamole.

First study	Second study	Dose sestamibi	Waiting period between injections (min)
Rest	Stress	Rest 259 MBq Stress 925 MBq	100
Stress	Rest	Stress 259 MBq Rest 925 MBq	100

Table 1.7
Schemata for one-day protocols. All scans are performed 60 min post injection. Each acquisition takes 30 min.

are not capable of adequate exercise may need to be switched to a dipyridamole study at the last moment. Prior preparation by caffeine withdrawal for a minimum of 4–6 h (preferably 18) will enable this to be performed without re-scheduling. Even small amounts of caffeine from drugs, food or drink may significantly impair the pharmacological action of dipyridamole.

Fasting The patient should arrive fasted or after having only a light breakfast.

Patient information Patients will be advised as to what will be involved in the test and to come suitably dressed (light clothing and trainers).

Exercise equipment

Generally, it is agreed that treadmill exercise is more physiological. More patients are able to achieve maximum exercise targets with treadmills than with bicycle ergometers, which are only really effective for individuals who have ridden bicycles regularly.

Choice of schedule

Sestamibi perfusion imaging can be performed either on one or two days.

Two-day protocol A basic protocol for sestamibi imaging is a two-day protocol in which patients have a maximum exercise or dipyridamole sestamibi study on the first day. This is compared with a rest study performed the following day when the sestamibi is injected at rest and imaging performed 1–2 h later. This has logistical and patient compliance problems and investigations have shown that a one-day protocol provides comparable information and is generally being adopted.

One-day protocol Both rest and stress studies may be performed on the same day. Depending on the scheduling and image processing logistics of a department the exercise study can be performed first. If this is entirely normal patients do not need to proceed to a rest study. Alternatively, it may be more convenient to perform the rest study, followed by the exercise test. In this case, all patients will have to undergo both studies. Table 1.7 compares protocols performing the exercise study first and rest study second and vice versa with the relevant doses and waiting times.

Assessing myocardial perfusion reserve

Establish free intravenous access in large forearm vein of right arm. Establish baseline ECG, heart rate and blood pressure and monitor during test.

Exercise testing Maximum achievable exercise should be undertaken according to a standard treadmill or ergometer protocol. The exercise end points are the same as standard exercise testing (chest pain, 90% maximal heart rate, excessive ST depression on ECG or fatigue/dyspnoea) as well as the contraindications. Inject 185–740 MBq as a bolus at 90% of maximum predicted heart rate using an indwelling intravenous catheter (one study = two injections, maximum of 1480 MBq). A first pass study can be performed with the sestamibi injection and provide added information of ejection fraction and ventricular function. In this case inject 740–925 MBq. Injection of sestamibi should be 60–90 s prior to cessation of exercise wherever possible.

Dipyridamole protocol Dipyridamole enables patients who cannot achieve maximum exercise to undergo myocardial perfusion imaging. The usual protocol is shown in Table 1.8. Dipyridamole stimulation differs from exercise testing in that it is predominantly based on coronary artery dilatation rather than increased oxygen demand. Exercise testing increases the uptake into skeletal muscle and hence lowers the blood background radioactivity at the time of imaging, improving image quality. In addition, performing dynamic exercise allows simultaneous assessment of the patient's exercise capacity. This is particularly relevant when perfusion abnormalities are associated with low levels of exercise. Dipyridamole is injected according to the standard protocol.

Image acquisition and processing

Planar or single photon emission computed tomography

Both planar or single photon emission computed tomography (SPECT) studies are appropriate and acceptable methods for imaging. Generally when SPECT is available and the quality control is adequate, this is to be preferred.

Time delay before imaging

The usual recommended time is to wait at least 1 h following the injection. In many patients the hepatobiliary clearance is sufficiently fast to undertake imaging within 15 or 30 min of the injection; this is particularly the case following exercise. Before imaging, a light meal should be eaten to empty the gallbladder and encourage clearance from the liver.

Role of cardiac gating in myocardial perfusion studies

ECG cardiac gating can become a normal part of myocardial imaging because of the improved count rates with the technetium-labelled compound, particularly with multiheaded cameras. Thallium studies have been performed with cardiac gating but have never shown significant advantage and therefore have not become routine practice. There are two benefits to gating myocardial perfusion studies. Firstly, by removing the blurring effect of the contracting myocardium the resolution is increased, and secondly, wall motion

1. Establish indication for dipyridamole and lack of contraindications (asthma, known hypersensitivity to dipyridamole, severe unstable angina, ingestion of xanthines/caffeine).
2. Insert large intravenous line into right antecubital fossa. Attach ECG leads and perform baseline ECG/blood pressure.
3. Draw up dose of dipyridamole: 0.56 mg/kg.
4. Inject slowly by manual injection or infuser pump over 4 min with continuous ECG monitoring. Blood pressure and full 12 lead ECG should be performed every 1–2 min.
5. Where possible perform low-grade dynamic exercise (e.g. walking on the spot) or isometric exercise (e.g.handgrip) for 6 min.
6. Inject 185–740 MBq sestamibi 4 min after completion of dipyridamole infusion. Continue exercise for a further 2 min.
7. Commence standard scanning protocol as soon as possible.

Table 1.8
Dipyridamole protocol. Note that if it is clinically necessary due to severe or continued chest pain, 125–250 mg aminophylline can be administered as a slow bolus. If possible, administration of aminophylline should be delayed for at least 1 min after the sestamibi injection. Aminophylline reverses the effect of dipyridamole.

and global function can be assessed. Functional data planar studies may be routinely gated without increasing the length of acquisition time. They can then be displayed in a cine mode for the assessment of global and wall motion or various algorithms may be used to display this information in a single functional image. Functional data from SPECT imaging are being investigated. Gating a SPECT study is technically more difficult but it is likely that this will become a routine part of SPECT myocardial imaging with technetium agents.

Planar method details

Non-gated

Collimator: High resolution parallel hole or low-energy all-purpose.
Matrix: 128 × 128
Zoom: 1.5 (range 1–2) 50% of diameter of field of view (depending on size of field of view)
Projections: LAO (30–45°) Ant, LAO 70° or LL
Window: Use 15–20% technetium-99m (140 keV) window

Gated

Collimator: High resolution parallel hole or low-energy all-purpose.
Matrix: 64 × 64 or 128 × 128
Frames: 16
Interval: R–R/16
Time: >10 min
Projections: LAO, Ant, LL
Window: Use 15–20% technetium-99m (140 keV) window
Zoom: 1.5 (range 1–2) 50% of diameter of field of view (depending on size of field of view)

Image processing

Qualitative imaging: With and without background subtraction
View black and white images (colour images optional)
Circumferential profile analysis
Normalize to maximum signal in myocardium
Amplitude, phase and ejection fraction optional if first-pass or gated acquisitions performed

SPECT method details

Image acquisition

Collimator: High resolution parallel hole or low-energy all-purpose
Matrix: 64 × 64
Timing: 30 s/stop (259 MBq: 7 mCi)
20 s/stop (925 MBq: 25 mCi)
Projections: 30–60
180° RAO (45°)–LPO (45°)
Slice thickness: 1 pixel
Filters: Butterworth – third-order 0.5 Nyquist frequency (NY)
Attenuation correction: None
Decay correction: Yes

Image processing

Filtering: Interplane or slice
Slice thickness: 1–2 pixels
Thresholding: None
Reconstruction: Double angle
Images: Horizontal long, vertical long and short axes

Displays A standard colour or black and white scale can be used, displaying to the maximum in each set of images. It is advised that once a satisfactory scale has been found this is then adhered to, as changing schemes tends to increase the risk of false-positive or -negative interpretations.

Quantitation

Both planar and SPECT studies can be displayed and assessed semi-quantitatively. For planar imaging isocount displays can be related to a normal patient database. The commonest method of quantification of SPECT studies uses polar maps, which can be qualitative or semi-quantitative and can also relate to a patient database. Quantitation and display background subtraction methods should be related to sestamibi and not to thallium protocols. Similarly the quantitative assessment should be compared to a database of normal studies with sestamibi rather than thallium.

Polar maps Polar maps are a diagrammatic way of displaying the distribution of the radiotracer in the myocardium in a standard format, which allows inter-subject comparisons. The maps are produced by a variety of softwares, using the short axis slices. The slices are re-sized and displayed as a series of concentric circles with the most apical slice in the centre, and the most basal outside (Figs. 1.12a.b). With this display, the same short axis orientation is kept, that is, septum on the left, anterior wall on top, etc. These are conventionally displayed in colour, normalizing for maximal counts in both the stress and rest studies. The stress and rest maps can be subtracted to produce a 're-perfusion map'. By comparing the normalized count distribution to a 'mean' polar map obtained from a series of age-matched volunteers, further maps can be produced showing areas of myocardium where perfusion is less

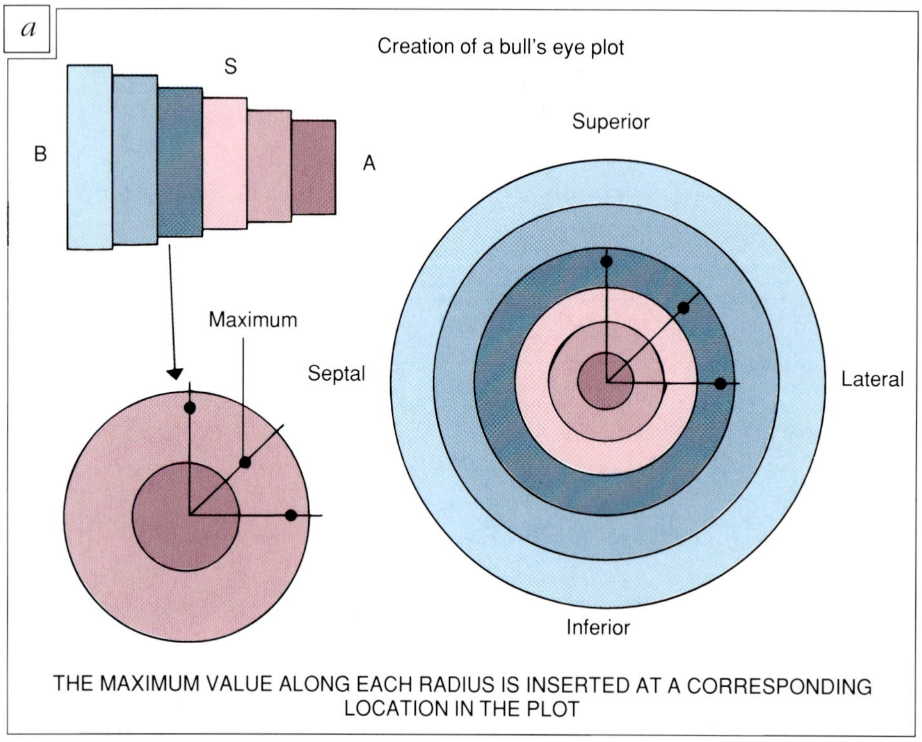

Figure 1.12a
Specific techniques have been developed which provide valuable quantification of abnormalities, for example the 'bull's eye technique' for the display of short axis SPECT images.

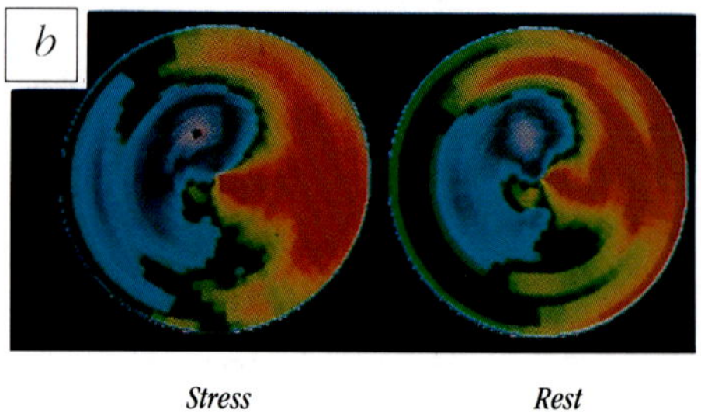

Figure 1.12b
In this case the blue represents decreased perfusion in the septum with very little change in total ischaemic area between rest and exercise.

than two standard deviations from the mean. While these displays are undoubtedly very useful, it must be noted that they should not be used alone without reference to the original images. In particular, due to the re-sizing of the slices, the extent of the lesions cannot be assessed.

Quality control

Centre of rotation and field uniformity With SPECT imaging, it is vitally important that regular centre of rotation checks and corrections are made, preferably weekly. High count (20 million) flood field uniformity checks should also be made regularly, with daily 1–5 million count floods. The variation for a SPECT flood field should be <2% to minimize artefact. Planar imaging will tolerate up to 5%.

2 BASIS OF IMAGE INTERPRETATION

This chapter will look at normal planar and single photon emission computed tomography (SPECT) myocardial perfusion images, as well as some of the normal variations that may be seen. Typical examples of commonly seen pathological abnormalities will be reviewed.

Normal Sestamibi Perfusion Study

Normal planar study

Figures 2.1a and 2.1b show a typical normal planar study using four views: anterior (ANT), left anterior oblique 40° (LAO 40°), left anterior oblique 60° (LAO 60°) and left lateral (LL), both after peak exercise and at rest. Alternatively, when only three views are recorded, the left lateral and the LAO 60° are replaced by a LAO 70° view (Figs. 2.1c,d). These images show the normal homogeneous distribution of tracer uptake in the left ventricle (LV) and the commonly seen appearance of the right ventricle (RV). Images are all shown in raw data as black and white displays with no background subtraction.

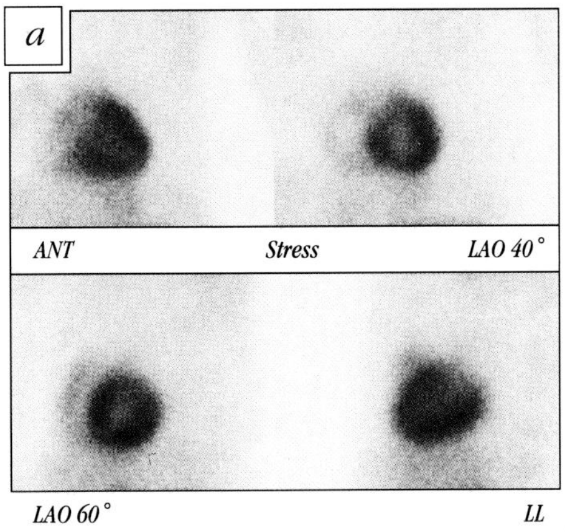

Figure 2.1a

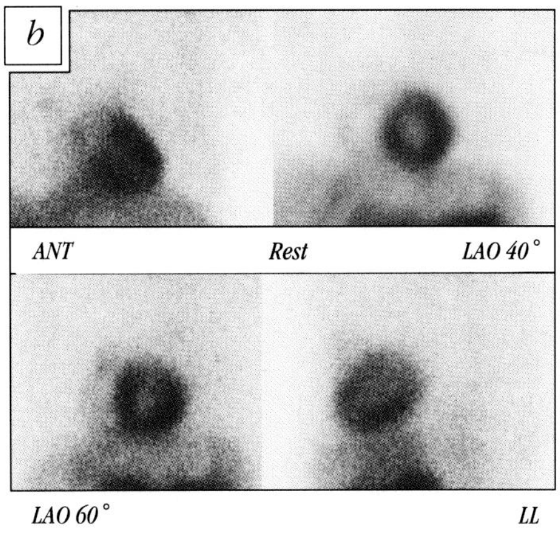

Figure 2.1b

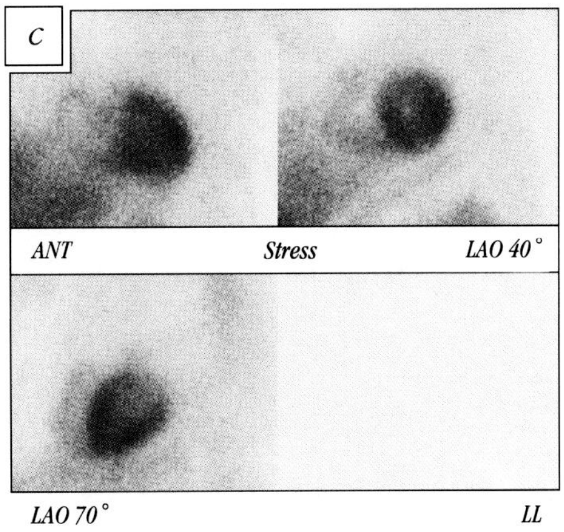

Figure 2.1c

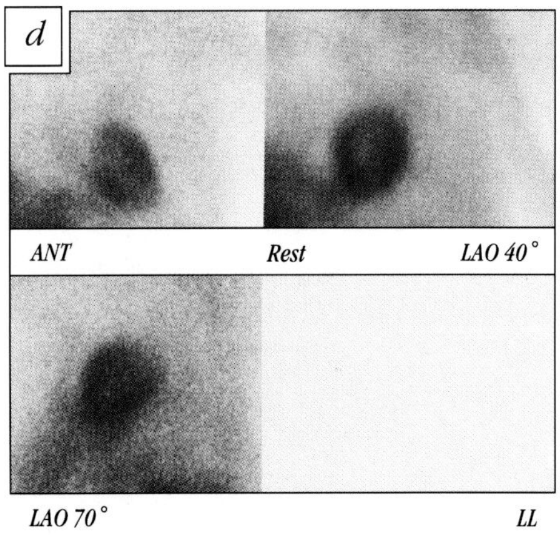

Figure 2.1d

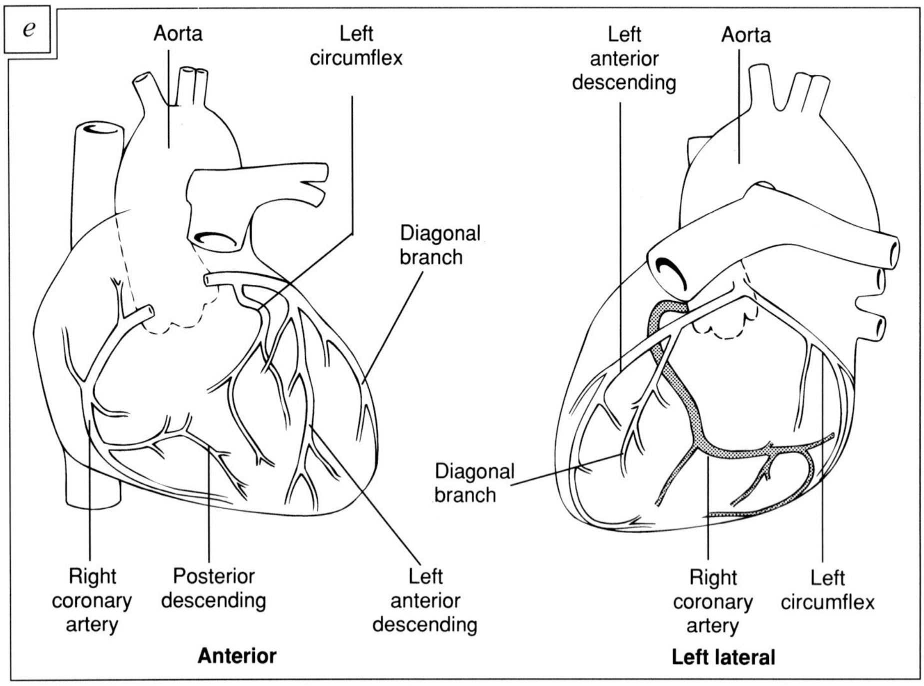

Figure 2.1e
Coronary circulation in anterior and left lateral views.

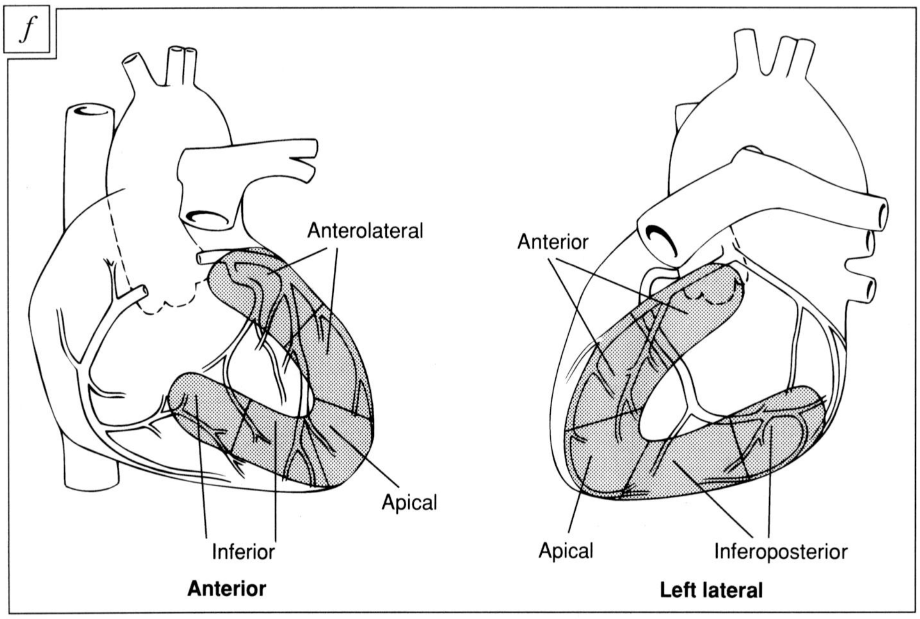

Figure 2.1f
Segmental representation of perfusion images to correspond with coronary anatomy.

Figures 2.1e and 2.1f show diagrammatically the normal coronary anatomy and the corresponding segmental representation of the perfusion images.

Figure 2.1g shows a typical appearance using the standard (Goris–Watson) method background corrected for sestamibi and Fig. 2.1h shows a normal isocount quantitation.

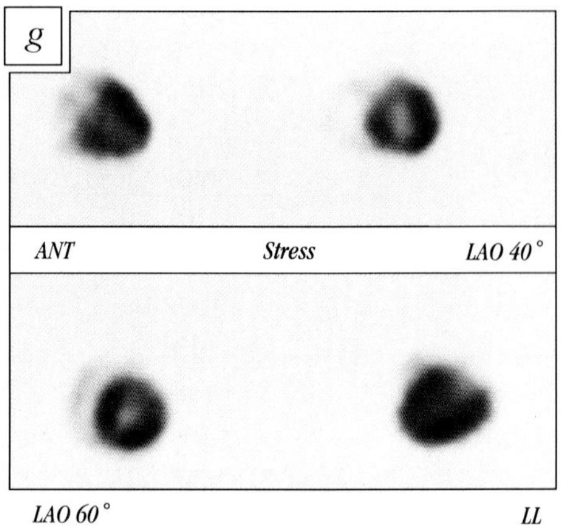

Figure 2.1g
Normal background subtracted planar study.

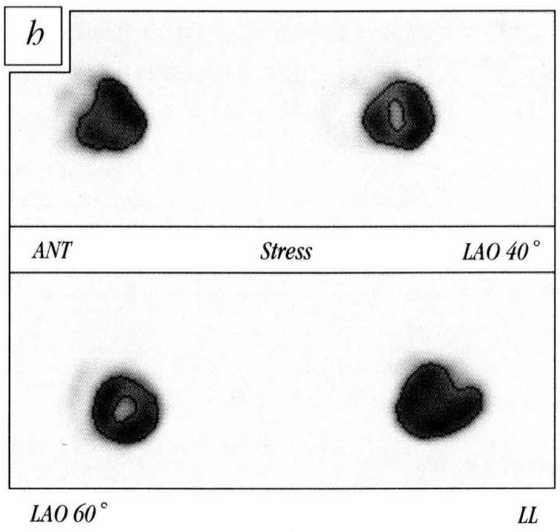

Figure 2.1h
Normal isocount contours.

Normal single photon emission computed tomography (SPECT)

Figures 2.2a and 2.2b show in colour typical myocardial slices of 2-pixel thick SPECT studies in the three usual orientations (horizontal long axis (HLA), vertical long axis (VLA) and short axis). This display represents a large portion of the myocardium and therefore allows the analysis of the extent of perfusion abnormalities. Figures 2.3a and 2.3b show the simplified way this is presented in exercise compared with rest, using single middle horizontal and vertical long axis views and two short axis views belonging to the apical and to the basal planes. This provides four views commonly used to illustrate an abnormality and to send to referring physicians. Quantitation is most commonly performed using the polar map method. Figure 2.4 shows a typical polar map of a normal sestamibi study comparing exercise with rest which shows a lack of any significant deviation from the normal database and a lack of any significant difference in distribution between exercise and rest.

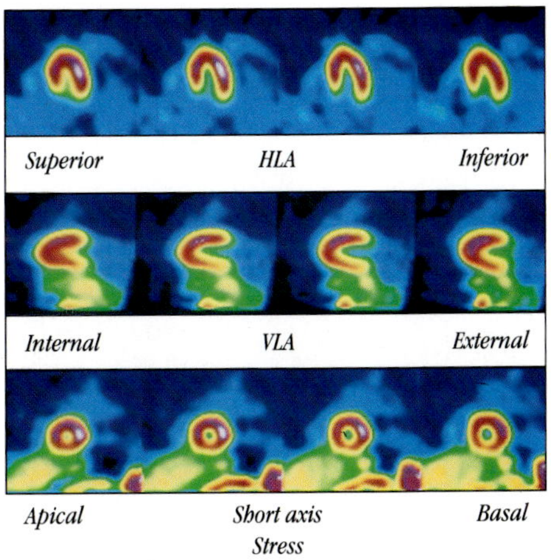

Figure 2.2a
Normal SPECT stress study (12 slices)

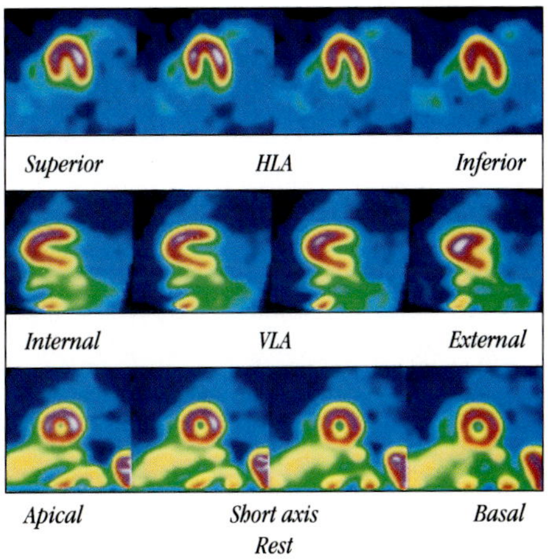

Figure 2.2b
Normal SPECT rest study (12 slices).

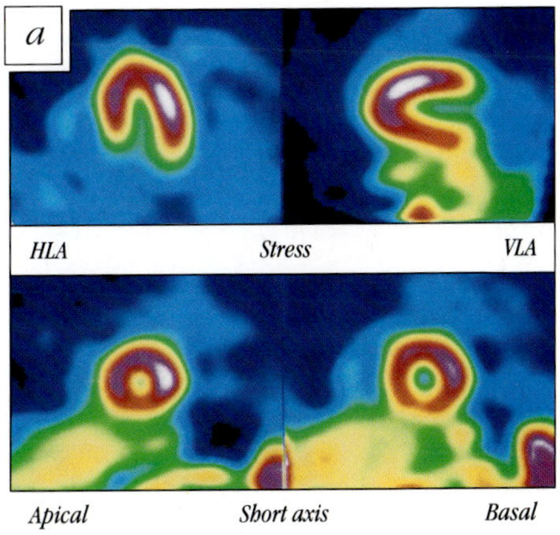

Figure 2.3a
Normal SPECT stress study (4 slices).

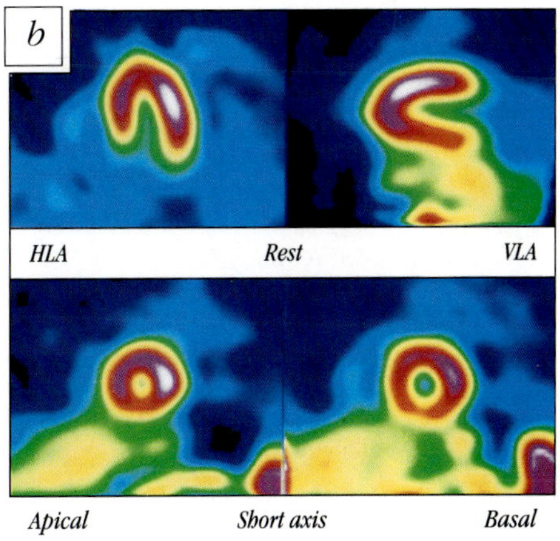

Figure 2.3b
Normal SPECT rest study (4 slices).

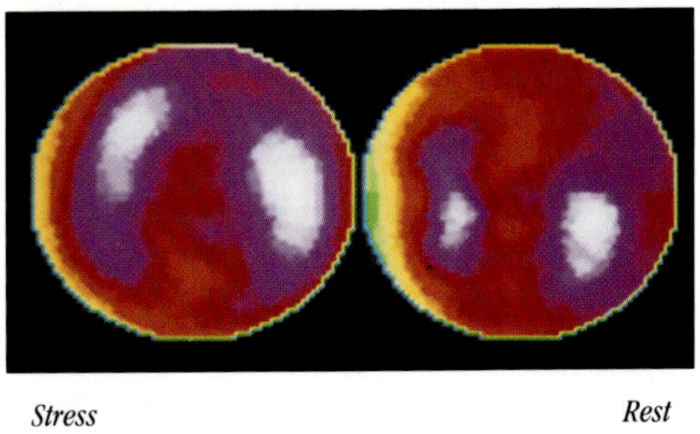

Figure 2.4
Normal polar maps comparing the stress with the rest study.

Non-pathological Variants

Apical thinning

The apex of the left ventricle commonly appears to be thin, which may be mistaken for a perfusion abnormality. Figures 2.5a and 2.5b show typical appearances of apical thinning.

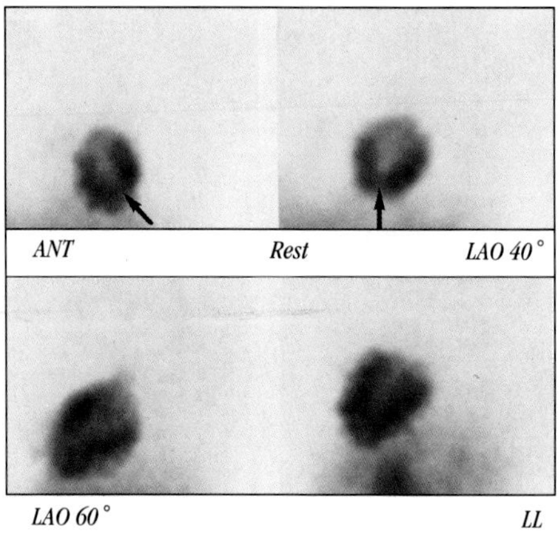

Figure 2.5a
Planar scintigraphy performed at rest in four projections, 1 h after injection of sestamibi, shows a relative photon deficient area in the apical region of the LV (arrows).

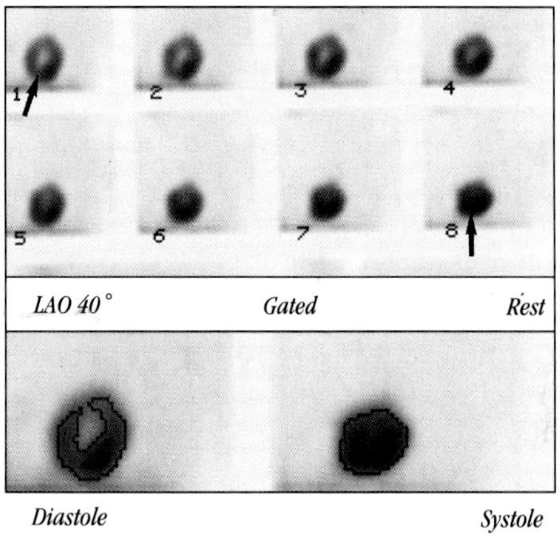

Figure 2.5b
In gated acquisition performed in the LAO 40 ° view, apical thinning is seen in the apical wall on diastolic frame (arrow) that disappears on systolic frame (arrow).

Gallbladder and gut

The typical appearance of gallbladder, liver and gut due to the excretion of sestamibi can be seen on (1) a planar image (Figs. 2.6a,b) and (2) a SPECT image (Figs. 2.6c,d). Only in a very few cases does this significantly interfere with the interpretation of the inferior wall of the LV due to upward scatter of radioactivity, and it is a less serious problem with SPECT studies.

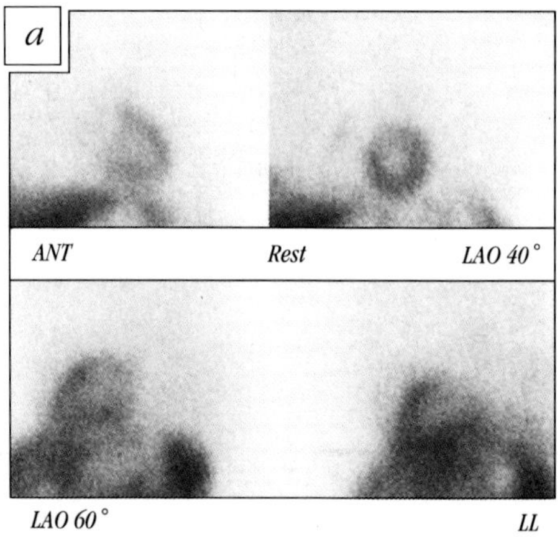

Figure 2.6a
Planar scintigraphy performed at rest 15 min after injection of sestamibi shows a great deal of background activity coming from the liver, the spleen and the intestines.

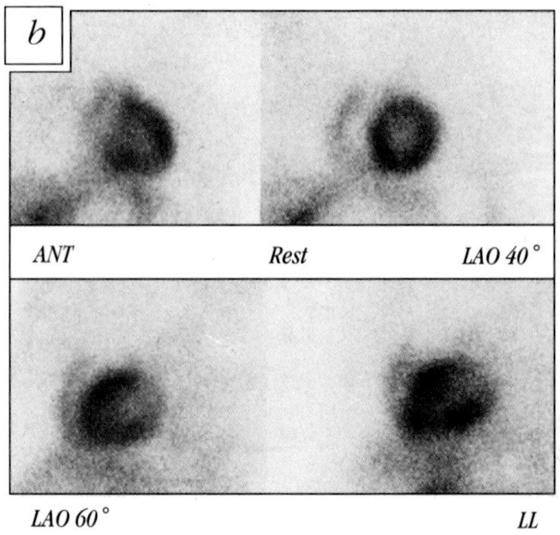

Figure 2.6b
Planar scintigraphy performed in the same patient 90 min after injection shows a considerable decrease in the background activity.

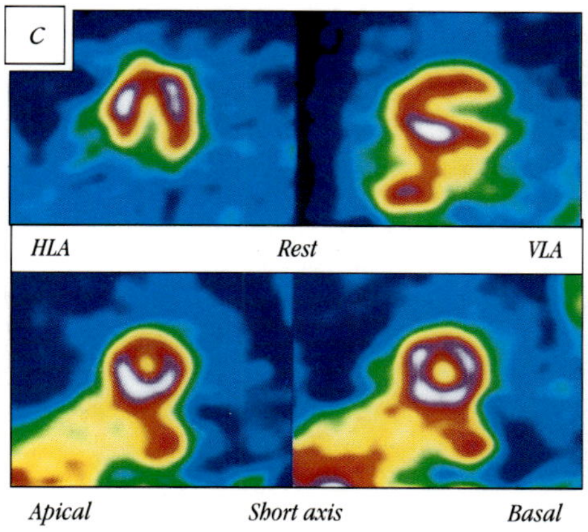

Figure 2.6c
SPECT study performed at rest in another patient 15 min after injection shows the presence of significant background activity coming from the liver and the gut.

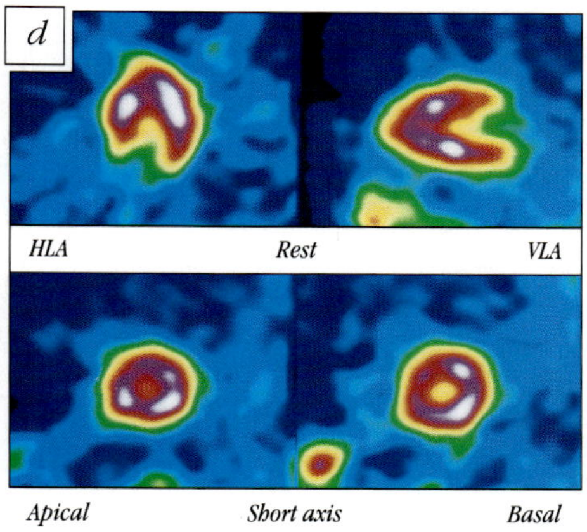

Figure 2.6d
A SPECT study performed in the same patient 60 min after injection shows the improvement of the ratio between myocardial activity and background, which are now clearly separated.

Septal thinning

Because the septum is short in patients with small hearts, it often appears to be 'thin' or hypoperfused (Fig. 2.7).

Short septal wall of the left ventricle

The upper part of the septum is fibrous rather than muscular and as a result the septum frequently appears short when compared to the lateral wall (Fig. 2.8).

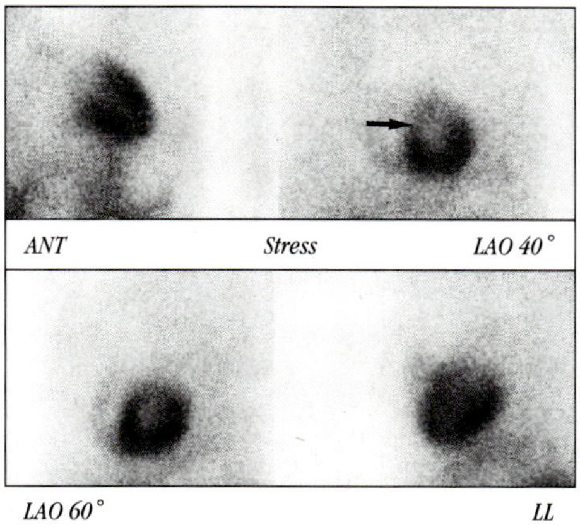

Figure 2.7
Planar scintigraphy performed at stress shows the presence of a thin left ventricular septal wall in the LAO 40° view without significant segmental perfusion abnormality (arrow). This phenomenon is related to overall motion of the heart during systole, which spreads the posterolateral wall activity but not the septal activity.

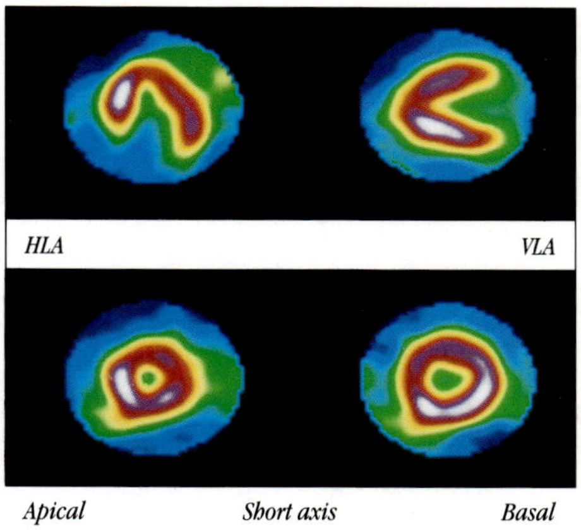

Figure 2.8
In SPECT studies, this asymmetry between the septum and the lateral wall is well defined on the horizontal long axis view (left upper panel).

Position of the heart

The position of the heart in the thorax may vary widely depending on the thorax configuration as well as on pathology (Figs. 2.9a,b).

Hypertrophy of the left ventricle

Hypertrophy of the LV can be idiopathic, or it can result from a volume, or a pressure overload (Fig. 2.10).

Right ventricular uptake

Right ventricular uptake varies significantly even in normal people. Figures 2.11a and 2.11b show the variation of right ventricular uptake from very little to a great deal of visualization in two normal people.

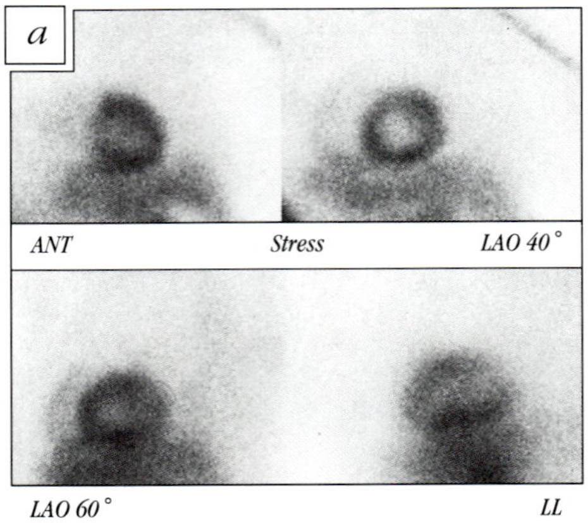

Figure 2.9a
A horizontal heart is characterized in planar scintigraphy by the shape of the LV representing a ring in the LAO 40° view.

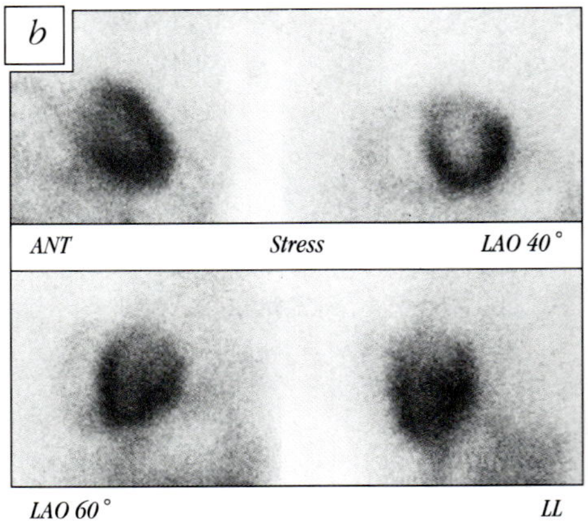

Figure 2.9b
When the heart is placed in the vertical position, the shape of the LV represents a horseshoe open in the region corresponding to the valvular plane, in the LAO 40° view.

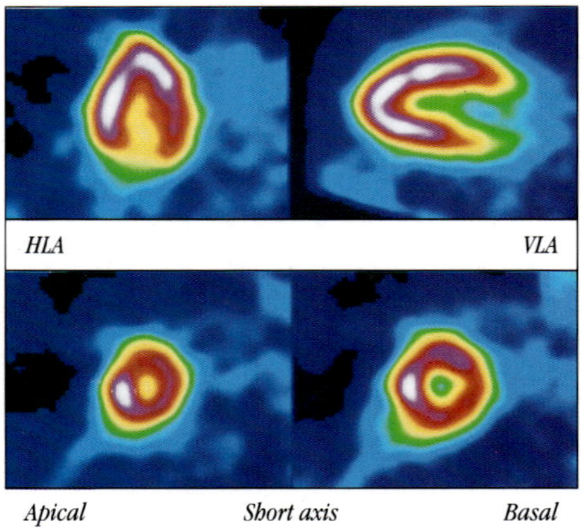

Figure 2.10
Tomography shows a small cavity and a thick myocardium in the three usual orientations (horizontal long axis, vertical long axis and short axis) due to LV hypertrophy.

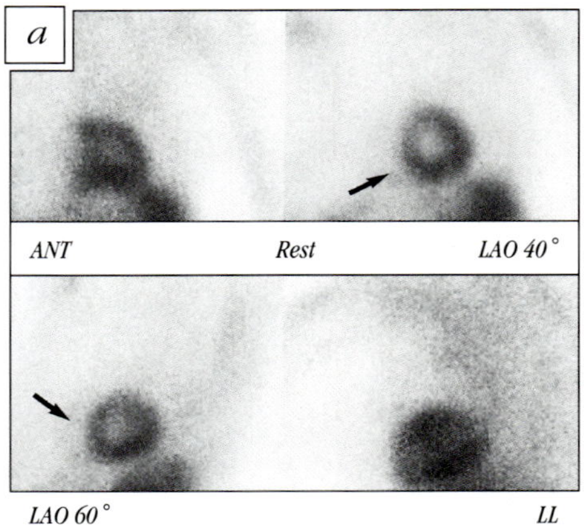

Figure 2.11a
Planar scintigraphy performed at rest in four projections shows very little right ventricular uptake of sestamibi in the LAO 40° and LAO 60° views (arrows) and a normal perfusion pattern for the LV.

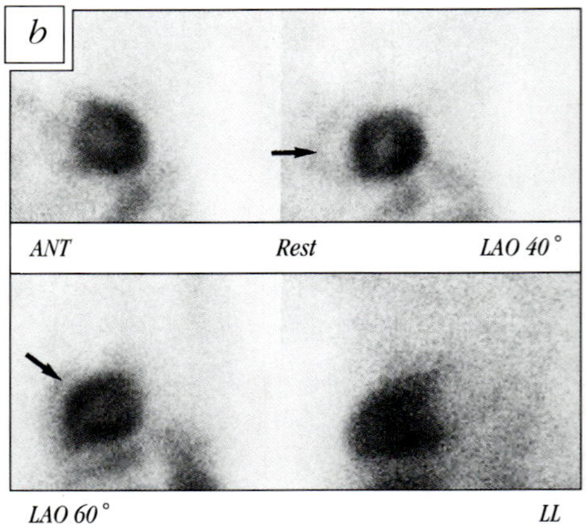

Figure 2.11b
In this other case, planar scintigraphy performed at rest demonstrates the presence of a more marked right ventricular uptake of sestamibi in the LAO 40° and LAO 60° views (arrows) and a normal left ventricular perfusion pattern.

Typical Patterns of Perfusion Abnormalities

Pattern of ischaemia

Myocardial ischaemia will normally be shown by areas of decreased sestamibi uptake or the post-stress scan. In all but the most severe examples of coronary artery stenosis the defects will not be apparent on the rest scan because the relative flow is only reduced during the coronary vasodilatation induced by exercise. The site of the defect will correspond to the coronary vessel involved. Figs 2.12a,b,c,d,e demonstrate examples of ischaemia.

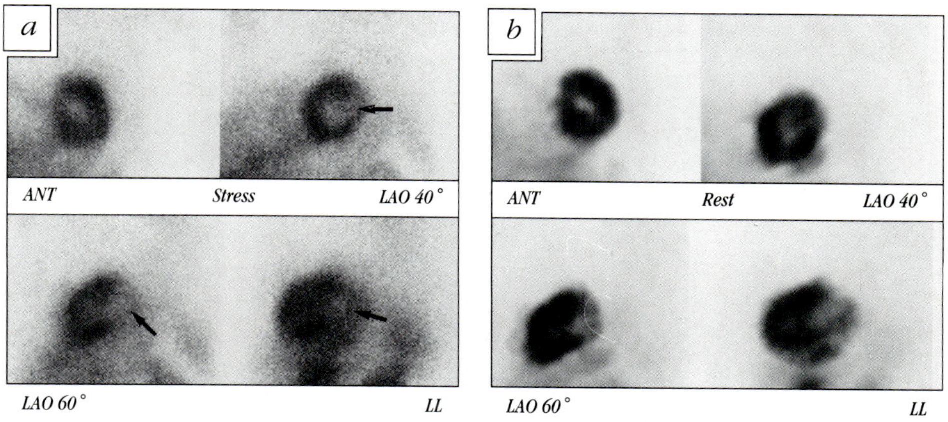

Figures 2.12a,b
Planar scintigraphy performed at stress in four projections shows sestamibi defects in the lateral and in the inferoposterior walls of the LV (arrows) in the left circumflex (LCx) vessel territory, while the comparative rest study shows a normal perfusion pattern.

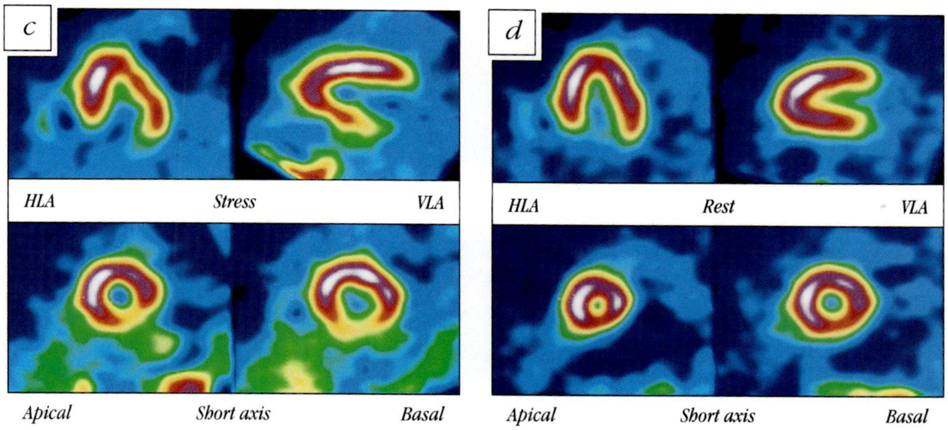

Figures 2.12c,d
SPECT studies performed at rest and at stress show perfusion abnormalities on stress tomograms, in the lateral wall of the left ventricle on the horizontal long axis view, and in the inferior wall on the short axis view and vertical long axis view corresponding to myocardial ischaemia in the left circumflex (LCx) or right coronary artery (RCA) vessel territories. The rest study shows a normal pattern.

Figure 2.12e
The electrocardiogram recorded during exercise shows ST depression appearing in the anterior lateral leads (V4–V5–V6) at a workload of 120 W. ST depression is still present during recovery, 4 min after interruption of the exercise.

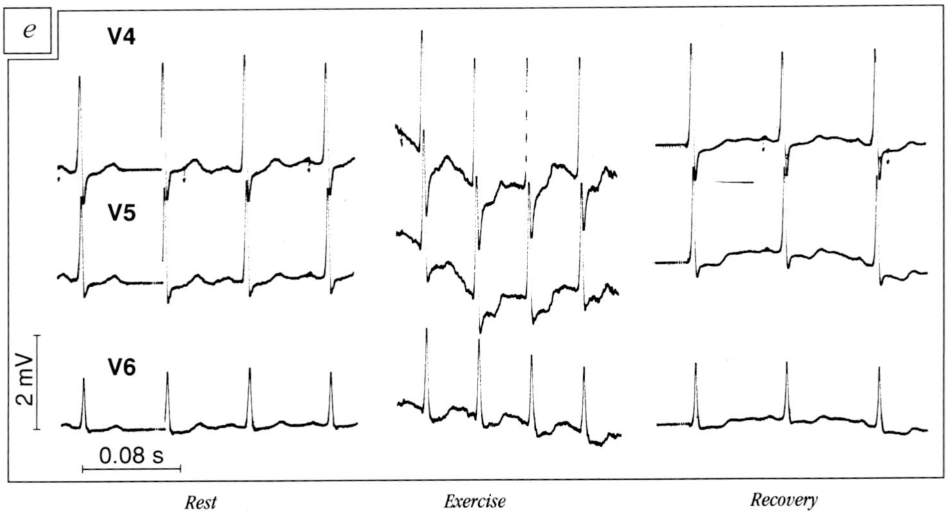

Pattern of necrosis

In comparison with ischaemia, necrosis or infarction will show the defect equally on both rest and stress scans (Figs. 2.13a,b,c,d,e).

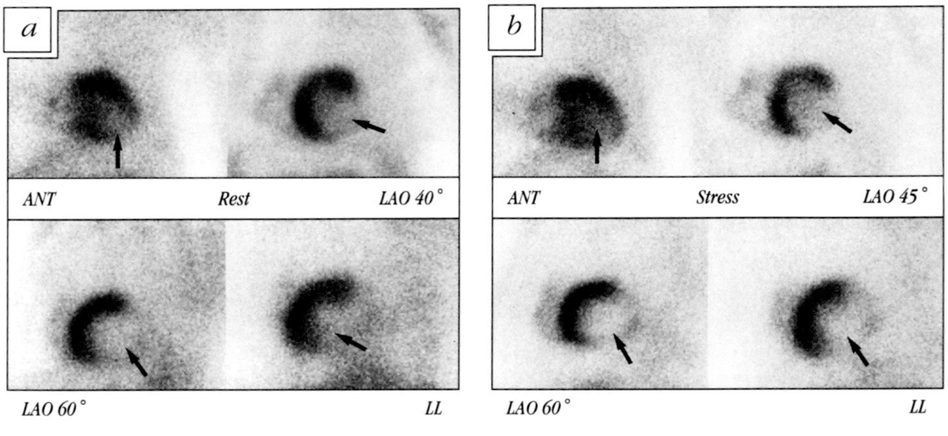

Figures 2.13a,b
Planar scintigraphy performed at rest and at stress shows identical sestamibi defects in extent and in severity, in the lateral, in the inferoposterior and in the inferoapical walls of the LV (arrows) corresponding to myocardial infarction. Planar images also demonstrate left ventricular dilatation.

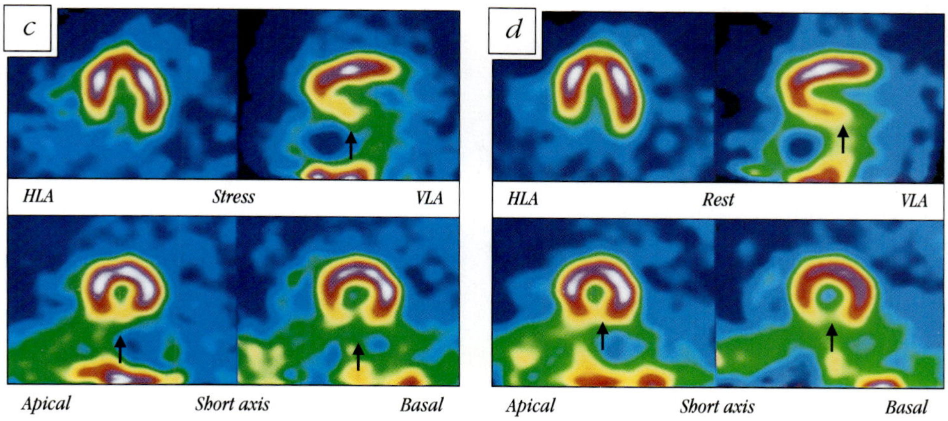

Figures 2.13c,d
These figures show an example of myocardial infarction in the inferior and inferoposterior walls of the LV, consecutive to right coronary occlusion. Perfusion abnormalities are well visualized on vertical and short axis views (arrows).

Figure 2.13e
The ECG performed at rest in this patient confirms the presence of inferior myocardial infarction with a Q-wave and a negative T-wave in leads DII, DIII and aVF.

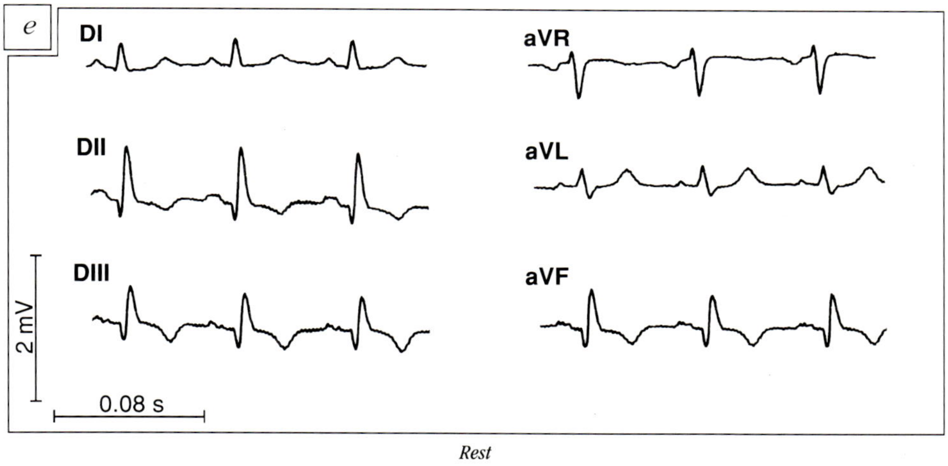

Pattern of proximal left anterior descending (LAD) disease

The pattern of proximal LAD disease is characterized by perfusion abnormalities involving the anteroseptal and the anterolateral walls of the LV (Figs. 2.14a,b,c,d).

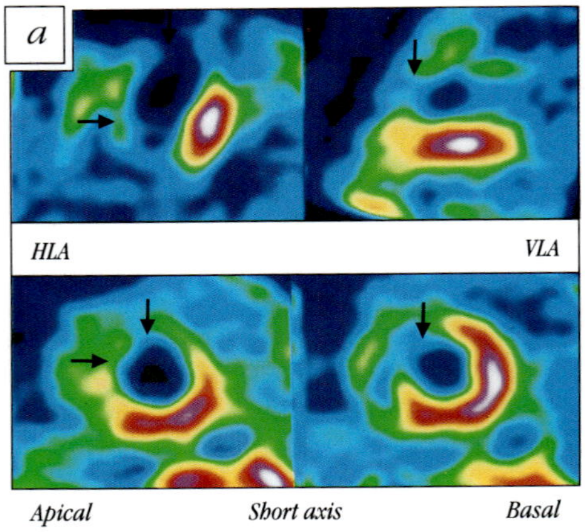

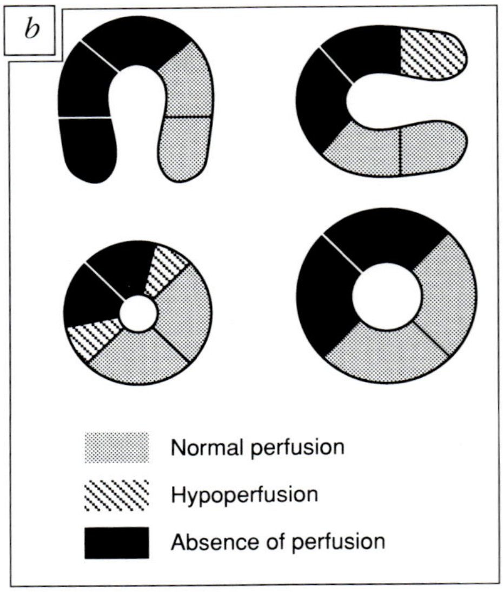

Figures 2.14a,b
On SPECT studies, these perfusion defects are visualized in the three usual orientations, involving the septum and the apex in the horizontal long axis (HLA) view, the antero-superior wall and the apex on the vertical long axis (VLA) view, and the septal and anterolateral quadrants in the short axis views (see arrows). The corresponding diagram is shown in (b).

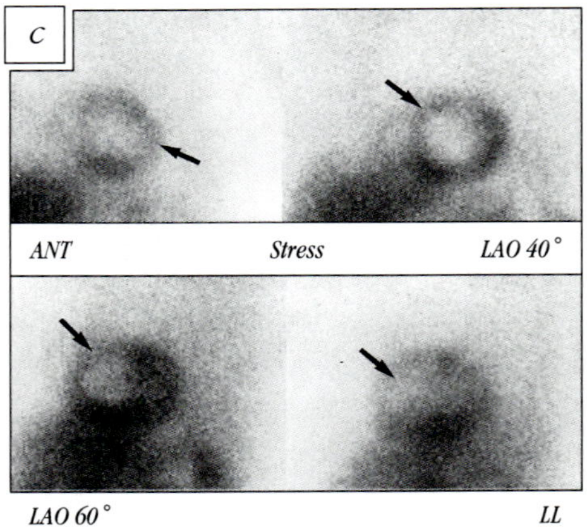

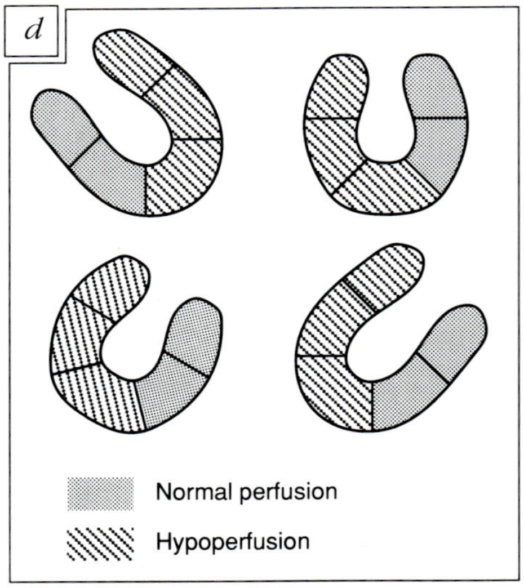

Figures 2.14c,d
In planar scintigraphy, defects are located on the anterolateral and on the anteroseptal walls of the LV. In this case, planar scintigraphy shows also left ventricular dilatation (see arrows). The corresponding diagram is shown in (d).

Pattern of middle left anterior descending disease

When the lesion is located after the main diagonal branch, defects involve the anteroseptal wall (Figs. 2.15a,b,c,d).

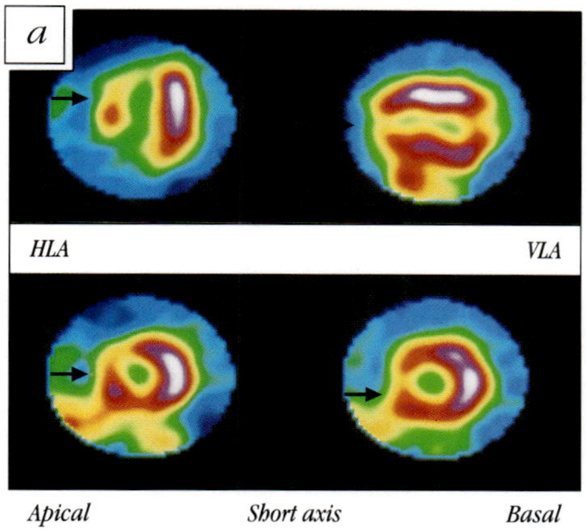

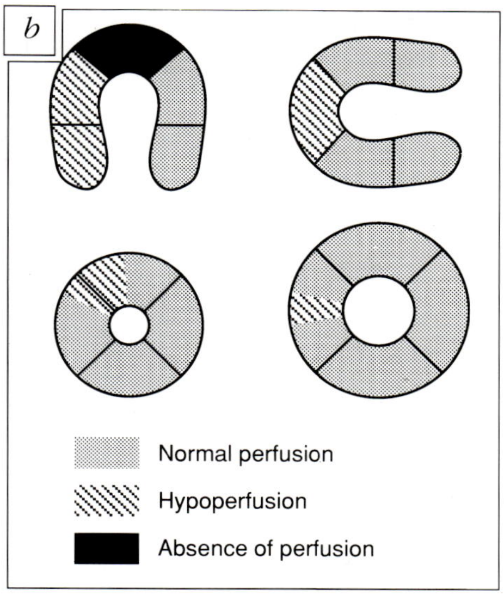

Figures 2.15a,b
These defects are visualized in this SPECT study on the horizontal and on the short axis views (see arrows). The corresponding diagram is shown in (b).

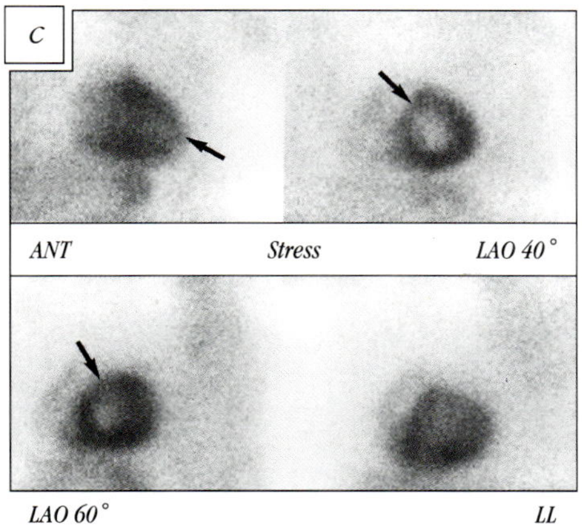

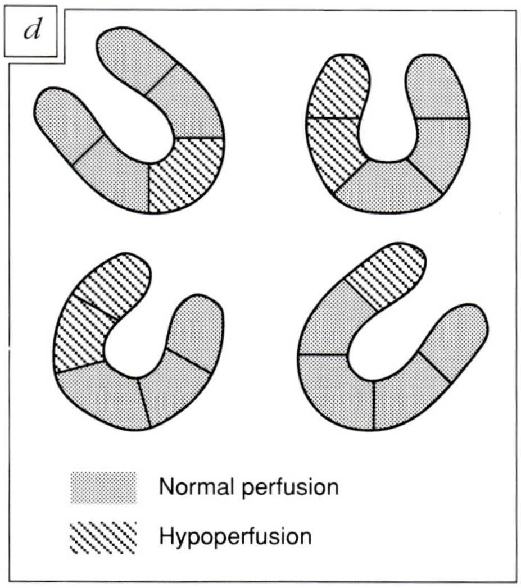

Figures 2.15c,d
In planar scintigraphy, sestamibi defects appear mainly in the anteroseptal wall on the LAO views (see arrows). The corresponding diagram is shown in (d).

Pattern of left circumflex disease

Perfusion abnormalities corresponding to left circumflex disease involve the lateral wall of the LV (Figs. 2.16a,b,c,d).

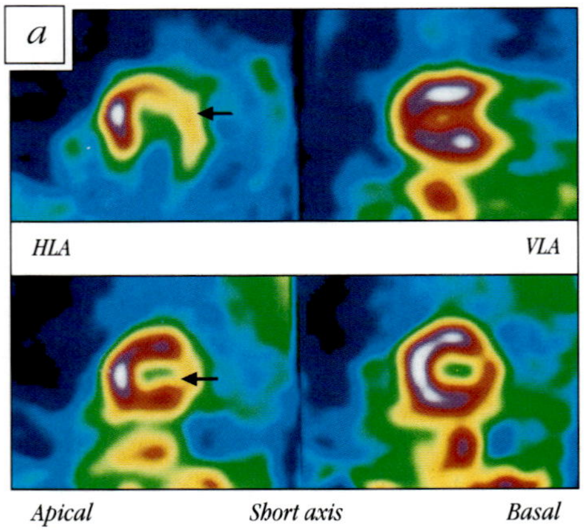

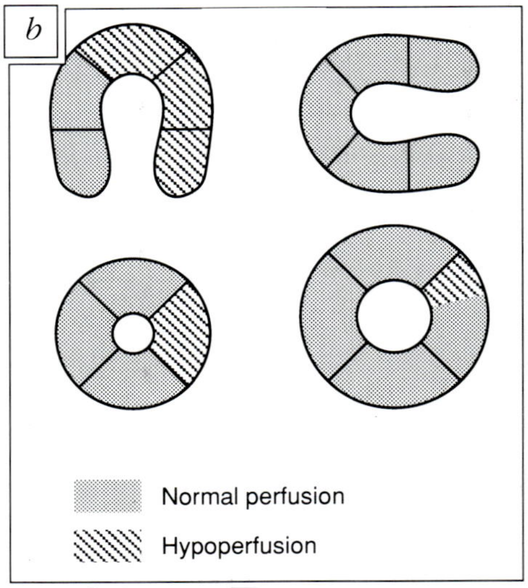

Figures 2.16a,b
This SPECT study shows sestamibi defects in the lateral wall of the left ventricle and illustrates the pattern of LCx coronary disease (see arrows). The corresponding diagram is shown in (b).

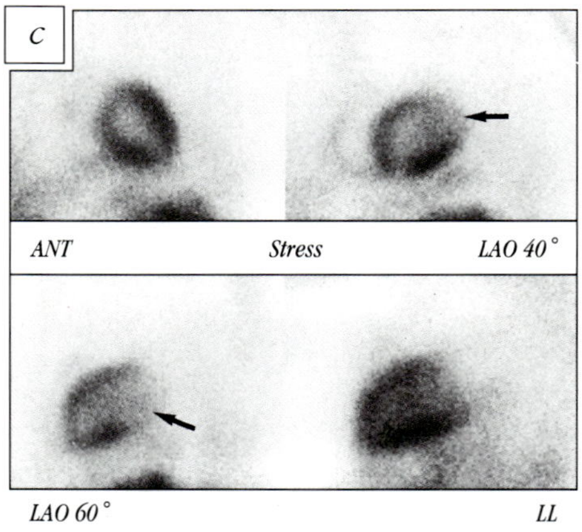

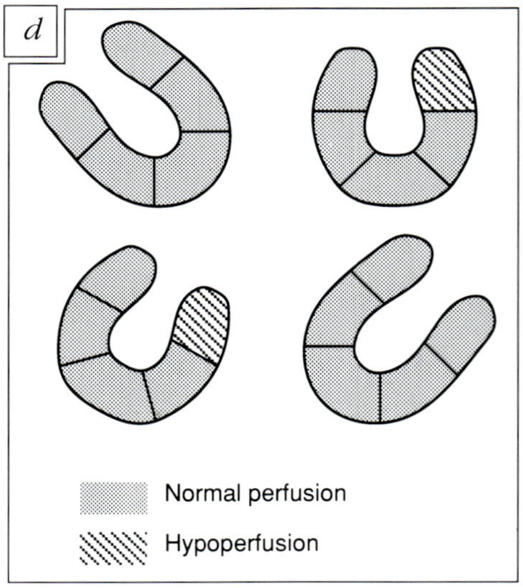

Figures 2.16c,d
In planar scintigraphy, the pattern of LCx disease is characterized by abnormal perfusion involving the lateral wall of the LV on the LAO 40° view (see arrow). The corresponding diagram is shown in (d).

Pattern of right coronary artery disease

Perfusion defects corresponding to right coronary artery disease involve the inferior wall and sometimes the inferoposterior wall of the LV (Figs. 2.17a,b,c,d).

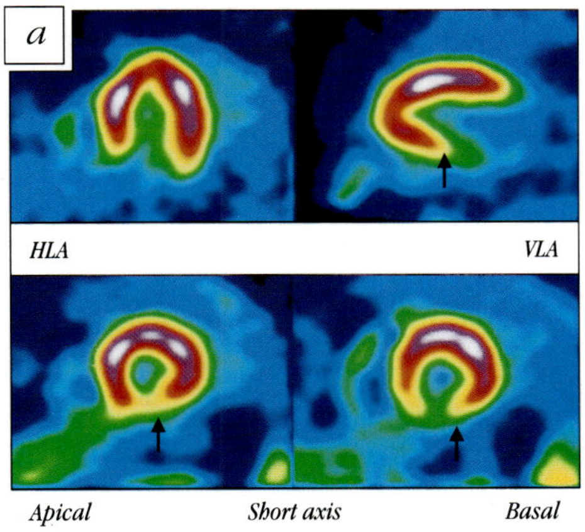

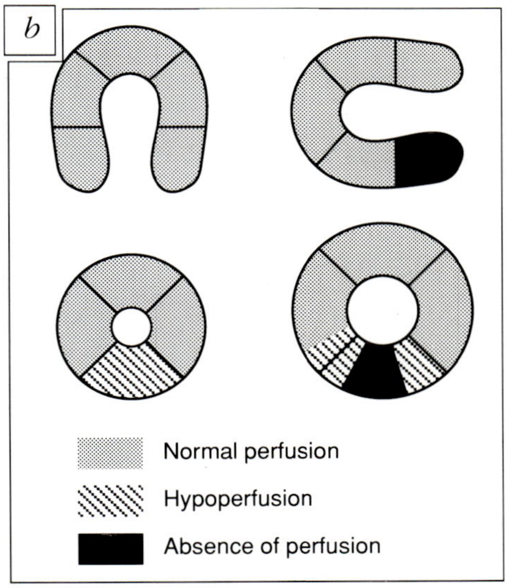

Figures 2.17a,b
In the presence of a RCA lesion, perfusion defects are located on sestamibi tomograms in the inferoposterior and in the inferior walls of the LV (a, arrows). The corresponding diagram of this lesion is shown in (b).

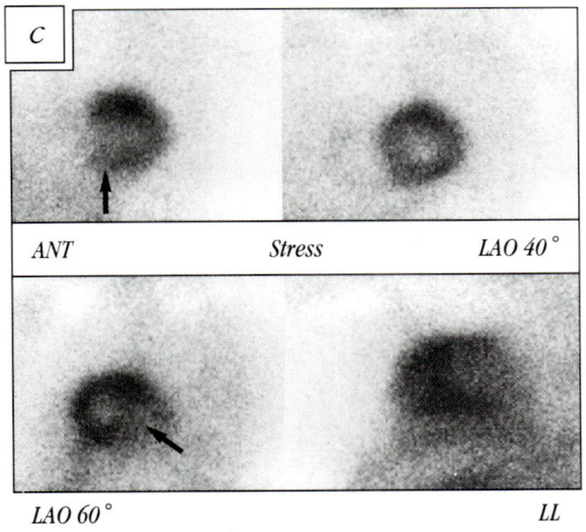

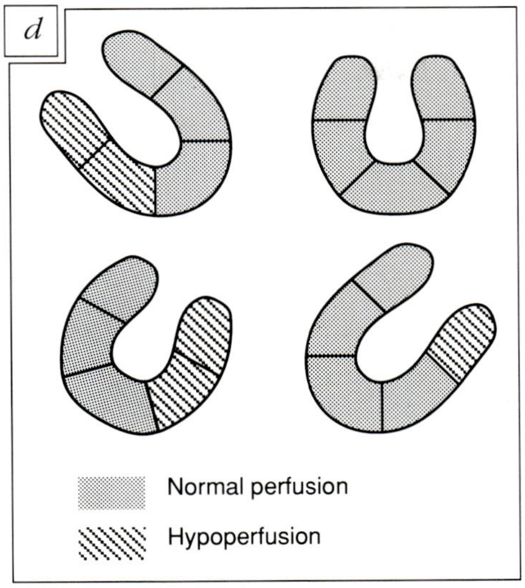

Figures 2.17c,d
In planar scintigraphy, perfusion defects involve the inferior wall of the LV in the anterior view and sometimes the inferoposterior wall (see arrows). The corresponding diagram of this lesion is shown in (d).

Multivessel disease

Multivessel disease pattern results from a combination of different vessel abnormalities (Figs. 2.18a,b,c,d).

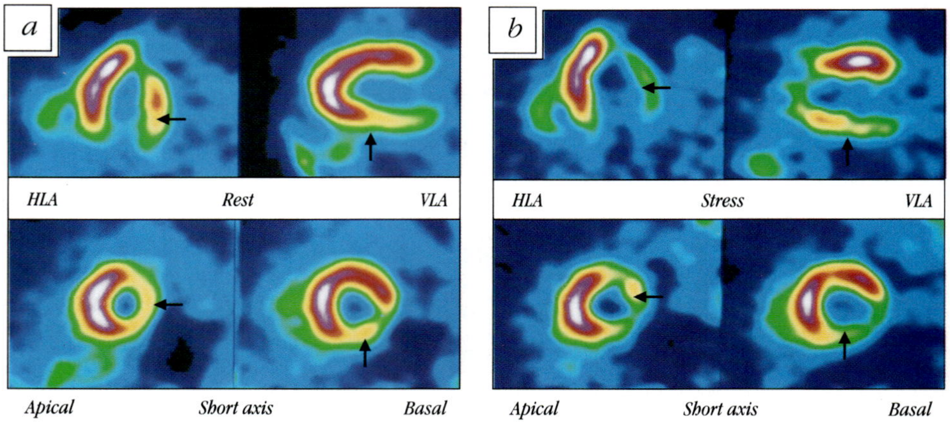

Figures 2.18a,b
Comparative rest/stress SPECT studies performed in a patient with multiple vessel disease. Perfusion defects described at rest (a, arrows) involve the lateral and inferoposterior walls of the LV and suggest myocardial scar. At stress, we observe an extension of perfusion defects in the lateral wall on the HLA and short axis views(b, arrow) as well as perfusion defects in the anterior wall on the VLA view (b, arrow). This comparative study illustrates a lateral myocardial infarction with residual ischaemia around the infarcted area and myocardial ischaemia in the LAD vessel territory.

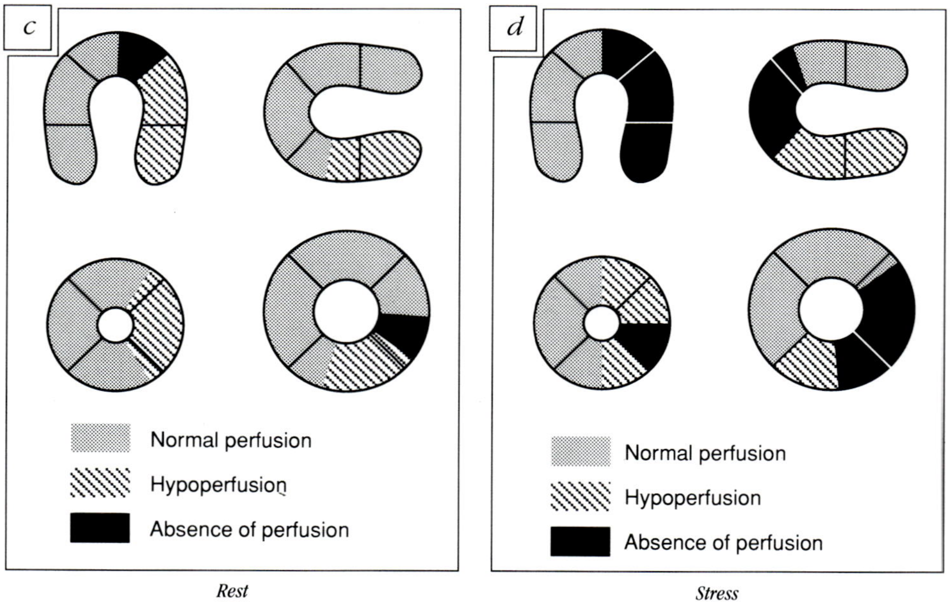

Figures 2.18c,d
The corresponding diagrams of this comparative rest/stress study.

Typical Patterns of Other Cardiac Abnormalities

Valvular disease

Valvular disease, depending on the type and site of the lesion, stenosis, regurgitation (mitral, aortic, etc), produces different combinations or auricular and ventricular dilatation and hypertrophy. Figs. 2.19a,b,c show an example of aortic regurgitation, while Table 2.1 lists the ventricular function data.

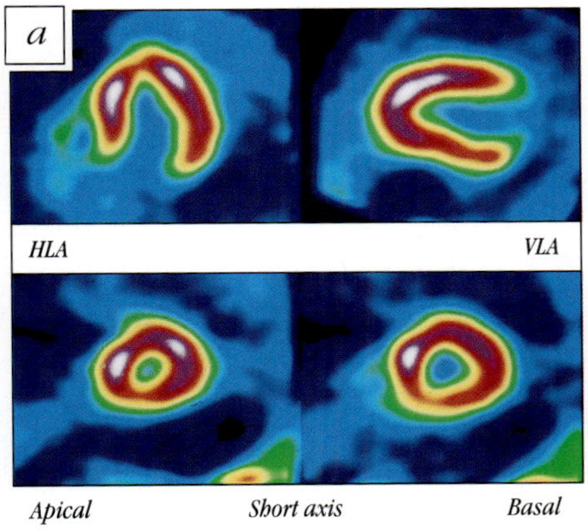

Figure 2.19a
Tomography performed at rest in a patient suffering from aortic regurgitation demonstrates a normal perfusion pattern associated with moderate left ventricular dilatation.

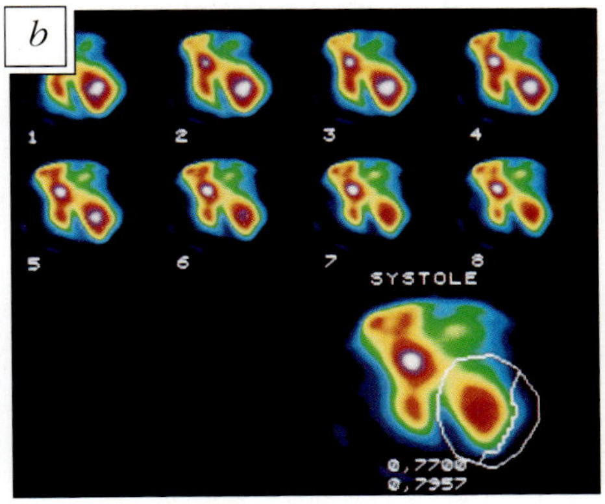

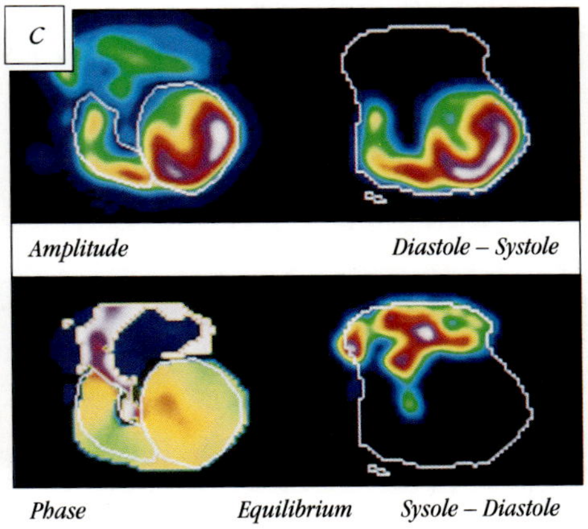

Figures 2.19b,c
Gated blood pool scintigraphy performed at equilibrium and at rest in the LAO 45° view with ^{99m}Tc confirms the presence of left ventricular dilatation more important in diastole (frame 1) than in systole (frame 8). This diastolic overload is also visualized on the amplitude and the phase images.

Left ventricular ejection fraction:	44%[a] (Normal value ≥ 50)
Regurgitation index (LV/RV):	3.63[a] (Normal value ≤ 1.5)
Regurgitation fraction:	67%[a]
Right ventricular ejection fraction:	44% (Normal value ≥ 40)

[a]Abnormal values.

Table 2.1 *Values obtained from the ventricular curves analysis.*

Chronic renal failure

In a patient with chronic renal failure, undergoing dialysis, sestamibi tomography shows dilatation and hypertrophy of the LV associated with a normal perfusion pattern (Fig. 2.20).

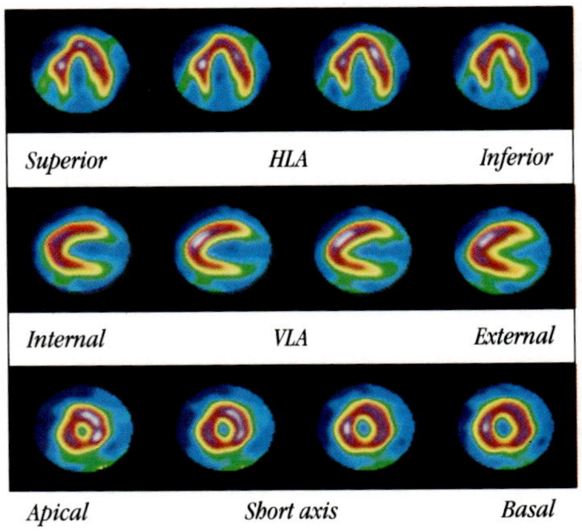

Figure 2.20

Left to right shunt

Left to right shunts increase pulmonary blood flow sometimes leading to pulmonary hypertension. Shunts at the pre-ventricular level produce volume overload of the right ventricle, while shunts at the ventricular and post-ventricular levels mainly overload the left ventricle. A case of atrial septal defect is illustrated with right ventricular dilatation and hypertrophy (Figs. 2.21a,b,c and Table 2.2).

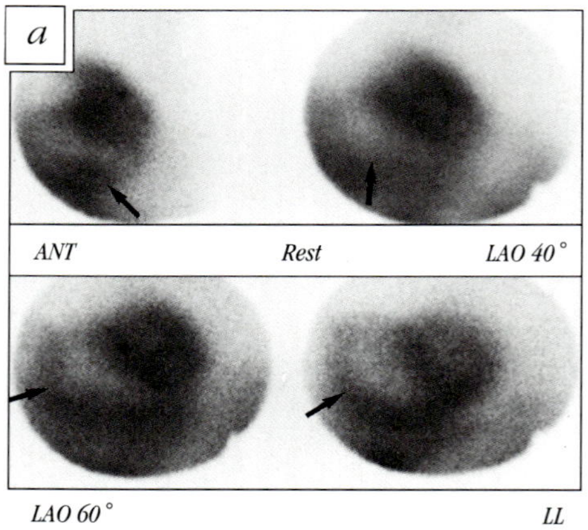

Figure 2.21a
Planar scintigraphy acquired at rest shows a normal perfusion pattern of the LV but a hypertrophy and dilatation of the RV (arrows) induced by right ventricular overload in a case of atrial septal defect.

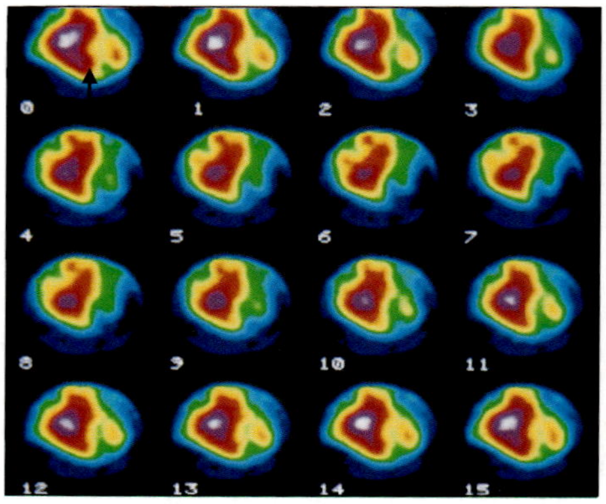

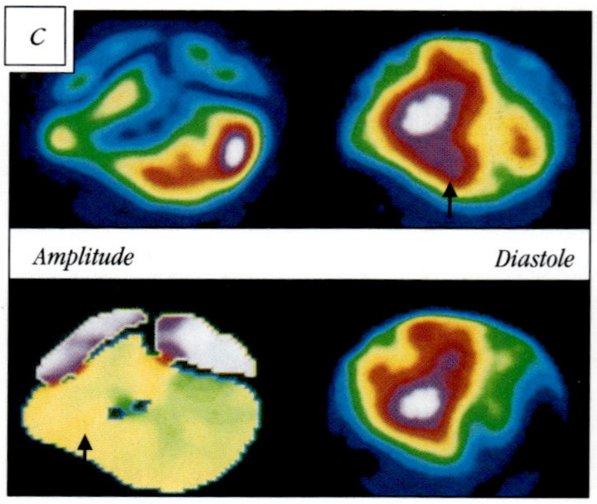

Figures 2.21b,c
Equilibrium blood pool scintigraphy performed at rest in the LAO 45° view shows diastolic overload of the RV (frame 1, arrow; diastole amplitude and phase images, arrows).

Left ventricular ejection fraction	70%
Right ventricular ejection fraction	44%
Right ventricular diastolic volume	162 ml/m^2 [a]
QP/QS (RV/LV)	1.83[a]
(Normal value ≤ 1.3)	
Shunt fraction	55%[a]

[a]Abnormal values.

Table 2.2 *Values obtained from the ventricular curves analysis.*

Left ventricular aneurysm

The extensive defect associated with left ventricular aneurysm distorts the LV silhouette on perfusion scintigraphy (Figs. 2.22a,b).

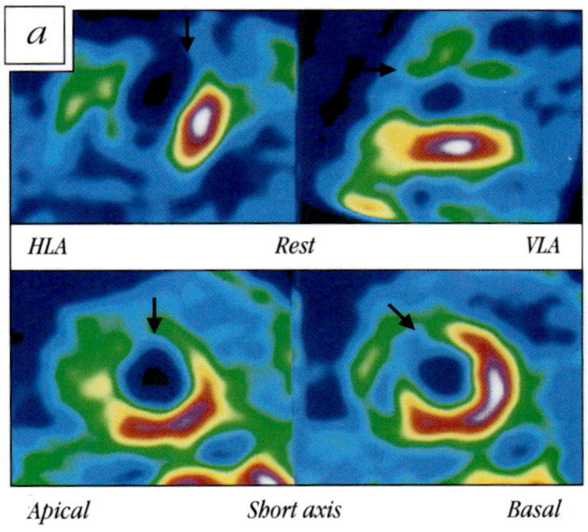

Figure 2.22a
SPECT performed at rest shows left ventricular dilatation and large sestamibi defects in the anteroseptal and apical walls of the LV, corresponding to necrosis. In this case, the infarction is complicated by left ventricular aneurysm responsible for the deformation and expansion of the anteroseptal and of the apical myocardial walls (arrows).

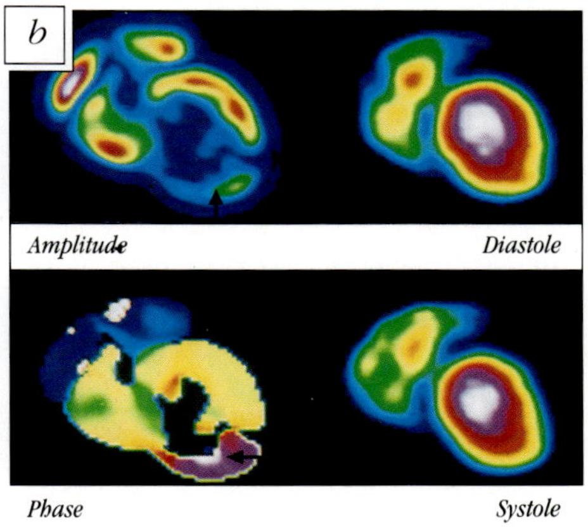

Figure 2.22b
On equilibrium gated blood pool scintigraphy performed at rest, left ventricular aneurysm is characterized by abnormal wall motion on the amplitude image (arrow) associated with a phase delay appearing in red on the phase image (arrow), corresponding to dyskinesia.

Congestive heart failure

Signs of congestive heart failure include left and right ventricular dilatation and persistent lung uptake of the tracer (Figs. 2.22c,d).

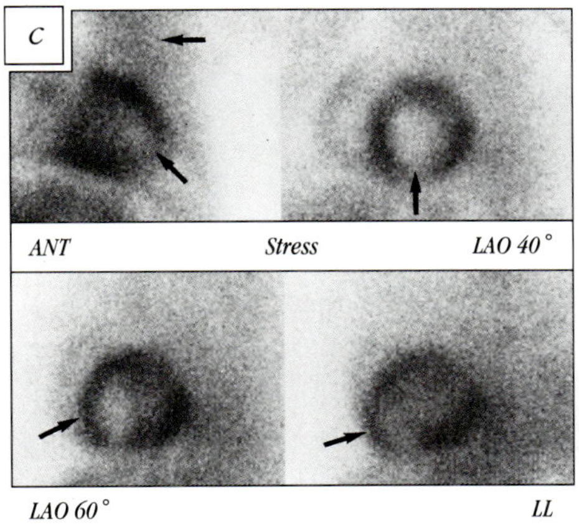

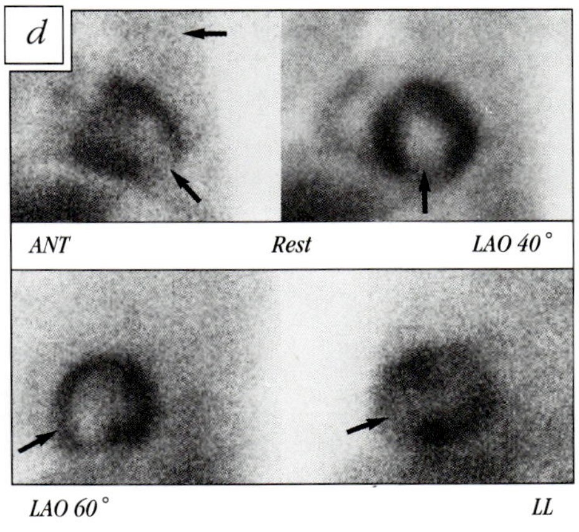

Figures 2.22c,d
Comparative stress/rest planar scintigraphy shows left ventricular dilatation, increased lung uptake of sestamibi and similar perfusion defects (arrows) in the anteroseptal and in the apical walls of the LV in a patient who developed congestive heart failure after myocardial infarction.

Hypertrophic cardiomyopathy

Different subsets of hypertrophic cardiomyopathy affect both the systolic and the diastolic ventricular function (Figs. 2.22e,f).

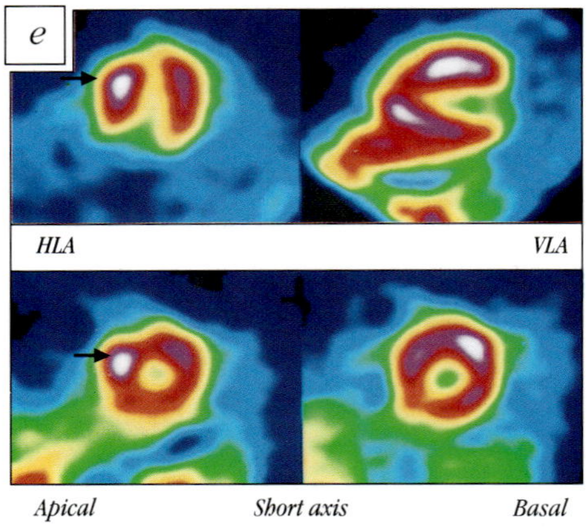

Figure 2.22e
In this SPECT study, obstructive hypertrophic cardiomyopathy is characterized by a great deal of septal wall thickening, visualized on the HLA view (left upper panel, arrow), and in this case also on the short axis view (lower panel, arrow). The cavity appears small.

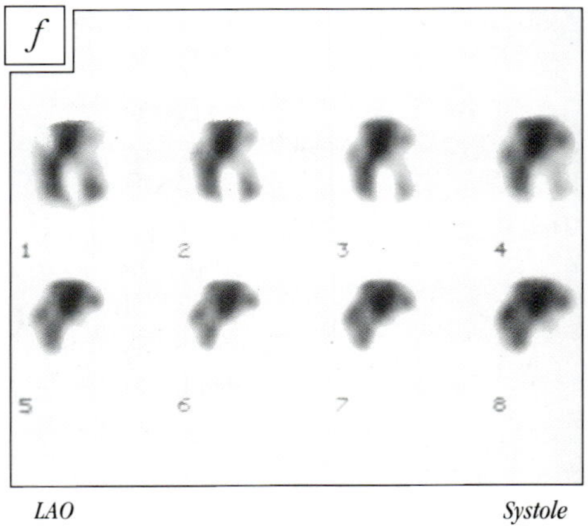

Figure 2.22f
The equilibrium gated blood pool study performed in this patient confirms the presence of a thick septum on the frames of the LAO 40° acquisition as well as of a small LV cavity.

Chronic obstructive pulmonary disease (COPD)

Pulmonary hypertension associated with COPD produces right ventricular hypertrophy then right ventricular dilatation (Figs. 2.22g,h).

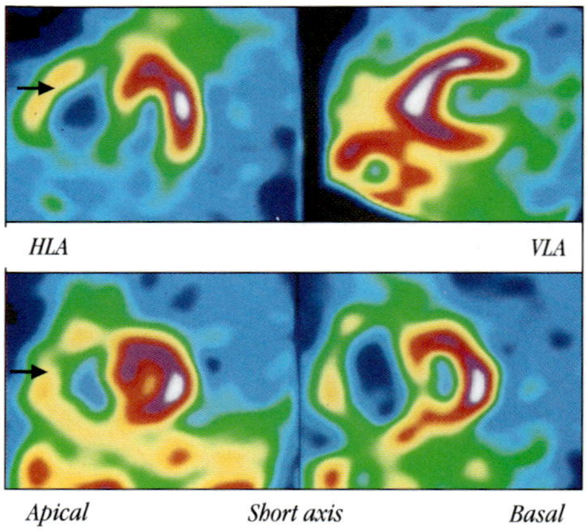

Figure 2.22g
Tomography performed at rest demonstrates deformation of the left ventricular perfusion pattern due to right ventricular hypertrophy and dilatation on the HLA and short axis views (arrows). The muscular septum is short and is incurvated towards the right ventricular cavity.

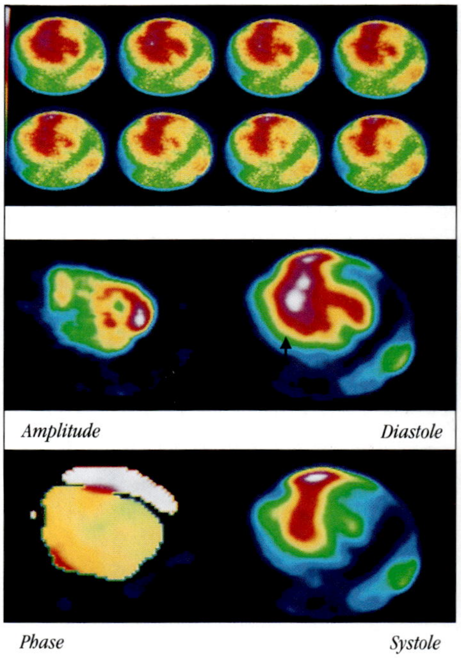

Figure 2.22h
Right ventricular dilatation is most evident on the blood pool equilibrium gated study performed at rest in the LAO view (arrow).

Image Artefacts

Soft tissue attenuation

The commonest attenuation artefact is breast attenuation, which is most marked on planar images (Fig. 2.23a) but still present on SPECT imaging (Fig. 2.23b). This is particularly important if the clothing results in the breast being in a different position for rest and stress studies. Taping the breast upwards for both studies reduces the problem. It is less important with sestamibi than with thallium due to the higher energy of technetium.

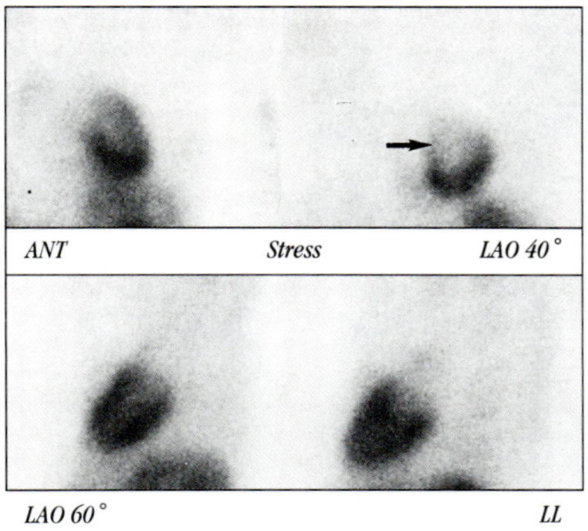

Figure 2.23a
Stress planar scintigraphy in a woman shows hypoperfusion in the septal wall on the LAO 40° view (arrow) corresponding to breast attenuation. Perfusion patterns are normal in the three other projections.

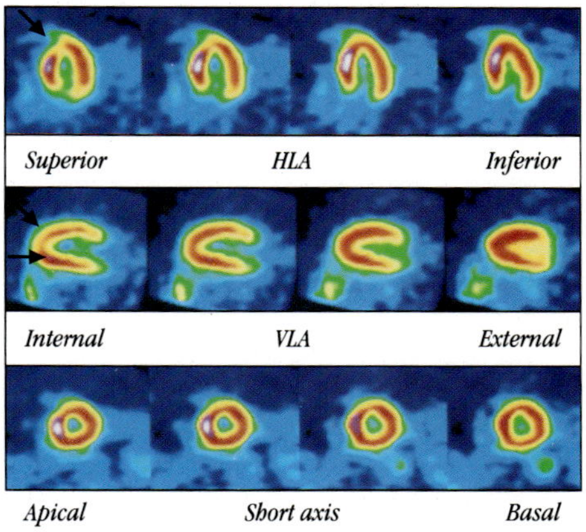

Figure 2.23b
Breast attenuation is also visualized on sestamibi tomography and may be responsible for false-positive results in the anteroseptal wall of the LV (arrows).

Movement of the patient

Each study should be reviewed by a cine display of the multiple planar images or of the sinogram to detect any movement artefact. Significant patient movement can cause image artefacts (Figs. 2.24a,b,c).

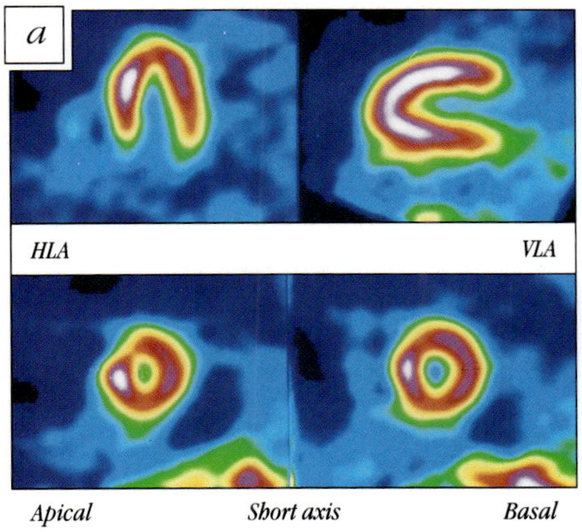

Figure 2.24a
Tomography acquired in absence of movement shows normal and homogeneous sestamibi uptake on tomographic slices.

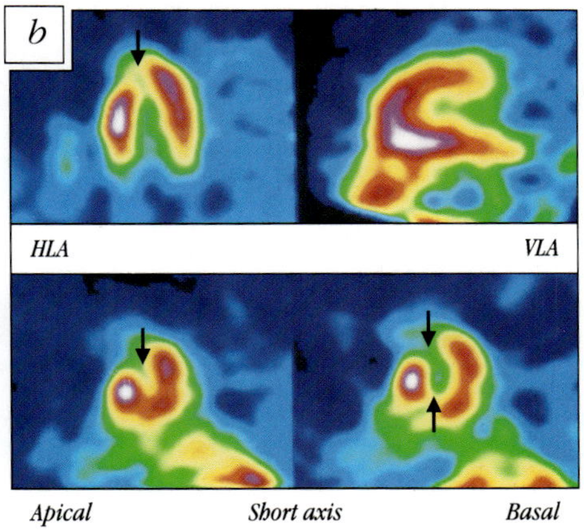

Figure 2.24b
When movement was present, sestamibi uptake is heterogeneous and artefacts may appear in the apical, anteroseptal and inferior walls of the HLA and short axis views (arrows).

A movement artefact which may be present on SPECT thallium studies is the upward creep artefact due to the changing position of the diaphragm and heart immediately after exercise. This is not a problem with sestamibi because imaging is delayed for at least 30 min after the exercise is discontinued. Software algorithms for motion detection and correction are being developed.

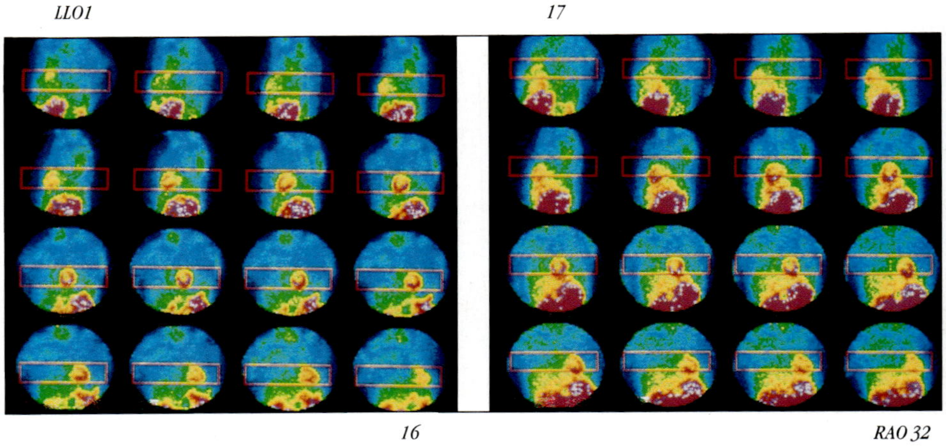

Figure 2.24c
The display represents the 32 projections from left lateral oblique (LLO) (frame 1) to right anterior oblique (RAO) view (frame 32). The heart normally stays inside the reference box during the whole acquisition. In this case, it moves outside the box from frame 17 to 32 as a result of patient movement. This movement is responsible for the artefacts observed.

Quality control artefacts

Adequate uniformity and centre of rotation corrections are prerequisites to obtain good quality. tomograms (Figs. 2.25a,b).

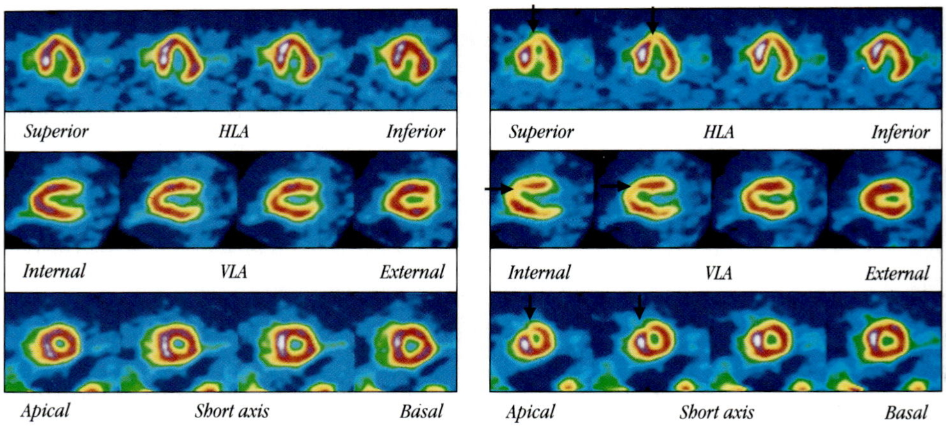

Figures 2.25a,b
Good uniformity correction is necessary to obtain good quality images and homogeneous sestamibi uptake on tomograms. This can be seen in (a). The absence of uniformity correction leads to artefacts, as illustrated by the arrows in (b).

Reconstruction artefacts

The resolution of the reconstruction filter modifies the shape and the thickness of myocardial walls and the size of the ventricular cavity as well as of the perfusion defects (Figs. 2.26a–h).

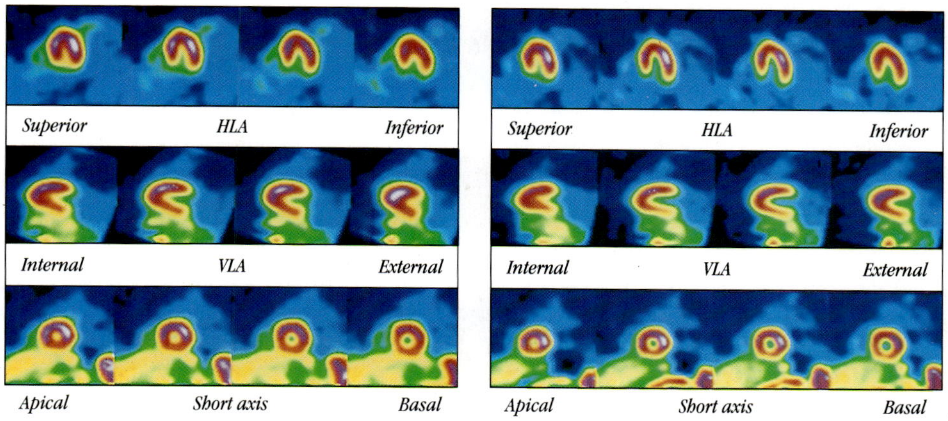

Figures 2.26a,b
In a normal subject, the apparent thickness of the myocardial wall is larger and the left ventricular cavity smaller with a lower resolution filter (a) than with a higher resolution filter (b).

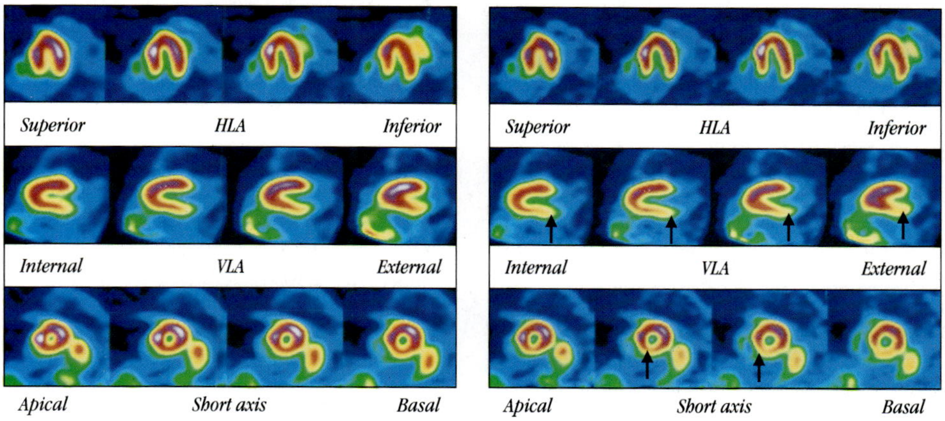

Figures 2.26c,d
The use of a higher resolution filter can induce artefactual sestamibi defects most often in the inferoposterior and in the inferior walls of the LV (d, arrow), as compared with a lower resolution filter (c).

Figures 2.26e,f
In a patient with an abnormal perfusion pattern, sestamibi defects in the inferoposterior and in the inferior walls of the LV (arrows) appear smaller with a lower resolution filter (e) than with a higher resolution filter (f).

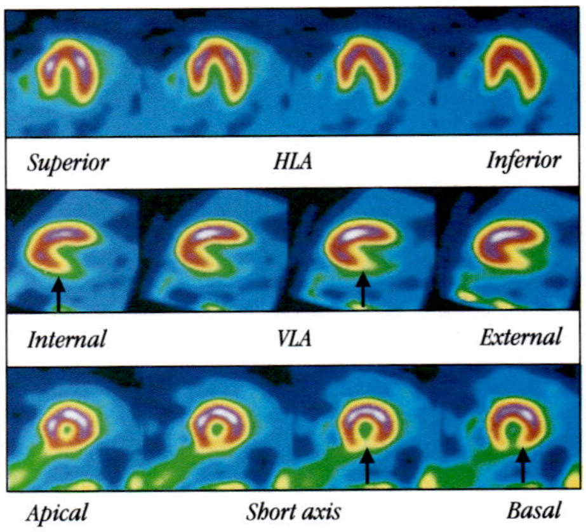

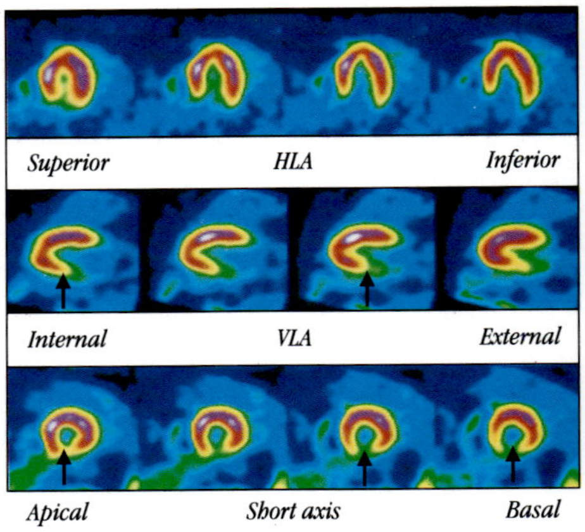

Figures 2.26g,h
Comparative results obtained after good (g) and bad reaxation of myocardial slices in control subject. Inadequate reaxation (h) alters the horseshoe symmetry of the HLA and VLA views (arrows) and creates inferoposterior and posteroseptal artefacts (arrows).

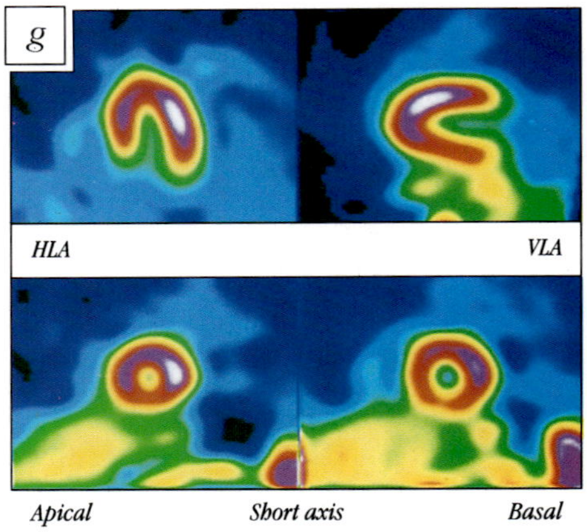

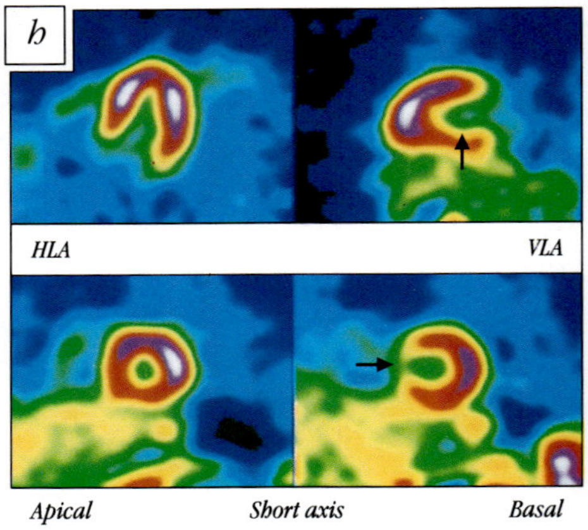

Normal Ventricular Function

First-pass images

Using a bolus injection of sestamibi routine first-pass ventricular function studies are possible (Figs. 2.27a,b,c,d).

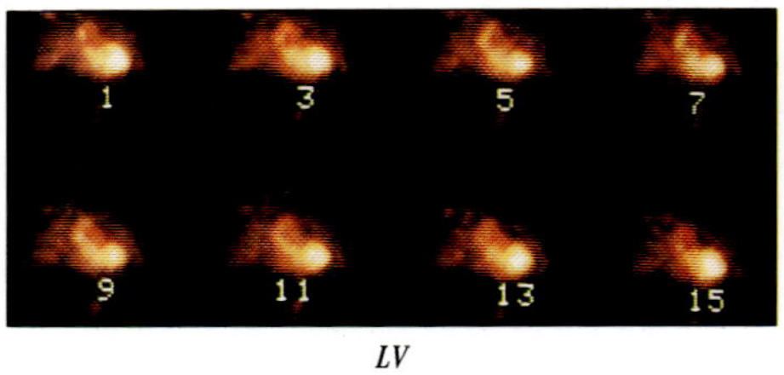

Figure 2.27a
Gated first-pass acquisition performed at rest in the anterior view after intravenous injection of 555 MBq sestamibi. Eight dynamic frames are visualized and represent an average cardiac cycle. Frame number 1 corresponds to diastole and frame number 9 to systole.

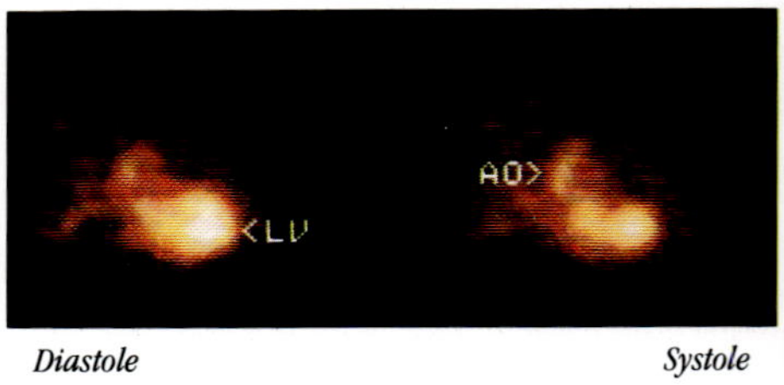

Figure 2.27b
Diastolic and systolic frames from which the evaluation of the left ventricular ejection fraction is obtained (LVEF = 51%).

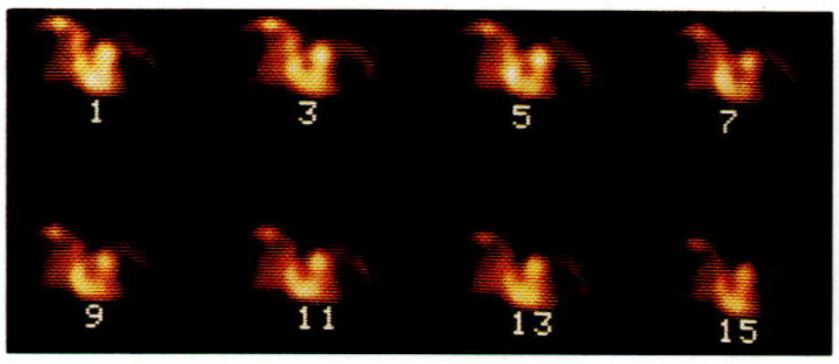

Figure 2.27c
Dynamic right ventricular frames obtained with the first-pass technique to assess global right ventricular function (anterior frame).

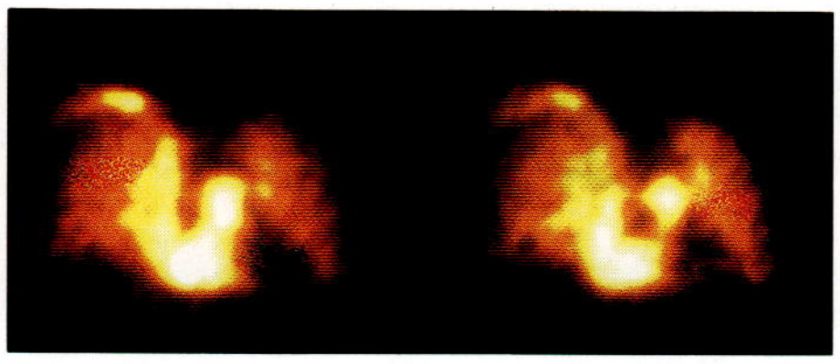

Figure 2.27d
As for the LV, right ventricular ejection fraction can be obtained from diastolic and systolic frames.

Gated planar and SPECT images

Synchronization of planar (Fig. 2.28a,b) and SPECT (Fig. 2.29a,b) perfusion images is an alternative method to obtain information on global and regional ventricular function.

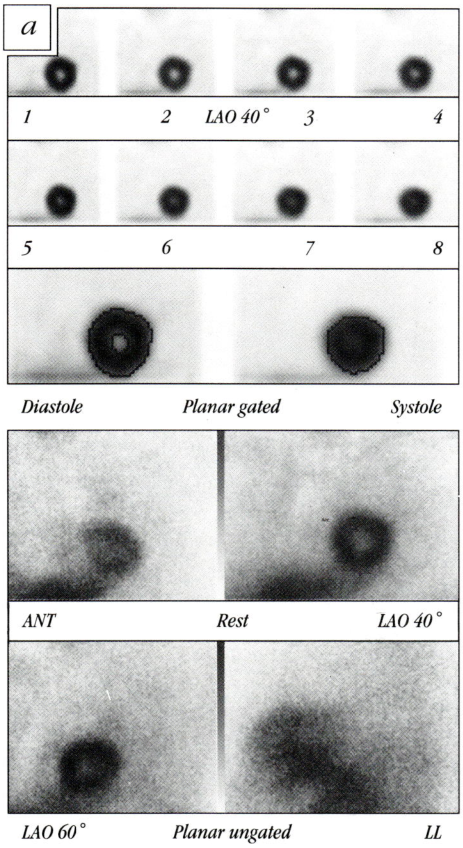

Figure 2.28a
Simultaneous analysis of myocardial perfusion and myocardial thickening after single injection of sestamibi. The LAO 40° frames are displayed from diastole to systole. Perfusion is normal and a good contraction pattern is evident. The gated study (top) is shown alongside the ungated study (bottom).

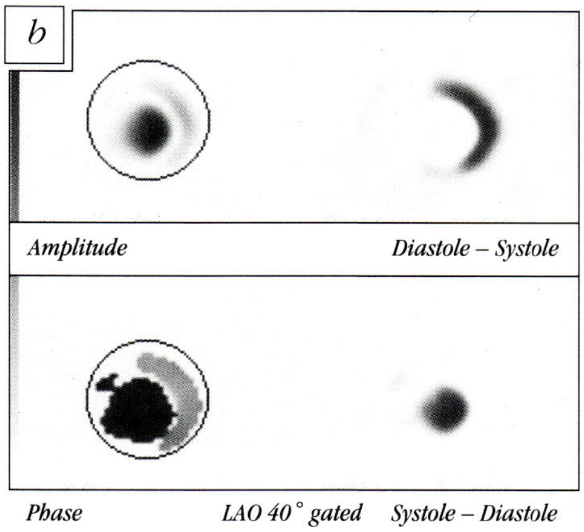

Figure 2.28b
The parametric images reflect both the overall cardiac displacement (from the posterolateral to the anteroseptal regions) and wall thickening. The epicardial motion best displayed on the phase image and the diastolic–systolic images mainly reflect overall cardiac displacement. The endocardial motion most evident on the amplitude and systolic–diastolic images mainly reflects wall thickening.

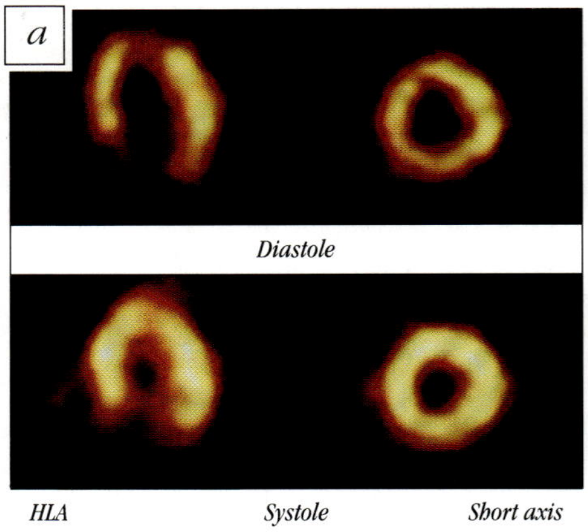

Figure 2.29a
Gated tomography performed at rest with sestamibi. Diastolic frames appear in the upper part of the panel and systolic frames in the lower part. The comparison between diastole and systole confirms the presence of good myocardial wall thickening of the LV.

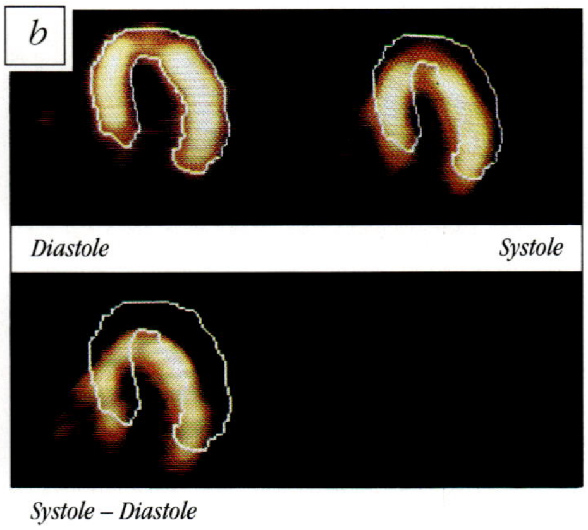

Figure 2.29b
Functional images of difference (S − D) displayed together with diastole (D) and systole (S) images as well as the diastolic outlines demonstrate good myocardial wall motion.

Clinical Indications for Sestamibi Imaging

Table 2.3 shows the main clinical indications for sestamibi imaging and the remainder of this book will address these individual clinical problems.

Patients with known ischaemic heart disease (IHD) Assessing the significance of mild/moderate coronary stenoses shown on angiography Assessing extent and distribution of disease in patients with known IHD Diagnosis of postinfarct ischaemia Diagnosis of myocardial viability in patients with cardiac failure *Atypical chest pain* Diagnosing/excluding ischaemic heart disease in patients with atypical chest pain	*Low-risk patients with positive or borderline exercise tests* Diagnosing/excluding IHD in patients in whom a false-positive exercise test is suspected *Baseline ECG abnormalities* Diagnosing/excluding IHD in patients with abnormal ECGs (left bundle branch block (LBBB), paced, etc.) in whom interpretation of the exercise test is not possible	*Low exercise tolerance* Diagnosing/excluding IHD in patients who cannot exercise (dipyridamole) *Therapeutic* Pre-streptokinase diagnosis of acute myocardial infarction Thrombolysis/angioplasty/coronary artery bypass graft follow-up Pre-surgical risk assessment for arteriopathic patients undergoing major surgery

Table 2.3 *Clinical indications for imaging with sestamibi.*

3 DIAGNOSIS OF CORONARY ARTERY DISEASE

Clinical Background

Coronary artery disease (CAD) is the major cause of premature death and disability in Western countries.[1,2] The risk factors for CAD have been clearly identified and include family history, age and sex, blood lipid disorders, smoking, hypertension and obesity. Correction of risk factors has been shown to improve prognosis both in the preclinical and clinical stages of the affection.

Initial manifestations of CAD consist of sudden death, myocardial infarction and angina (Fig. 3.1). Early diagnosis is therefore mandatory to decrease mortality and avoid permanent sequelae of the disease. Diagnosis relies on subjective or objective signs of myocardial ischaemia or infarction or on angiographic evidence of coronary obstructions.[3,4]

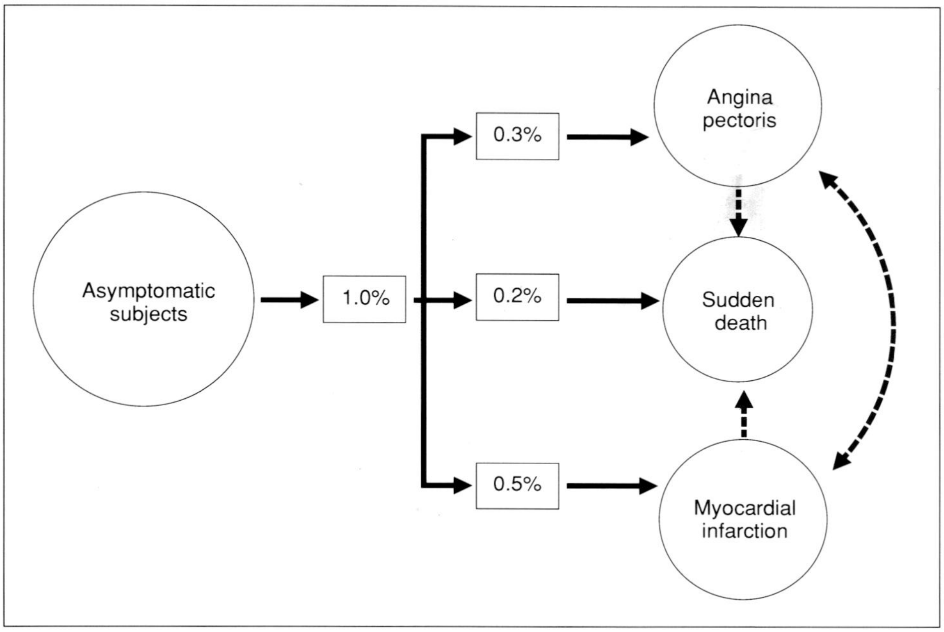

Figure 3.1
Initial presentation in CAD (Framingham Study: male subjects 45–54 years old). (Modified from Ross[3].)

Clinical history provides the first and most important information. Patients usually complain of chest pain classified as typical or atypical for angina pectoris or as non-cardiac pain. Typical chest pain has a pressure-like character, is induced by exercise, is localized in the mid-sternal region, and is often radiated to the jaw or to the left arm (Fig. 3.2). It is relieved by cessation of exercise and by nitrates. Atypical chest pain lacks some of those key elements; frequently it occurs at rest. Non-cardiac pain is clearly suggestive of a parietal origin or of visceral origin different from the heart. Dyspnoea can be an anginal equivalent sign of ischaemia.

The prevalence of CAD has been shown to vary with the clinical presentation and tables are available predicting the percentage prevalence of disease according to age, sex and clinical presentation (Table 3.1). Physical examination can provide evidence of ventricular dysfunction in patients with infarction or acute ischaemia, but is frequently non-contributing in patients with chronic CAD.

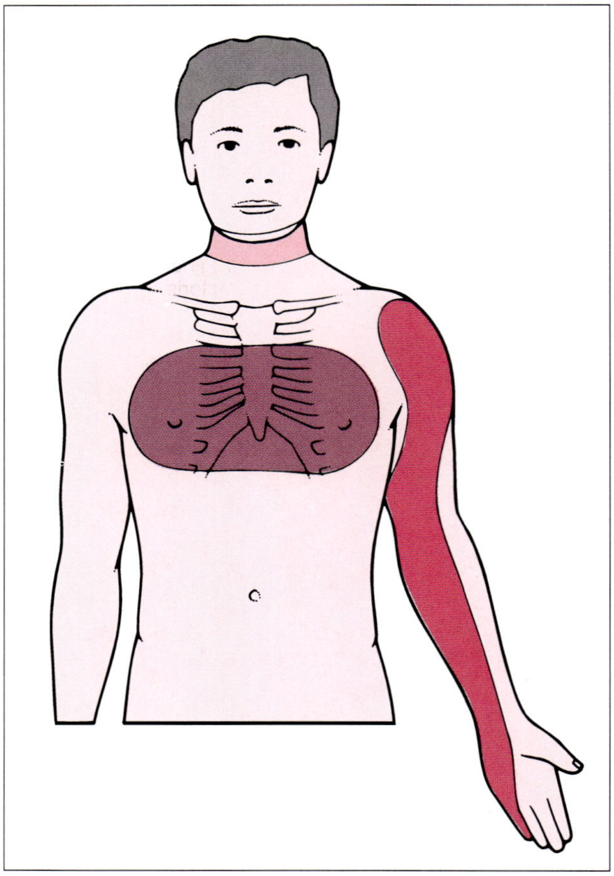

Figure 3.2
Localization and principal radiations of anginal pain.

Exercise ECG provides the next step for diagnosis. Exercise can elicit typical chest pain or demonstrate reduced exercise tolerance or ECG changes 'typical' for CAD (Fig. 3.3). Exercise ECG will, however, give both false-negative and false-positive results, as its sensitivity and specificity are not perfect (Table 3.2). False-positive results are more frequent in women.[5]

The increased efficacy of combining diagnostic information from independent tests simultaneously, or in cascade, using a bayesian approach, has been demonstrated. Myocardial perfusion imaging is such a test. It provides information not only on the presence, but also on the site and extent of stress-induced perfusion abnormalities and their reversibility at rest.

Myocardial imaging is both more sensitive and more specific than exercise ECG for the diagnosis of CAD (Table 3.3).[6–10]

Age	Non-anginal chest pain		Atypical angina		Typical angina	
(years)	Men	Women	Men	Women	Men	Women
30–39	5.2±0.8	0.8±0.3	21.8±2.4	4.2±1.3	69.7±3.2	25.8±6.6
40–49	14.1±1.3	2.8±0.7	46.1±1.8	13.3±2.9	87.3±1.0	55.2±6.5
50–59	21.5±1.7	8.4±1.2	58.9±1.5	32.4±3.0	92.0±0.6	79.4±2.4
60–69	28.1±1.9	18.6±1.9	67.1±1.3	54.4±2.4	94.3±0.4	90.6±1.0

Table 3.1
Pre-test likelihood of coronary artery disease in symptomatic patients according to age and sex.[4]

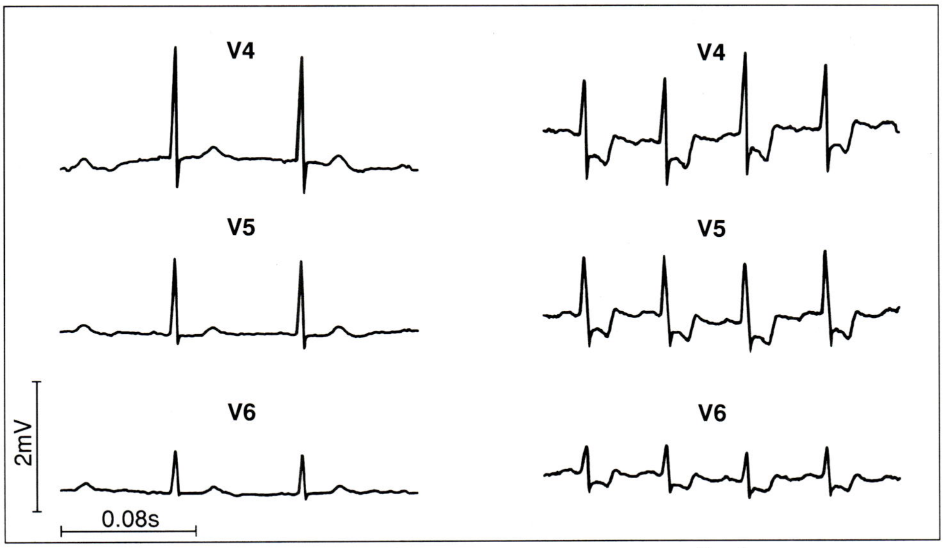

Rest Exercise

Figure 3.3
Rest and exercise ECG in a patient with typical angina pectoris (typical ST depression).

Table 3.2
Sensitivity and specificity of exercise ECG and visual planar thallium imaging.

	Sensitivity	Specificity
Gianrossi et al[5]	66%	77%
Kotler and Diamond[6]	84%	87%

Clinical Problems

Indications for myocardial imaging

Diagnostic work-up including myocardial imaging is most often required in patients with low or intermediate probability for CAD, that is in patients with atypical chest pain and/or absence or low incidence of risk factors, as well as in women. Myocardial imaging is also frequently requested in patients with non-diagnostic ECGs (hypertension, patients on digitalis, patients with pacemaker or conduction disturbances) or in patients unable to exercise properly. Pharmacological stress (dipyridamole or dobutamine) is frequently proposed as an alternative to exercise in combination with myocardial imaging in these patients (Fig. 3.4).[11]

Patients with a high probability for CAD (a typical history combined with positive risk factors) require imaging for diagnosis less often. However, imaging will frequently be performed

Table 3.3
Sensitivity and specificity of ^{99m}Tc sestamibi and thallium by SPECT imaging.

	Sensitivity		Specificity	
	Thallium	Sestamibi	Thallium	Sestamibi
Detection of CAD				
Kiat et al[12]	80%	93%	75%	75%
Iskandrian et al[14]	82%	82%	82%	100%
Detection of individual vessel disease				
Kiat et al[12]	77%	87%	86%	86%
Khan et al[13]	60%	79%	69%	72%

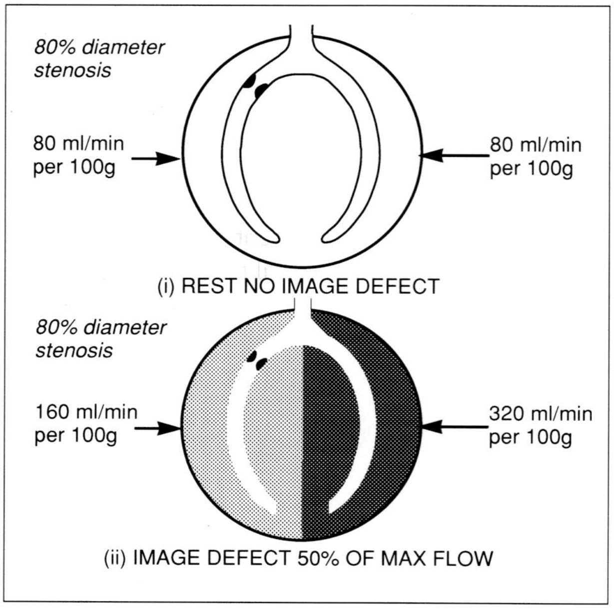

Figure 3.4
Mechanism of dipyridamole myocardial imaging in patients with CAD.

in these patients to assess the location and extent of the disease and to aid the planning of the therapeutic course.

Coronary angiography

Systematic performance of diagnostic coronary angiography in patients with suspected CAD has been advocated in the past. However, this approach is more costly, it carries more risk to the patient, and in fact provides no more or perhaps less prognostic information than is available by the use of stress myocardial perfusion imaging. Furthermore, coronary angiography shows the coronary anatomy – not the hydraulic and functional consequences of the lesions.

Identification of a coronary stenosis, especially of mild or moderate degree, does not prove that this stenosis is responsible for the patient's symptoms. Numerous studies have highlighted that the so-called 'gold standard' is frequently a false idol!

Aims of sestamibi studies

Sestamibi stress perfusion studies are indicated to diagnose CAD in symptomatic patients with low to moderate probability of the disease or in patients with higher probability in whom initial testing has failed to confirm presence of the disease. Sestamibi studies are also indicated to define the extent of CAD (see Chapter 4) during the diagnostic phase and to assess the need for angiography and invasive therapeutic planning. The increased sensitivity of tomographic imaging to detect multiple vessel disease has increased the importance of this indication.[12–14]

The value of using myocardial imaging and sestamibi to screen asymptomatic patients with low disease probability has not yet been established. Indeed, in these groups of patients, the false-positive rate can be higher than the true-positive rate and diagnostic accuracy is lower unless the test has almost perfect specificity.

Myocardial infarction can sometimes remain silent and go completely unnoticed, especially in diabetic patients. Myocardial imaging is useful in these patients to confirm the presence of necrosis and to evaluate the extent of the disease.

Conclusion

Myocardial imaging is playing an increasing role in the non-invasive diagnosis of CAD. The improved sensitivity and specificity of sestamibi is likely to further extend the indications of the test.

Clinical Points

- Myocardial perfusion imaging is both more sensitive and more specific than exercise ECG for the diagnosis of coronary heart disease.
- Maximal benefit is observed in patients with intermediate probability of the disease, and in patients with non-diagnostic ECGs.
- Patients with a high probability for coronary heart disease require imaging to aid in the planning of the therapeutic course rather than for diagnosis.
- Myocardial imaging is particularly useful to confirm silent myocardial ischaemia or infarction.
- The value of myocardial imaging to screen asymptomatic patients with low disease probability has not yet been established. A test with very high specificity is needed for this purpose.

References

1 KULLER LH, Epidemiology of cardiovascular disease: current perspectives, *Am J Epidemiol* (1976) **104**:425.

2 KANNEL WB, GORDON T, *The Framingham Study: an epidemiological investigation of cardiovascular disease* (Dept. of Health, Education and Welfare: Washington DC 1974) Publication No. (NIH) 174-599.

3 ROSS RS, Surgery for coronary artery disease placed in perspective, *Bull NY Acad Med* (1982) **48**:1163.

4 DIAMOND GA, FORRESTER J, Analysis of probability as an aid in the clinical diagnosis of coronary-artery disease, *N Eng J Med* (1979) **300**:1350.

5 GIANROSSI R, DETRANO R, MULVIHILL D et al, Exercise-induced ST depression in the diagnosis of coronary artery disease: a meta-analysis, *Circulation* (1989) **80**:87.

6 KOTLER TS, DIAMOND GA, Exercise thallium-201 scintigraphy in the diagnosis and prognosis of coronary artery disease, *Ann Inter Med* (1990) **113**:684.

7 GERSON M, Test accuracy, test selection and test result interpretation in chronic coronary artery disease. In: Gerson M, ed, *Cardiac nuclear medicine* (McGraw-Hill Book Co: New York 1987) 309.

8 POHOST GM, ZIR LM, MOORE RH et al, Differentiation of transiently ischemic from infarcted myocardium by serial imaging after a single dose of thallium-201, *Circulation* (1977) **55**:294.

9 FINTEL DJ, LINKS JM, BRINKER JA et al, Improved diagnostic performance of exercise thallium-201 single photon emission computed tomography over planar imaging in the diagnosis of coronary artery disease: a receiver operating characteristic analysis, *J Am Coll Cardiol* (1989) **14**:1477.

10 VAN TRAIN KF, MADDAHI J, BERMAN DS et al, Quantitative analysis of tomographic stress thallium-201 myocardial scintigrams: a multicenter trial, *J Nucl Med* (1990) **31**:1168.
11 TAILLEFER R, Technetium-99m Sestamibi myocardial imaging: same day rest–stress studies and dipyridamole, *Am J Cardiol* (1990) **66**:80E.
12 KIAT H, MADDAHI J, ROY L et al, Comparison of Tc-99m methoxy isobutyl isonitrile with thallium-201 imaging by planar and SPECT techniques for assessment of coronary disease, *Am Heart J* (1989) **117**:1.
13 KAHN J, MCGHIE I, AKERS M et al, Quantitative rotational tomography with thallium and Tc-99m 2-methoxy-isobutyl-isonitrile: a direct comparison in normal individuals and patients with coronary artery disease, *Circulation* (1989) **79**:1282.
14 ISKANDRIAN AS, HEO J, KONG B et al, Use of technetium-99m isonitrile (RP-30A) in assessing left ventricular perfusion and function at rest and during exercise in coronary artery disease, and comparison with coronary arteriography and exercise thallium-201 SPECT imaging, *Am J Cardiol* (1989) **64**:270.

Case Study III.1

Usefulness of myocardial imaging in the presence of false-negative ECG

Mr SL is a 50-year-old man. He smokes, and presents hypertension as well as dyslipaemia. He was admitted to the cardiology department for the occurrence of typical chest pain induced by moderate efforts such as walking quickly or climbing up stairs. Pain is relieved by nitrates.

An exercise test was performed on a bicycle up to a load of 90 W and a maximum heart rate of 140 beats/min. The exercise test was interrupted for precordial chest pain but the ECG remained normal during exercise and during recovery (Fig. III.1a).

Sestamibi was injected intravenously at peak exercise and images were acquired 1 h later. Tomography at stress demonstrated the presence of defects in the lateral wall of the left ventricle (LV) (horizontal long axis (HLA) view), in the inferoposterior wall (vertical long axis (VLA) view) and in the inferolateral wall (short axis view) (Fig. III.1b, arrows). The comparative rest study revealed a normal perfusion pattern (Fig. III.1c). This comparison strongly suggested the presence of myocardial ischaemia in the left circumflex (LCx) territory, as confirmed by angiography (Fig. III.1d).

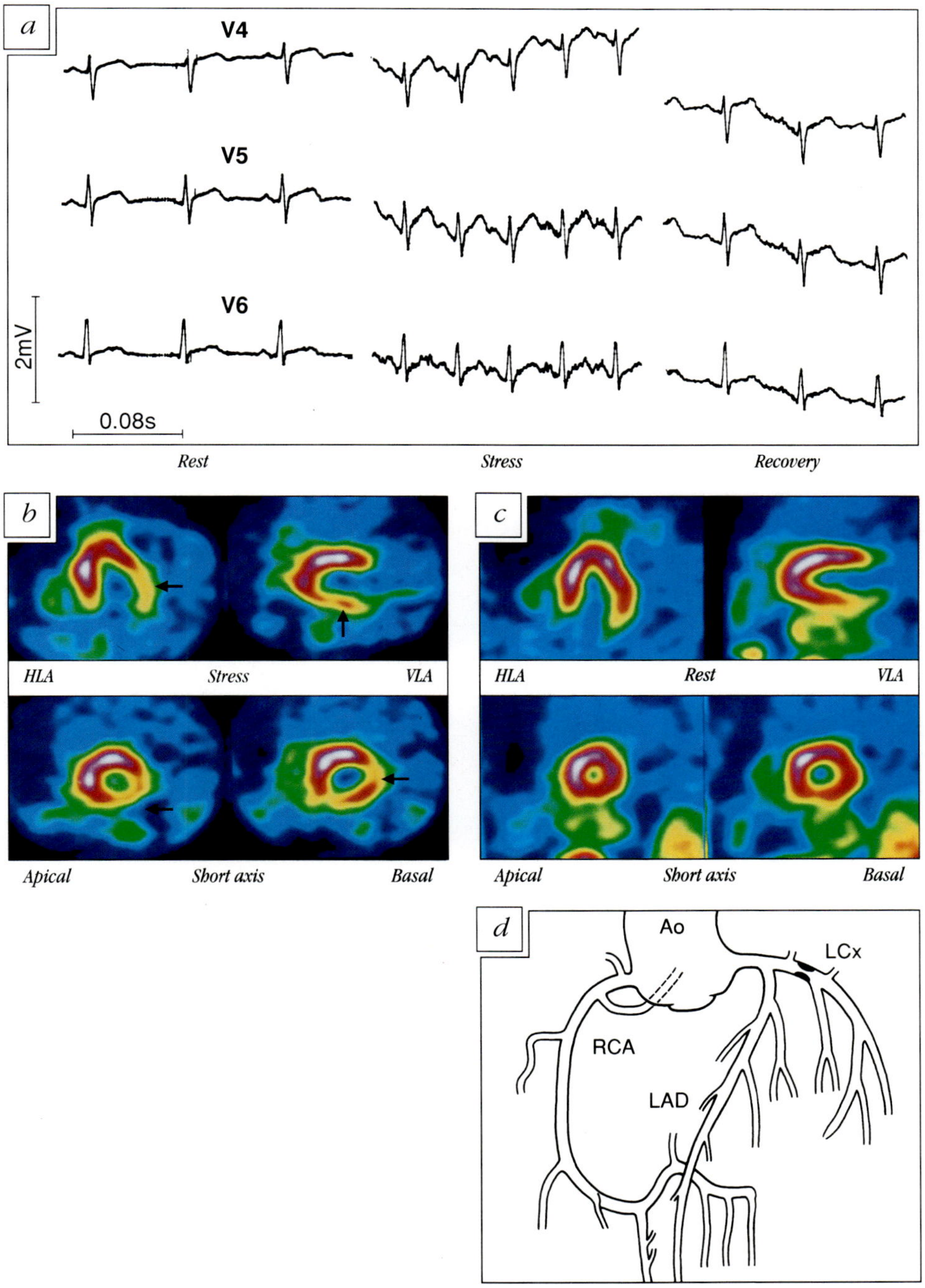

Ao, aorta; RCA, right coronary artery; LAD, left anterior descending; LCx, left circumflex.

Case Study III.2

Interest of perfusion imaging in a patient with a probable false-positive ECG

Mr BM (60 years old) was admitted to the cardiovascular care unit to explore events similar to transient ischaemic attacks. His cardiovascular risk factors include smoking and hypertension.

He exercised on a bicycle at an increasing load of 30 W every 2 min from 30 to 90 W, reaching a heart rate of 130 beats/min at maximum exercise. From 60 W, a significant ST depression appeared in the precordial leads (V3,V4,V5 and V6). This ST depression disappeared during recovery. The patient did not feel chest pain (Fig. III.2a).

Tomography showed homogeneous and normal myocardial uptake in the different myocardial segments (Fig. III.2b). The ECG was considered to be probably false positive, and as the patient had no cardiac symptoms he was not referred for invasive cardiac investigations.

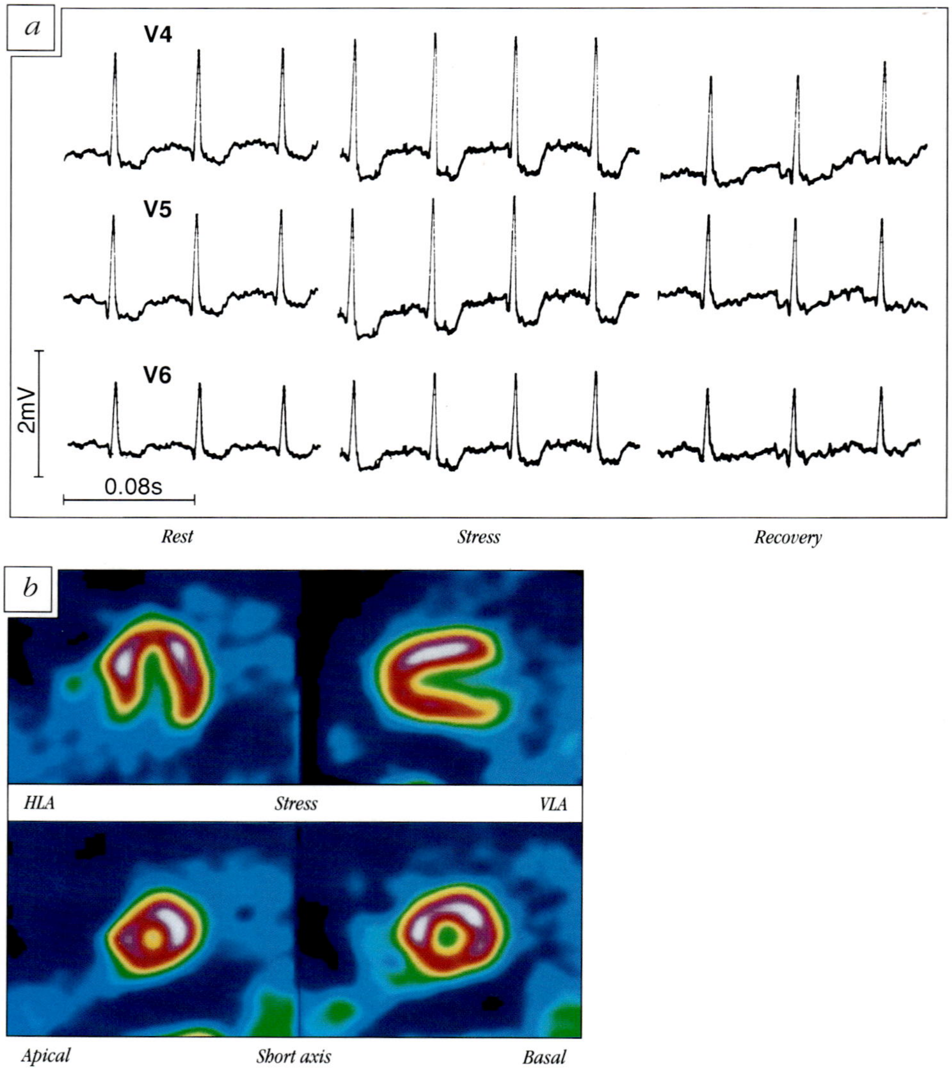

Case Study III.3

Diagnosis of CAD in a patient with mild to moderate probability of disease

The patient is a 41-year-old man, a smoker with no complaint of chest pain but presenting an abnormal resting ECG (presence of RSR' in lead V2) compatible with a posterior necrosis (Fig. III.3a).

The patient underwent maximal bicycle exercise, reaching a load of 280 W and a heart rate of 180 beats/min. The exercise test was interrupted for exhaustion, without occurrence of chest pain.

Planar scintigraphy performed in four projections 1 h after intravenous injection of 555 MBq ^{99m}Tc sestamibi showed normal myocardial uptake of the tracer in the different walls of the LV (Fig. III.3b).

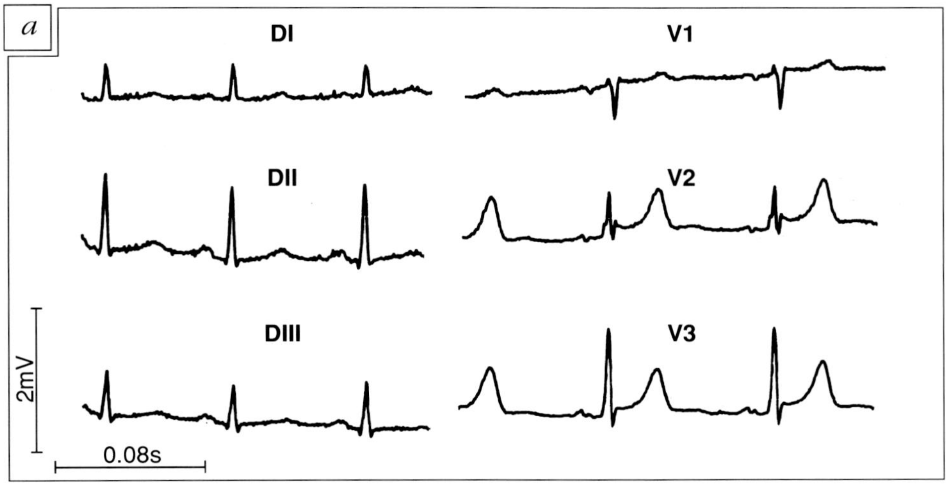

Rest

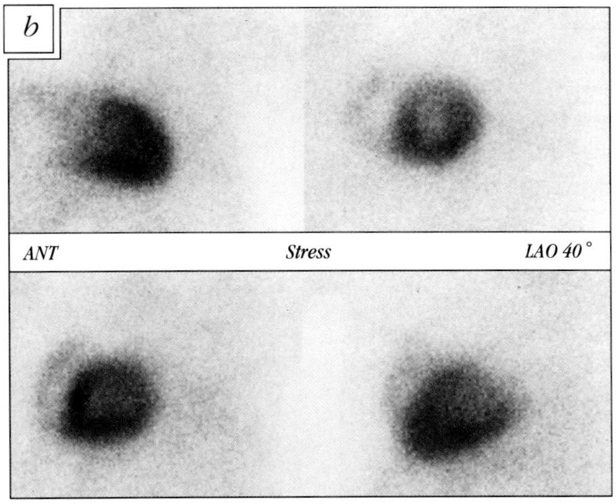

LAO 60° LL

Case Study III.4

Absence of CAD in a woman with atypical chest pain

Mrs PM is a 53-year-old woman who complains of precordial chest pain occurring mainly when tired. Pain is lateralized, non-radiated and not typically induced by exercise such as walking. The patient presents chronic hypertension and has an abnormal ECG (Fig. III.4a).

The patient exercised on a bicycle for 7 min (with load increments of 30 W every 2 min) up to a load of 120 W and a heart rate of 150 beats/min without chest pain.

Myocardial imaging showed a completely normal perfusion pattern at exercise (Fig. III.4b). No sign of ischaemic heart disease developed during 2 years' follow-up.

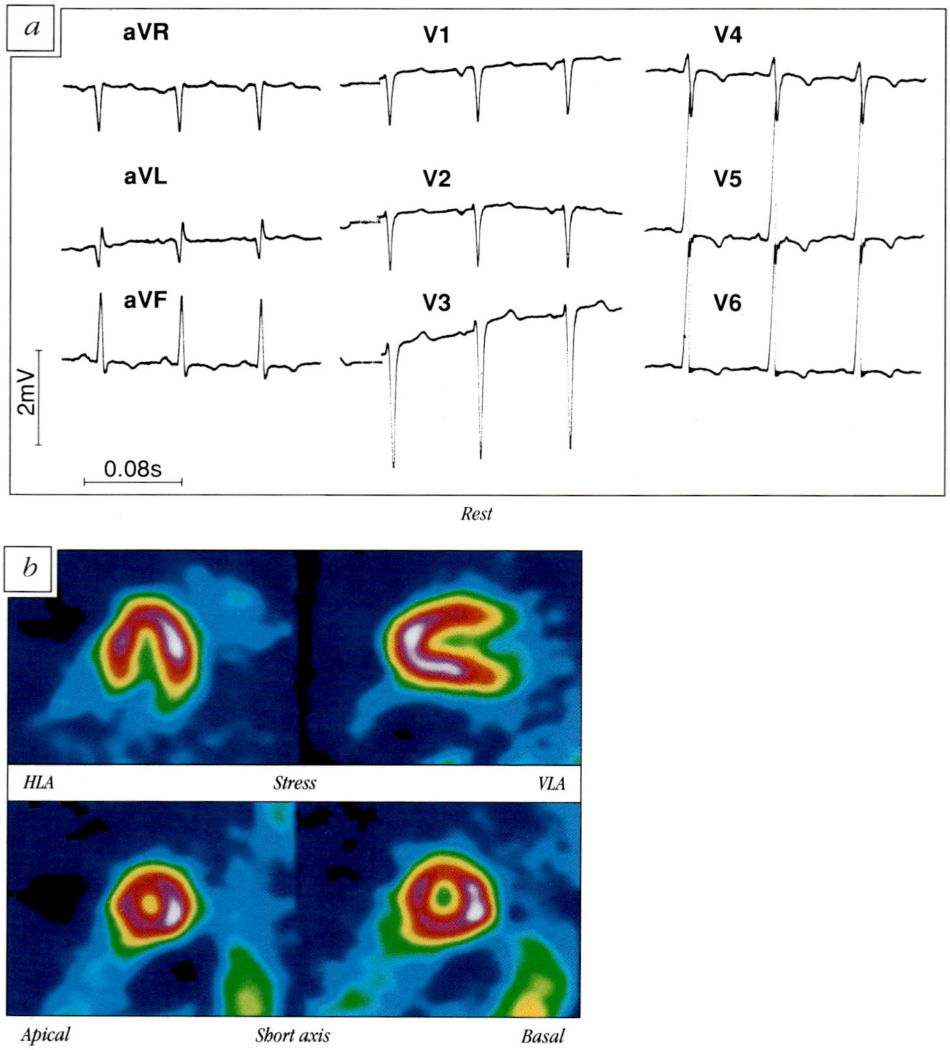

Case Study III.5

Usefulness of perfusion imaging in a patient with a non-diagnostic ECG

Mr MP is a 77-year-old man who has developed a complete atrioventricular block requiring electrostimulation. He has a double chamber pacemaker. He recently presented precordial chest pain of more than 1 h duration, radiated to the left arm. The pain was not relieved by nitrates.

ECG interpretation was difficult in the presence of a pacemaker (Fig. III.5a). Therefore a tomographic study was performed and revealed left ventricular dilatation and a severe sestamibi hypofixation in the anterior wall of the LV, corresponding to a myocardial scar (Fig. III.5b, arrows).

A dipyridamole study demonstrated the presence of mild ischaemia around the infarcted area as well as in the inferoposterior wall of the LV (Fig. III.5c, arrows).

The coronary angiogram showed an occlusion of the middle left anterior descending (LAD), a severe stenosis of the diagonal branch, and a significant stenosis of the right coronary artery (RCA) (Figs. III.5d,e).

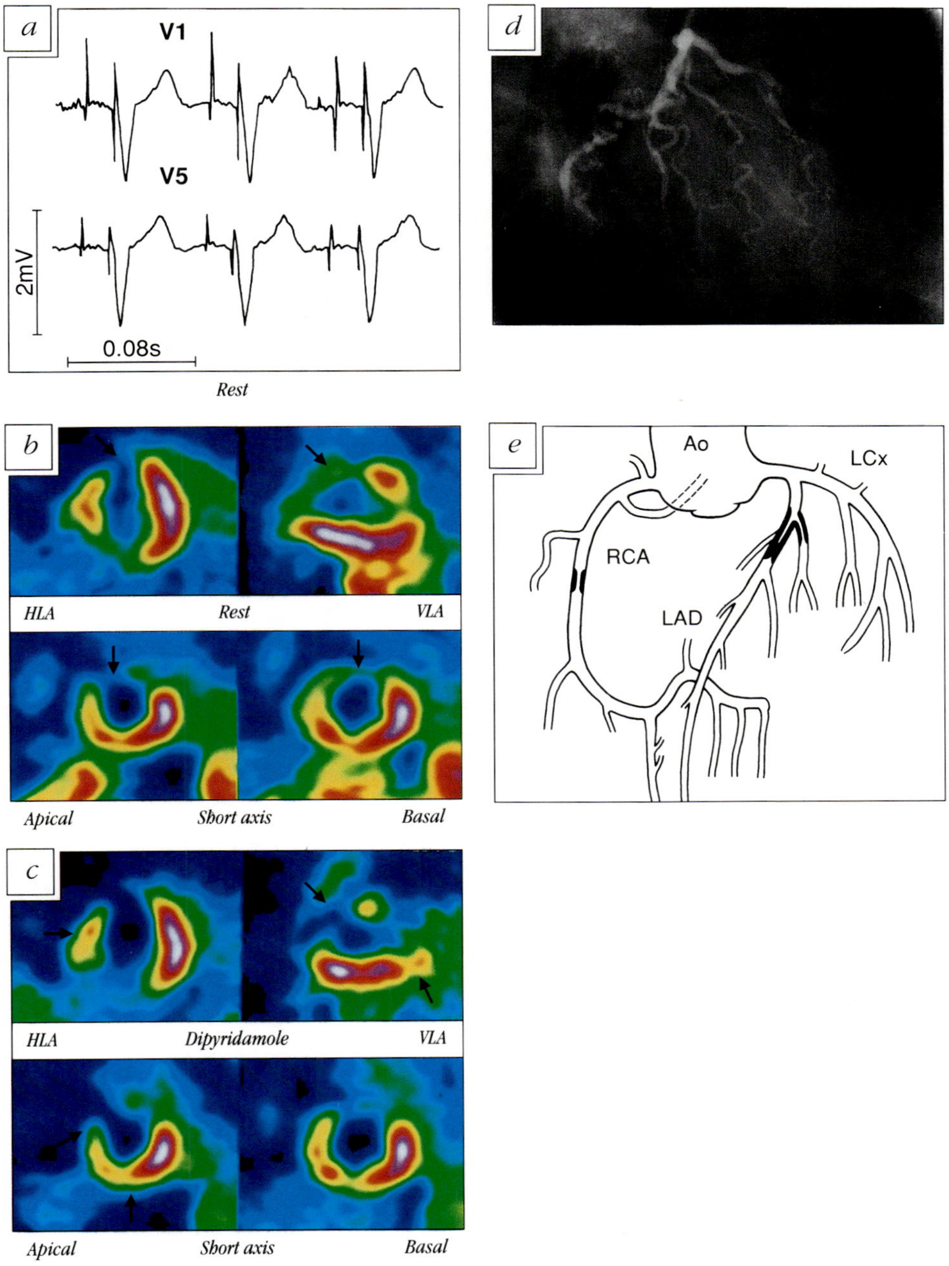

Case Study III.6

Non-diagnostic ECG

This young male patient (30 years old) is a smoker and his father suffers from CAD. He recently developed chest pain, not induced by stress, nor by walking or running, and non-radiated.

The patient's symptoms did not respond to nitrates administered sublingually. His ECG revealed a left bundle branch block (LBBB). He bicycled up to a load of 120 W and reached a heart rate of 145 beats/min (Fig. III.6a). The exercise was interrupted for dyspnoea but not for chest pain.

Planar images showed homogeneous sestamibi uptake in the different walls of the LV. Perfusion imaging in this case did not confirm significant CAD and allowed angiography to be deferred (Fig. III.6b).

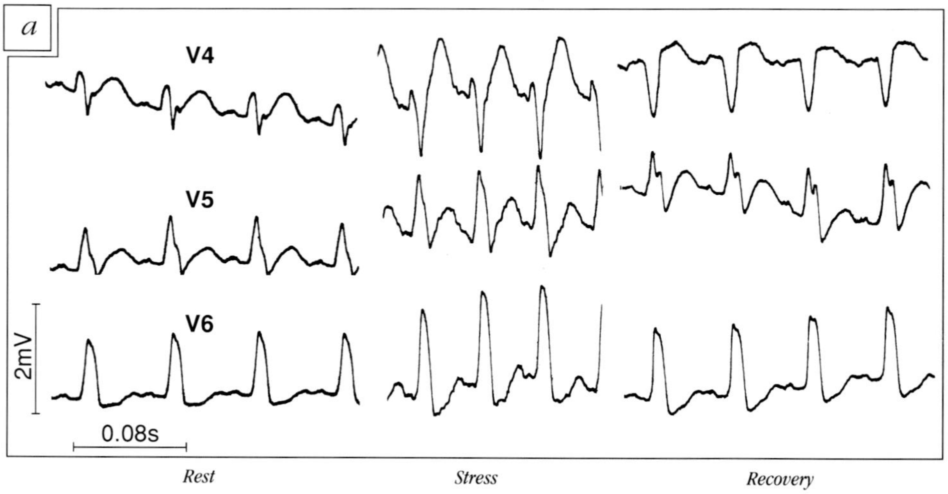

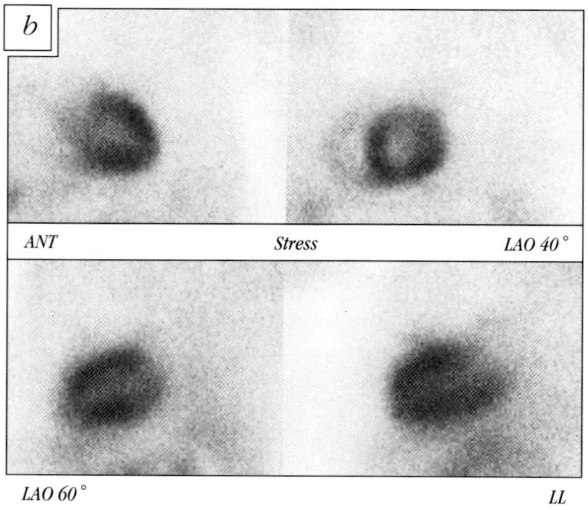

Case Study III.7

Non-diagnostic ECG consecutive to the presence of LBBB

Mr MH is a 70-year-old man admitted to hospital for unstable angina pectoris. Episodes of chest pain are frequent and present at rest. His resting ECG shows LBBB (Fig. III.7a).

A few days after admission of the patient to the intensive care unit, a dipyridamole tomographic study was performed to assess the location and extent of myocardial ischaemia. This study demonstrated the presence of sestamibi defects in the anteroseptal wall of the LV (HLA and short axis views) and also defects in the inferoposterior and inferior walls of the LV, corresponding to significant stenosis of the LAD and of the right coronary arteries which were confirmed by angiography (Figs. III.7b,c, arrows).

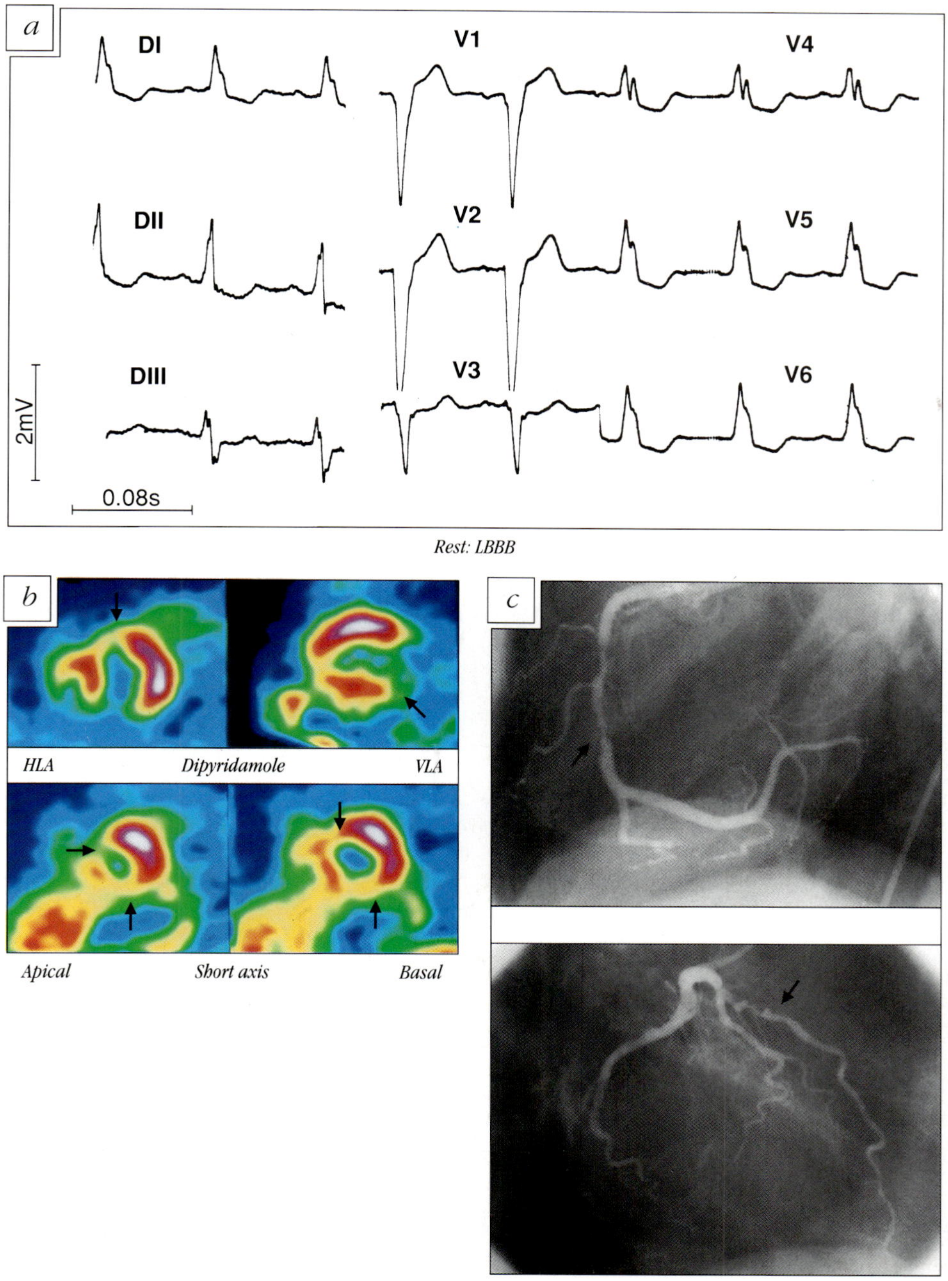

Case Study III.8

Diagnostic study in the presence of LBBB

Mr DC is a 70-year-old man describing precordial chest pain induced by stress but not by walking. He has no previous cardiovascular risk factor.

The patient exercised up to a load of 150 W, reaching a heart rate of 170 beats/min. During exercise, he described dyspnoea and precordial chest pain, but the ECG was difficult to interpret because of an LBBB (Fig. III.8a).

At peak exercise 555 MBq sestamibi was injected for perfusion imaging. Planar scintigraphy performed in four projections 1 h after injection showed moderate left ventricular dilatation and a slightly heterogeneous myocardial uptake (Fig. III.8b, arrow).

Comparative rest scintigraphy 1 day later demonstrated persistent heterogeneity in the uptake of sestamibi (Fig. III.8c, arrow).

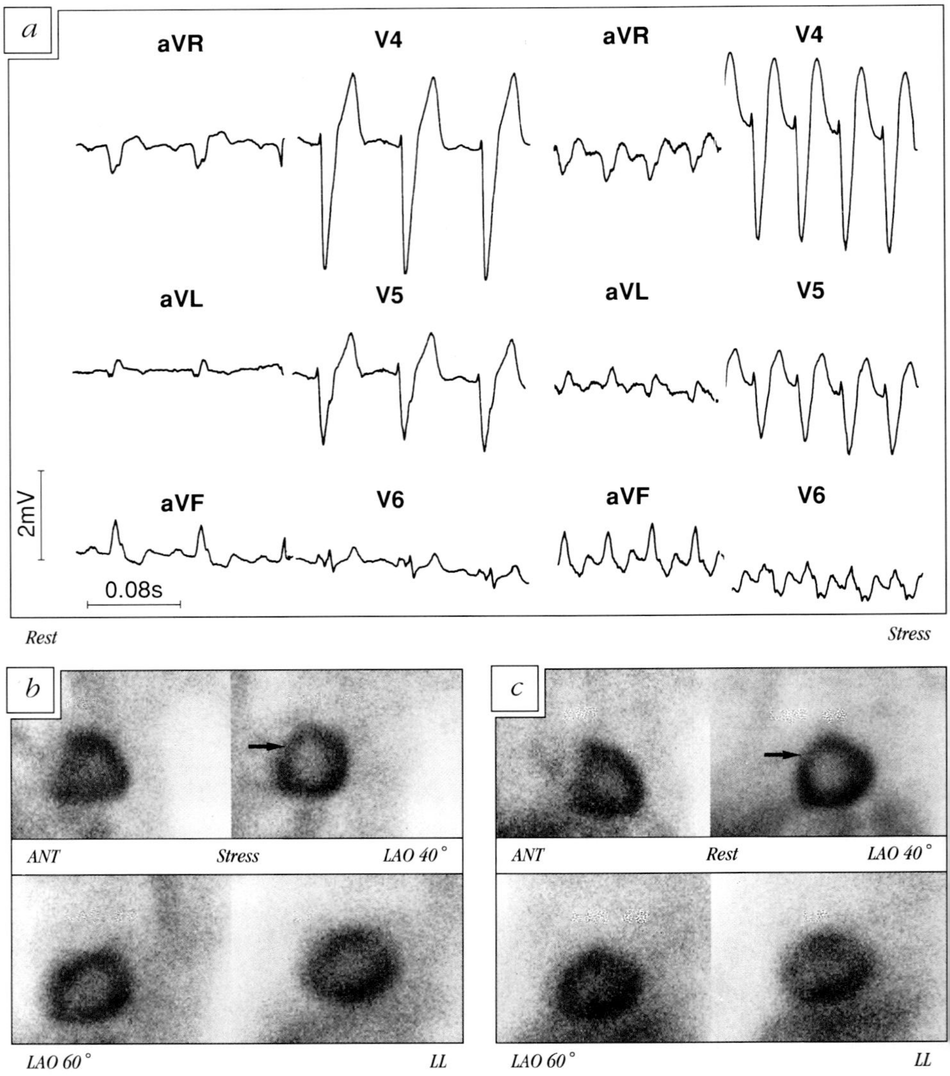

A gated LAO acquisition combined with the classical perfusion images and functional images demonstrated abnormal wall motion in the left ventricular septum (amplitude image) (Figs. III.8d,e). Coronary angiogram confirmed the absence of CAD in this patient (Fig. III.8f). Heterogeneity of myocardial uptake of sestamibi and abnormal septal motion are therefore related to the presence of LBBB.

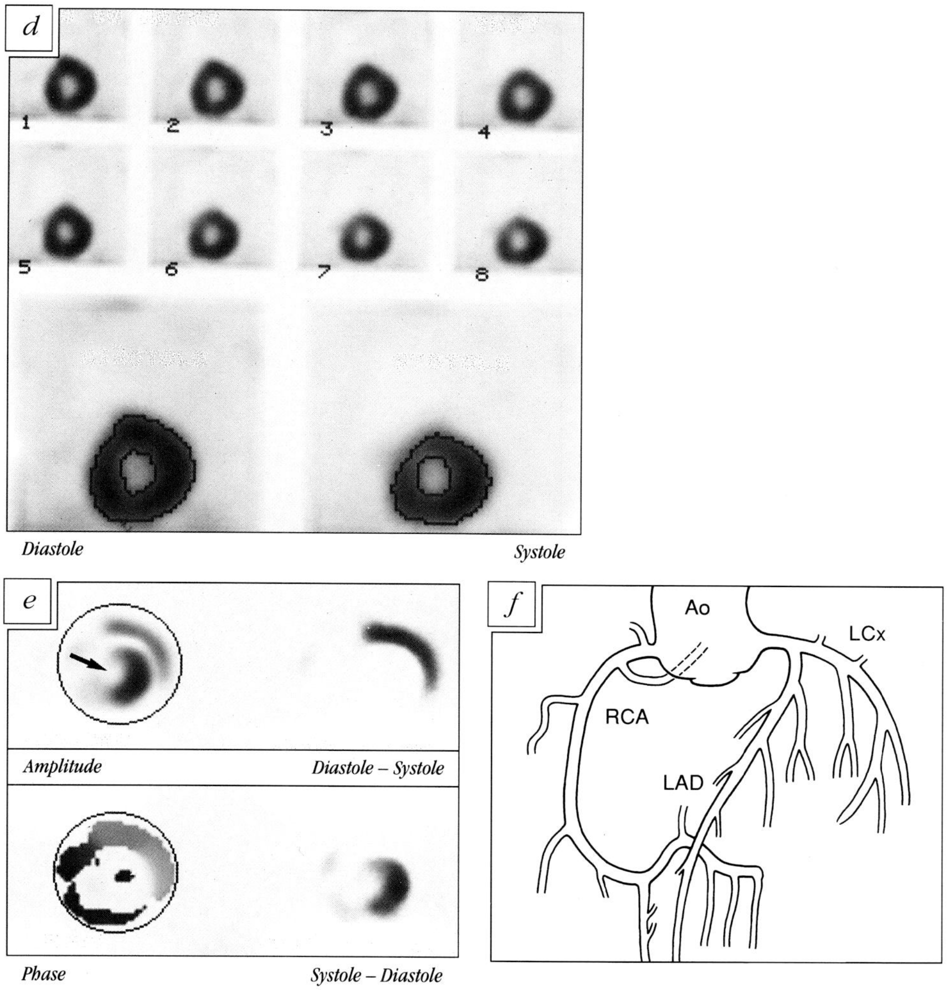

Case Study III.9

Usefulness of perfusion imaging associated with dipyridamole test

This case in an 84-year-old man illustrates the interest of dipyridamole as an alternative to stress in patients who cannot exercise. Dipyridamole is slowly injected intravenously at the dose of 0.146 mg/kg per min over a period of 4 min. Cardiovascular parameters such as blood pressure and heart rate are regularly checked. At the end of the infusion, the patient performs an isometric exercise such as handgrip for a period of 2 min. Thirty seconds before the end of handgrip, sestamibi is injected.

Two minutes after the beginning of the test, the patient described chest pain, but non-conclusive ST depression in leads V4 and V5 was observed on the ECG (Fig. III.9a).

Tomographic images showed sestamibi defects in the inferoposterior and inferior walls of the LV (Fig. III.9b, arrows). The comparative rest study demonstrated normal myocardial perfusion (Fig. III.9c). The comparison established the presence of myocardial ischaemia in the RCA territory. Considering the age of the patient, medical therapy was preferred to invasive explorations.

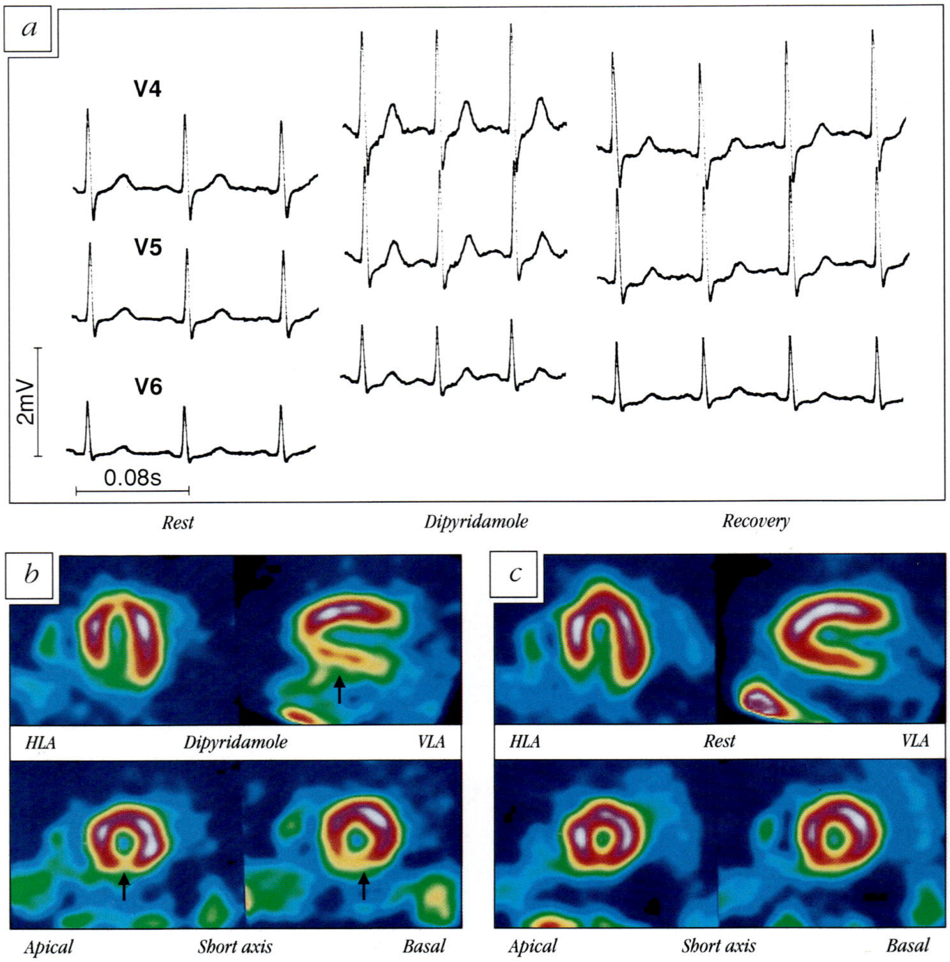

Case Study III.10

Interest of perfusion imaging combined with dipyridamole in a patient unable to exercise

Miss GG is a 69-year-old woman. She describes typical chest pain radiated to her left arm; this pain occurs on walking and sometimes at rest. As she could not easily exercise, dipyridamole perfusion imaging was used to detect myocardial ischaemia.

The ECG recorded during dipyridamole injection was not contributive (Fig. III.10a), but tomography performed 1 h after injection showed sestamibi defects in the anteroseptal wall of the LV (Fig. III.10b), while the comparative rest study showed a normal perfusion pattern (Fig. III.10c).

The angiogram performed a few days later confirmed the presence of significant LAD stenosis (Fig. III.10d) and the patient was referred for transluminal angioplasty.

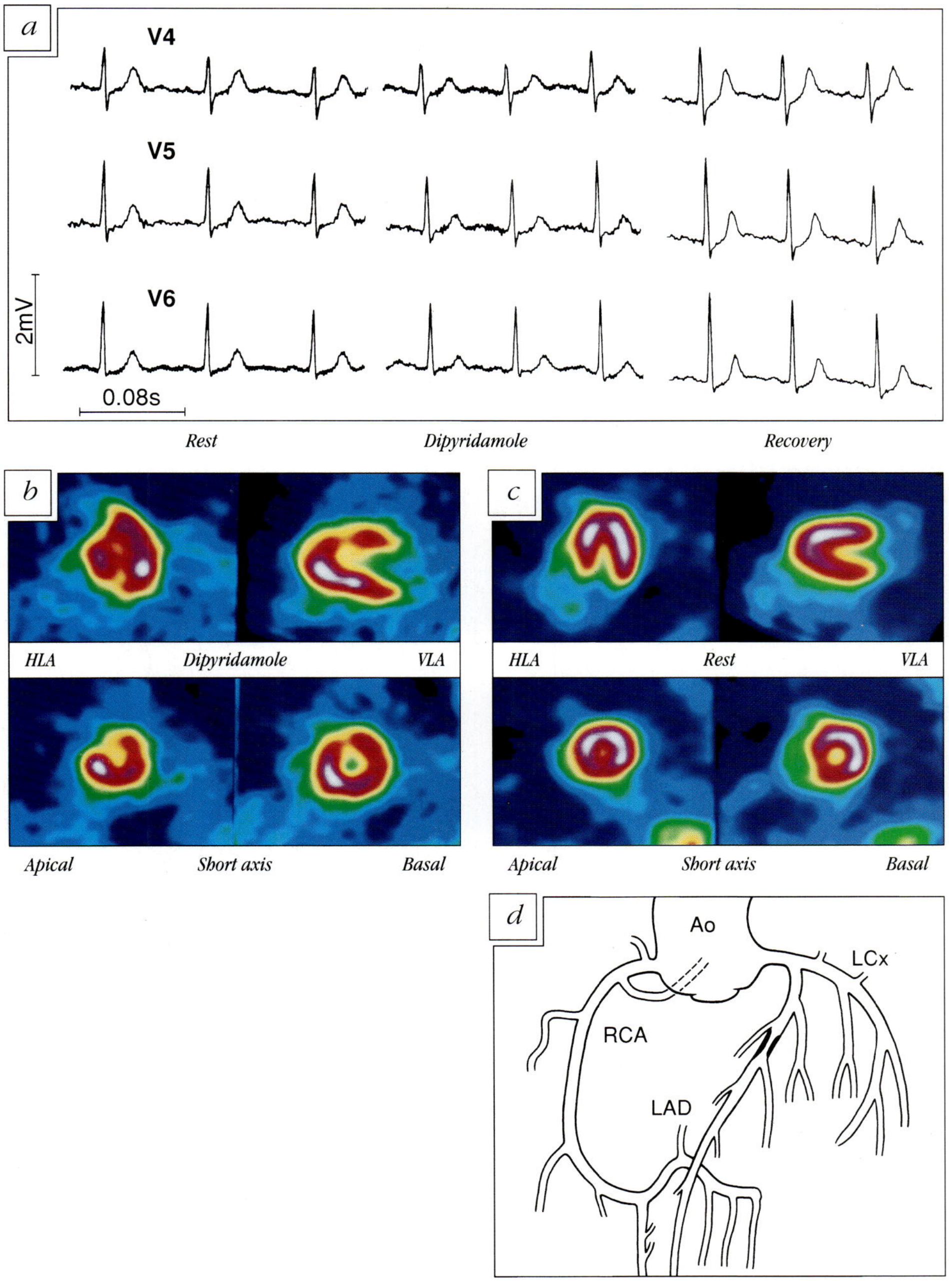

Case Study III.11

Indication of perfusion imaging combined with dipyridamole test

Mrs LM is an 83-year-old woman complaining of left precordial atypical chest pain not induced by exercise and not radiated. She has no history of cardiovascular disease. She cannot exercise because of a prosthetic hip.

A dipyridamole study was performed. A slight ST depression in leads V4 and V5 was observed 3 min after the beginning of injection that disappeared during recovery. The patient felt no typical chest pain (Fig. III.11a).

Tomography showed normal myocardial uptake of sestamibi in the LV (Fig. III.10b). The patient was not referred for coronary angiography.

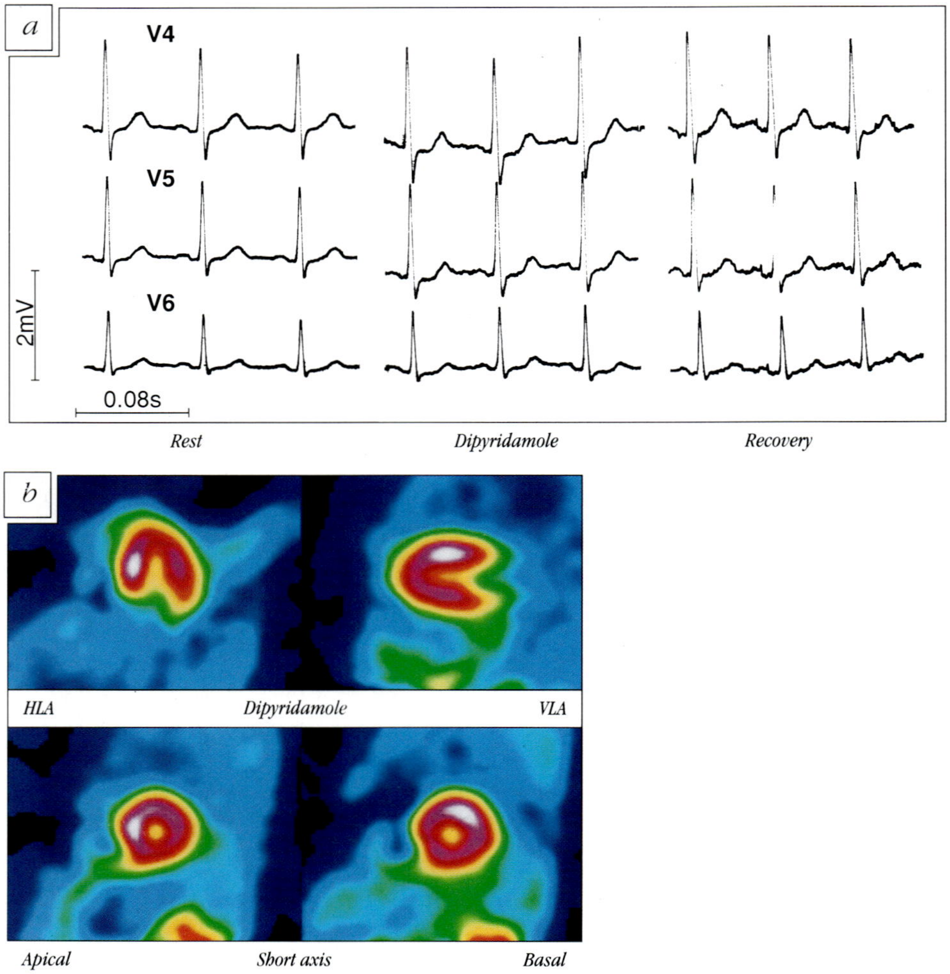

Case Study III.12

Usefulness of tomographic imaging after perfusion of dobutamine at ischaemic dose

Mr DR is a 66-year-old man with chronic renal failure requiring haemodialysis. He has suffered from hypertension for several years with an increased cardiac output and has progressively developed hypertrophy and dilatation of the LV.

Perfusion imaging was requested because of chest pain occurring during haemodialysis. As the patient could not exercise easily on a bicycle, the cardiologist decided to perform echocardiography during incremental infusion of dobutamine in order to assess left ventricular dysfunction and abnormal myocardial contraction corresponding to ischaemia.

Sestamibi was injected during dobutamine infusion and tomographic images were acquired 2 h later.

Tomograms showed the presence of severe sestamibi defects in the anteroseptal and anterior walls. Left ventricular dilatation was also present (Fig. III.12a, arrows).

The comparative rest study demonstrated a persistent left ventricular dilatation and improvement of sestamibi uptake in the LAD territory (Fig. III.12b). Angiographic control in this patient confirmed the presence of a significant stenosis of the LAD after the first diagonal branch (Fig. III.12c).

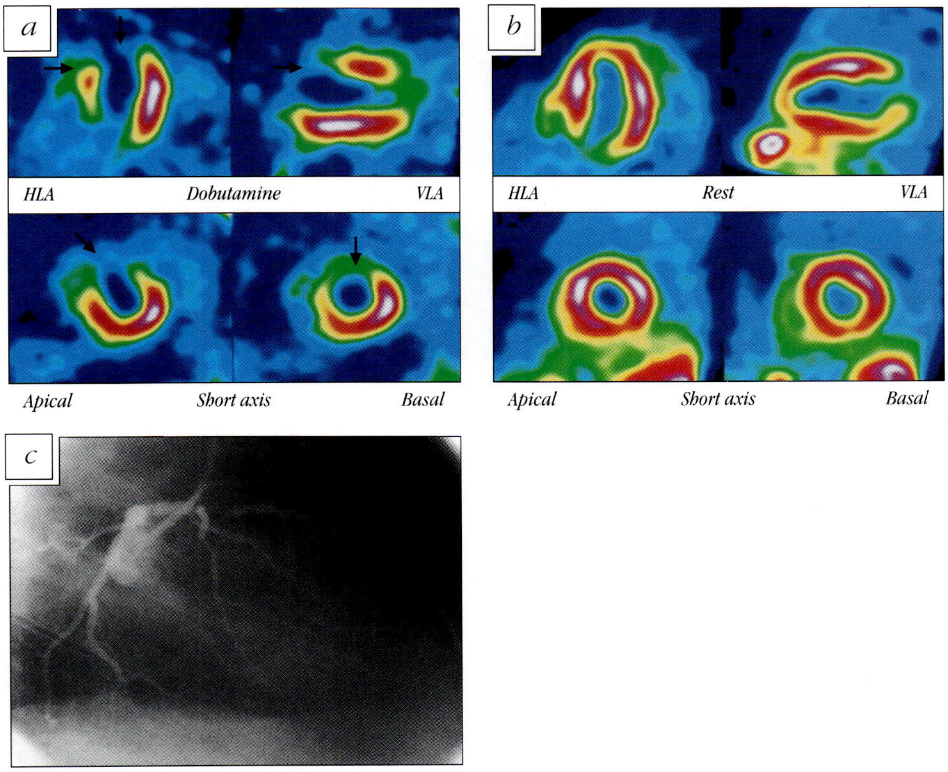

Case Study III.13

Perfusion imaging in a patient with a high probability of CAD

Mr JJ is a 68-year-old man describing precordial chest pain occurring at stress and radiated to the shoulders and the left arm. Pain quickly disappears when he stops walking. His main cardiovascular risk factor is the presence of systolic and diastolic hypertension for several years.

An exercise test was performed on a bicycle lasting 4 min up to a load of 60 W. The heart rate at peak exercise was 130 beats/min (more than 85% of the maximum predicted heart rate). The exercise was interrupted for angina pectoris and ST depression in leads V4, V5 and V6. Abnormal repolarization persisted for 4 min during recovery (Fig. III.13a). Myocardial imaging was performed 1 h later.

The tomograms demonstrated the presence of severe sestamibi hypofixation in the inferior and inferoposterior walls of the LV (Fig. III.13b, arrows). The comparative resting study showed an improved perfusion pattern (Fig. III.13c). This indicated the presence of myocardial ischaemia in the RCA territory. Coronary angiography showed the presence of a significant stenosis of the RCA. The patient underwent successful transluminal angioplasty (Fig. III.13d).

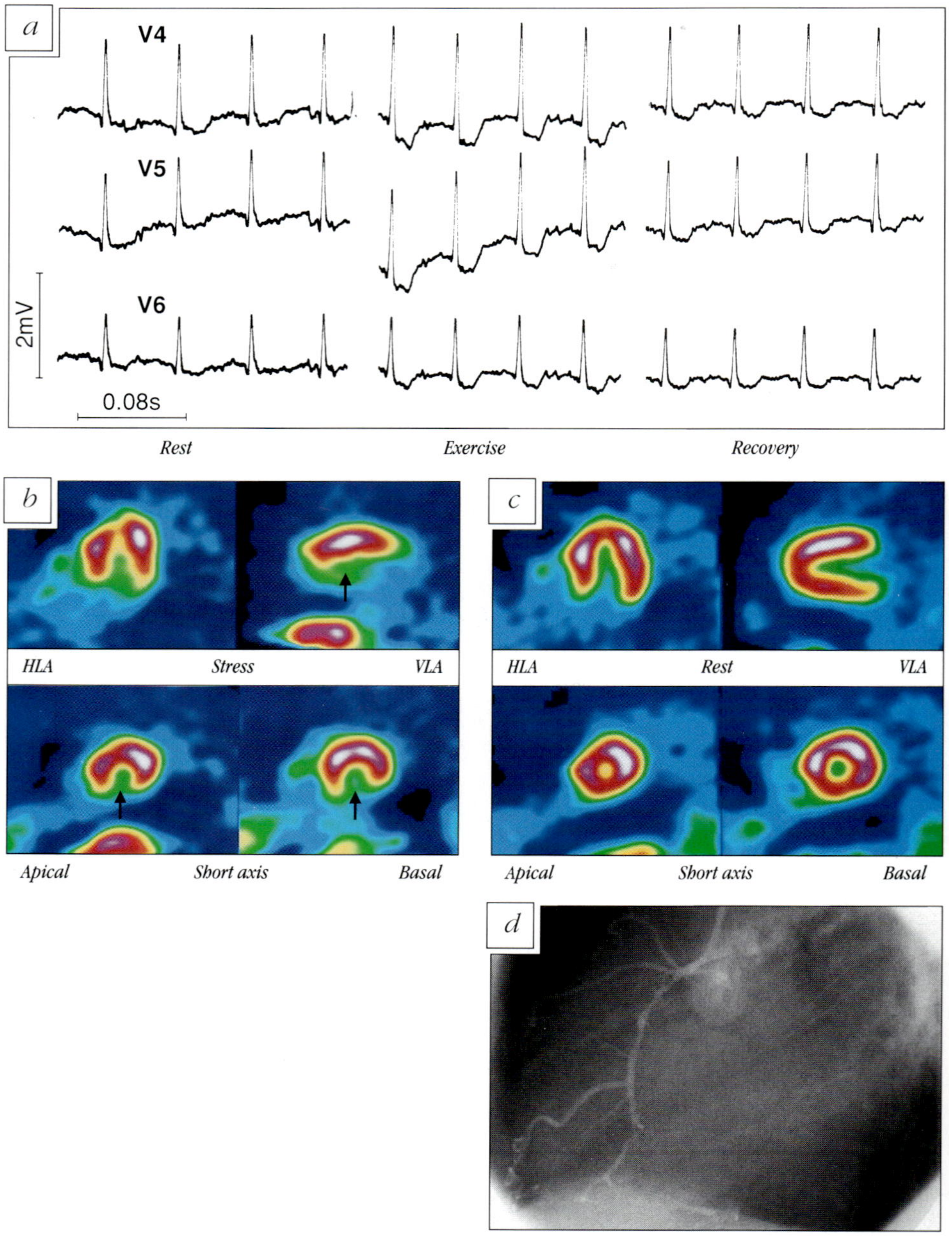

4 EXTENT OF CORONARY ARTERY DISEASE

Clinical Background

Diagnosis of the presence of coronary artery disease (CAD) is clinically and prognostically important. A more complete evaluation of the patient with suspected ischaemic heart disease should include assessing the extent of disease. This is especially true in patients with overt clinical signs of CAD and in patients with known disease, including patients with previous infarction. Indeed, extent of disease and its functional repercussions are the principal factors determining prognosis and influencing therapy selection.[1–3]

Extent of CAD needs to be defined in a broad sense. It includes the severity of coronary stenosis, from minimal plaque with little stenotic repercussions to complete occlusion; the site of the lesion and its relation to the anatomical variations and the functional perfusion bed (area at risk), including the repercussions of the presence or absence of collaterals; the number of lesions, taking into consideration the special significance of left main disease as it is greater than that of combined left anterior descending (LAD) and left circumflex (LCx) disease.

Extent of CAD should also cover the functional consequences of the lesions, whether potential, transient or fixed, and investigations should be carried out to assess exercise-inducible ischaemic dysfunction and global or regional dysfunction corresponding to stunned or hibernating myocardium or permanent scar.

Finally, evaluation of potential complications such as mitral regurgitation, septal rupture or ventricular aneurysm should also be performed.

Clinical Problems

Non-invasive assessment of the extent of CAD is difficult despite the presence of some clinical clues. The incidence of CAD increases with age, but this has no direct influence on the extent of the disease, even though the presence of anginal symptoms of long duration favours multiple vessel disease. Functional impairment and reduced exercise tolerance also increase the probability of multiple vessel or proximal lesions, as does the magnitude of the ST segment changes, especially if they occur at a low exercise level.[4]

Electrocardiographic changes, however, are neither sensitive nor specific enough to detect multiple vessel or proximal disease, or even left main disease, and the localizing value of the electrocardiogram is poor.[5,6] Concomitant consideration of exercise tolerance and haemodynamic changes (such as blood pressure) improves the value of the information provided.

Imaging of regional myocardial function and perfusion are the techniques of choice to define the extent of disease.[7–10] Imaging of function can be performed using radionuclide ventriculography or echocardiography. Both approaches, however, require actual malperfusion or malfunction of all individual jeopardized areas to provide a complete description of the extent of the disease, which is unlikely to occur in all cases as the patient will stop exercising as soon as ischaemic symptoms related to the area of the most critical lesion become evident.

While the sensitivity of criteria based on function or perfusion is probably similar, the specificity of perfusion abnormalities is probably higher as functional changes are modulated by changes in loading conditions (preload and afterload), by global changes in function and by the behaviour of contiguous regions. In some cases, however, patients with multiple vessel disease have balanced perfusion abnormalities that may complicate evaluation. Evidence of some perfusion heterogeneity together with ventricular dilatation usually serves as a clue to recognizing these patients, but diagnostic errors are occasionally possible. The sensitivity to detect multiple vessel disease using perfusion imaging is influenced by the presence of a previous myocardial infarction (MI). Although detection of a second lesion is enhanced overall when the first lesion corresponds to infarction rather than to another ischaemic lesion, the presence of a large infarct complicates visualization of further ischaemia.[11–13]

The use of single photon emission computed tomography (SPECT) as compared to planar imaging has considerably improved the ability of perfusion imaging to define the extent of the disease. Indeed, SPECT diminishes the overlap between vascular territories as compared to projections. It also provides more specific views to help identify different vascular lesions. While the advantages of SPECT do not appear overriding for diagnostic purposes, for defining the extent of disease SPECT definitely has an edge.[14,15]

Patients with left main disease, multiple vessel disease and probably also with severe proximal disease, especially when associated with mild or moderate ventricular dysfunction, are at increased risk of MI or death and should be revascularized. The optimal revascularization procedure has not yet been defined, but the choice of surgery versus angioplasty should be made primarily on the basis of angiography, although the relative experience of the angioplasty and surgical teams also plays a role.

Selection of patients for angiography can be done quite effectively and results in a high proportion of patients treated by revascularization, thus making optimal use of generally limited resources. Performance of angiography in all patients with CAD to confirm diagnosis and define disease extent has been advocated but does not seem warranted as it is a more costly strategy and results in more iatrogenic problems. Experience has also shown a tendency to intervene on anatomical lesions regardless of symptoms, natural history data or functional significance, when angiography has been performed first.

Aims of Sestamibi Study

Myocardial imaging to define the extent of disease should be performed in all patients with CAD, either at the time of diagnostic evaluation or later to assess prognosis and plan therapy.

The use of SPECT is particularly suited to a technetium-labelled agent as the higher photon flux and physical properties of technetium considerably improve the quality of the images.

In these conditions, sestamibi adequately defines the extent of disease (presence or absence of multiple vessel disease) in the majority of patients. Recognition of left main disease remains difficult, however. While patients with left main disease usually have abnormal scans, the incidence of a typical scintigraphic pattern associating defects in the proximal LAD distribution with a defect in the LCx distribution remains low (possibly because patients with such a pattern would be at very high risk). The importance of detecting signs of multiple vessel disease and of proximal LAD disease should not be underestimated, however, as patients with these patterns are at increased risk and can benefit from the diagnosis through revascularization.

Clinical Points

- Defining the extent of CAD has important therapeutic and prognostic implications.
- Diagnostic techniques based on evaluation of perfusion or function at stress have a tendency to underestimate the extent of the disease as the patients stop exercising when ischaemia occurs in the region supplied by the most critical stenosis.
- SPECT is the preferred technique to assess disease extent using myocardial perfusion imaging.
- Evaluation of the functional repercussions of previous damage is an important step in the definition of disease extent.

References

1 SCHULZE RA, STRAUSS HW, PITT B, Sudden death in the year following myocardial infarction. Relation to ventricular premature contractions in the late hospital phase and left ventricular ejection fraction, *Am J Med* (1977) **62**:192.

2 MOCK M, RINGQVIST I, FISHER L et al, Survival of medically treated patients in the coronary artery surgery study CASS registry, *Circulation* (1982) **66**:562.

3 GIBSON RS, WATSON DD, CRADDOCK GB et al, Prediction of cardiac events after uncomplicated myocardial infarction: a prospective study comparing predischarge exercise thallium-201 scintigraphy and coronary angiography, *Circulation* (1983) **68**:321.

4 MICHAELIDES AP, TRIPOSKIADIS FK, BOUDOULAS H et al, New coronary artery disease index based on exercise-induced QRS changes, *Am Heart J* (1990) **120**:292.

5 MEYERS DG, BENDON KA, HANKINS JH et al, The effect of baseline electrocardiographic abnormalities in the diagnostic accuracy of exercise-induced ST segment changes, *Am Heart J* (1990) **119**:272.

6 KOTLER TS, DIAMOND GA, Exercise thallium-201 scintigraphy in the diagnosis and prognosis of coronary artery disease, *Ann Intern Med* (1990) **113**:684.

7 GIBBONS RJ, Rest and exercise radionuclide angiography for diagnosis in chronic ischemic heart disease, *Circulation* (1991) **84**:I93.

8 CALDWELL JH, HAMILTON GW, SORENSEN SG et al, The detection of coronary artery disease with radionuclide techniques. A comparison of rest-exercise thallium imaging and ejection fraction response, *Circulation* (1980) **61**:610.

9 BELLER GA, Diagnostic accuracy of thallium-201 myocardial perfusion imaging, *Circulation* (1991) **84**:I1.

10 BROWN KA, Prognostic value of thallium-201 myocardial perfusion imaging. A diagnostic tool comes of age, *Circulation* (1991) **83**:363.

11 RIGO P, BAILEY IK, GRIFFITH LS et al, Value of limitations of segmental analysis of stress thallium myocardial imaging for localization of coronary artery disease, *Circulation* (1980) **61**:973.

12 RIGO P, BAILEY IK, GRIFFITH LS et al, Stress thallium-201 myocardial scintigraphy for the detection of individual coronary arterial lesions in patients with and without previous myocardial infarction, *Am J Cardiol* (1981) **48**:209.

13 LAROCK MP, CANTINEAU R, LEGRAND V et al, 99mTc-MIBI (RP-30) to define the extent of myocardial ischemia and evaluation ventricular function, *Eur J Nucl Med* (1990) **16**:223.

14 BERMAN DS, KIAT H, VAN TRAIN KF et al, Comparison of SPECT using technetium-99m agents and thallium-201 and PET for the assessment of myocardial perfusion and viability, *Am J Cardiol* (1990) **66**:72E.

15 BERMAN DS, KIAT H, MADDAHI J, The new 99mTc myocardial perfusion imaging agents: 99mTc Sestamibi and 99mTc Teboroxime, *Circulation* (1991) **84**:I7.

Case Study IV.1

Assessment of the risk area in a patient with LAD disease

Mr JG, a 55-year-old male, complained of left precordial pain with activities such as driving his car. During the last few months pain was getting more frequent and more severe.

A sestamibi study was performed to assess the presence and the extent of CAD. Tomograms showed a large perfusion defect at stress in the anteroseptal and in the anterolateral walls of the left ventricle (LV) (Fig. IV.1a, arrows; HLA, horizontal long axis; VLA, vertical long axis) while the perfusion pattern was normal at rest (Fig. IV.1b). The perfusion abnormalities suggested severe and extended myocardial ischaemia in the proximal LAD territory, confirmed by angiography (Fig. IV.1c, arrow).

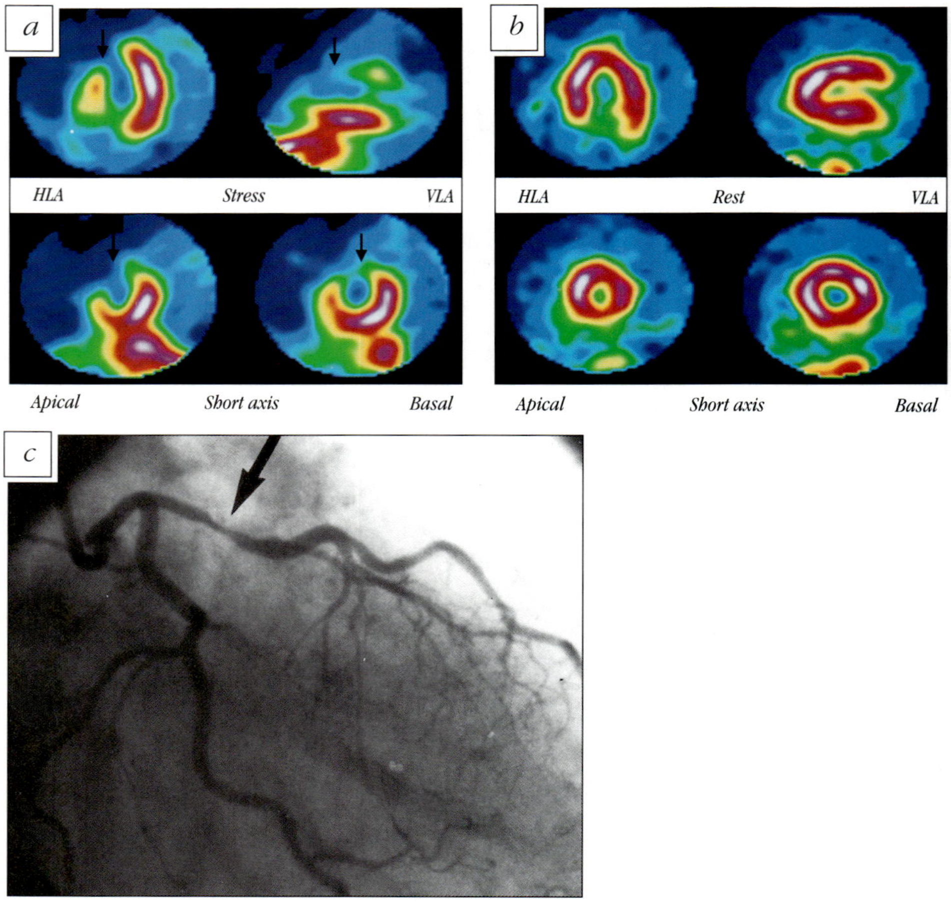

Case Study IV.2

Assessment of the risk area in a patient with LAD disease

This 56-year-old female patient came to the out-patient clinic for recent precordial chest pain radiated to her shoulders and to her throat which was induced by housework. Pain was relieved by nitrates.

The resting ECG was normal. She exercised on a bicycle up to a load of 120 W and complained of chest pain although the ECG remained normal.

Sestamibi tomography demonstrated the presence of a small stress defect in the anteroseptal wall of the LV (Fig. IV.2a, arrows) and a normal perfusion pattern at rest one day later (Fig. IV.2b).

The angiogram confirmed the presence of a distal isolated 90% LAD stenosis (Fig. IV.2c, arrows).

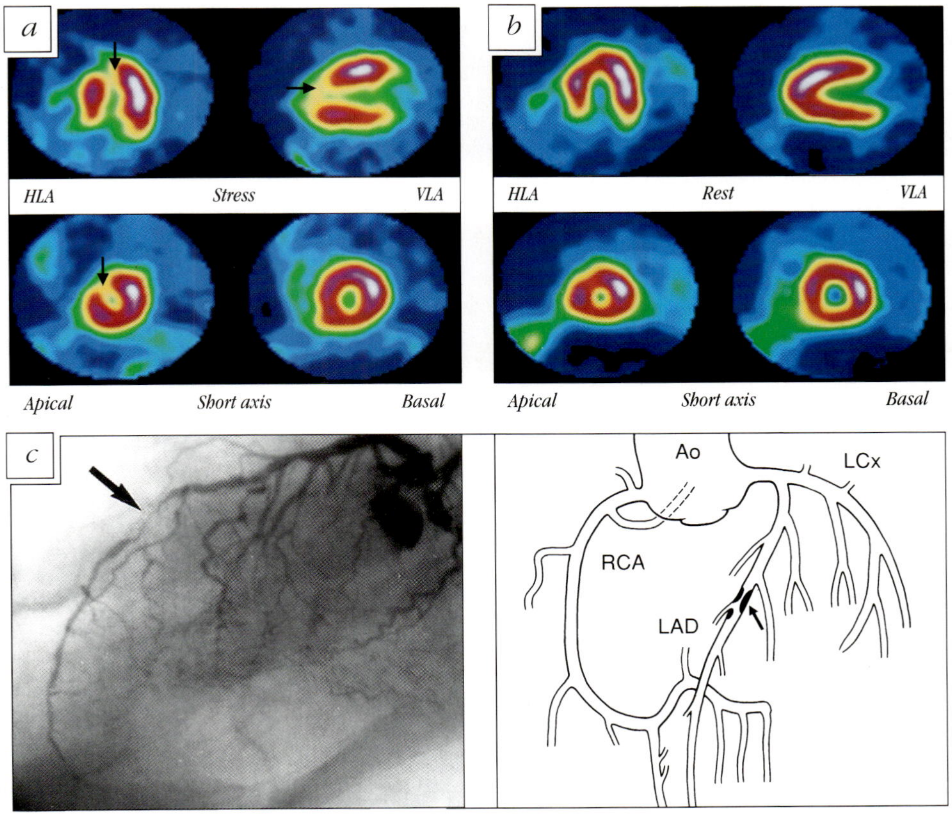

Case Study IV.3

Assessment of multiple vessel disease with sestamibi myocardial perfusion imaging

Mr VG suffered from angina pectoris for several years and had remained under successful medical management. For one month, he complained of more frequent pain and was therefore re-evaluated.

Myocardial perfusion imaging at stress demonstrated the presence of perfusion defects involving the anteroseptal, apical and inferoposterior walls of the LV (Fig. IV.3a, arrows). At rest, sestamibi myocardial uptake was normal and the LV less dilated (Fig. IV.3b).

Coronary angiography confirmed the presence of severe coronary lesions on the LAD and right coronary artery (RCA) requiring reperfusion (Figs. IV.3c,d, arrows).

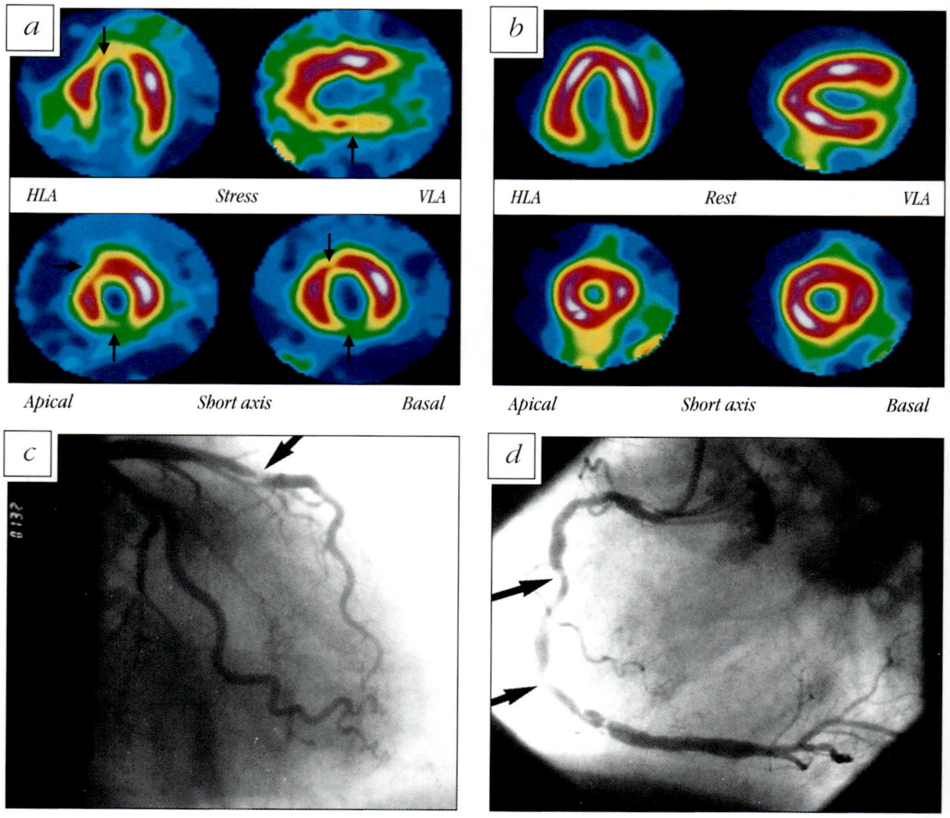

Case Study IV.4

Myocardial perfusion imaging with sestamibi in a patient with left main disease

Mr PM (53 years old) first developed left precordial chest pain radiated to his arms and to his throat while he was arguing in his office. The patient is a smoker and has suffered from hypertension for six years. The pain came back on similar occasions during the following weeks and his doctor asked for further investigations.

The bicycle exercise test was interrupted at 100 W for anginal pain and significant ST–T changes in the precordial leads (2.5 mm ST depression in leads V4, V5 and V6).

Sestamibi demonstrated a perfusion defect in the anterior, the lateral, the apical and the inferoposterior walls of the LV suggesting extensive CAD (Fig. IV.4a, arrows).

Angiography revealed the presence of a left main disease (70%) as well as an 80% RCA stenosis (Fig. IV.4b, arrows) and the patient underwent coronary artery bypass grafting (CABG).

The postoperative study revealed an almost normal myocardial uptake (small apical defect remaining) (Fig. IV.4c, arrow).

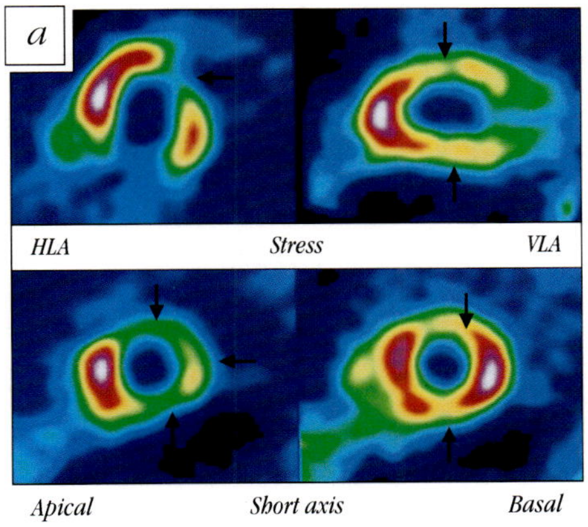

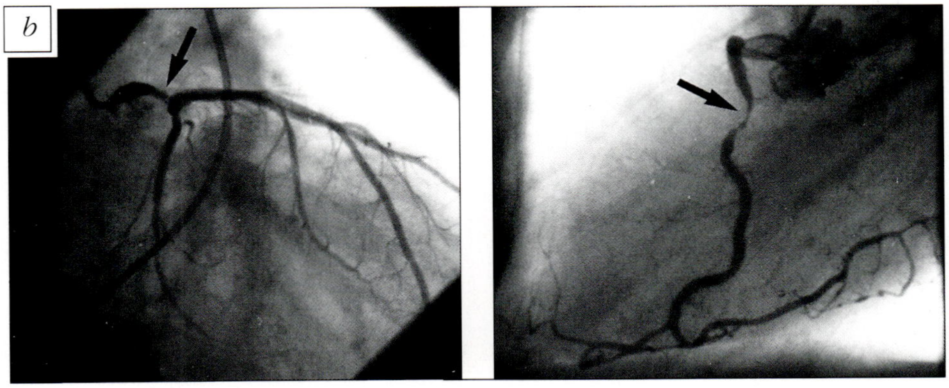

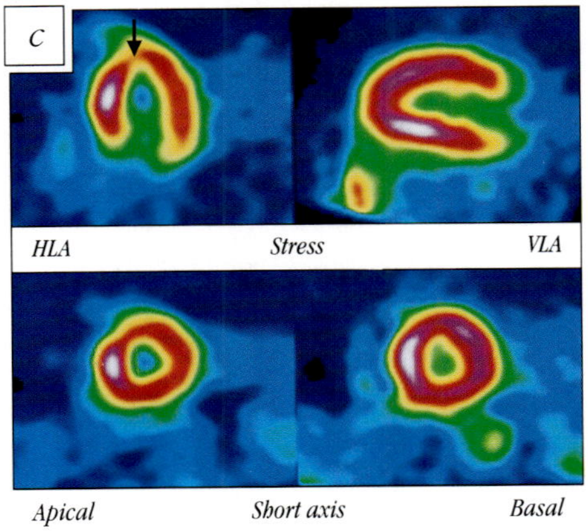

Case Study IV.5

Assessment of the extent of CAD after previous myocardial infarction

This patient was admitted to the coronary care unit 12 h after the occurrence of a prolonged episode of chest pain. The ECG at rest showed acute anteroseptal MI (Fig. IV.5a).

Because of the long delay the patient did not receive fibrinolysis and he later developed transient signs of left-sided failure with ventricular arrhythmias. Myocardial perfusion and function were evaluated before discharge to assess prognosis.

The equilibrium radionuclide ventriculography revealed a left ventricular systolic aneurysmal deformation and an anteroapical dyskinesia appearing in red on the phase image (Fig. IV.5b). The first-pass ejection fraction evaluated with sestamibi was decreased and calculated to be 28% (Fig. IV.5c).

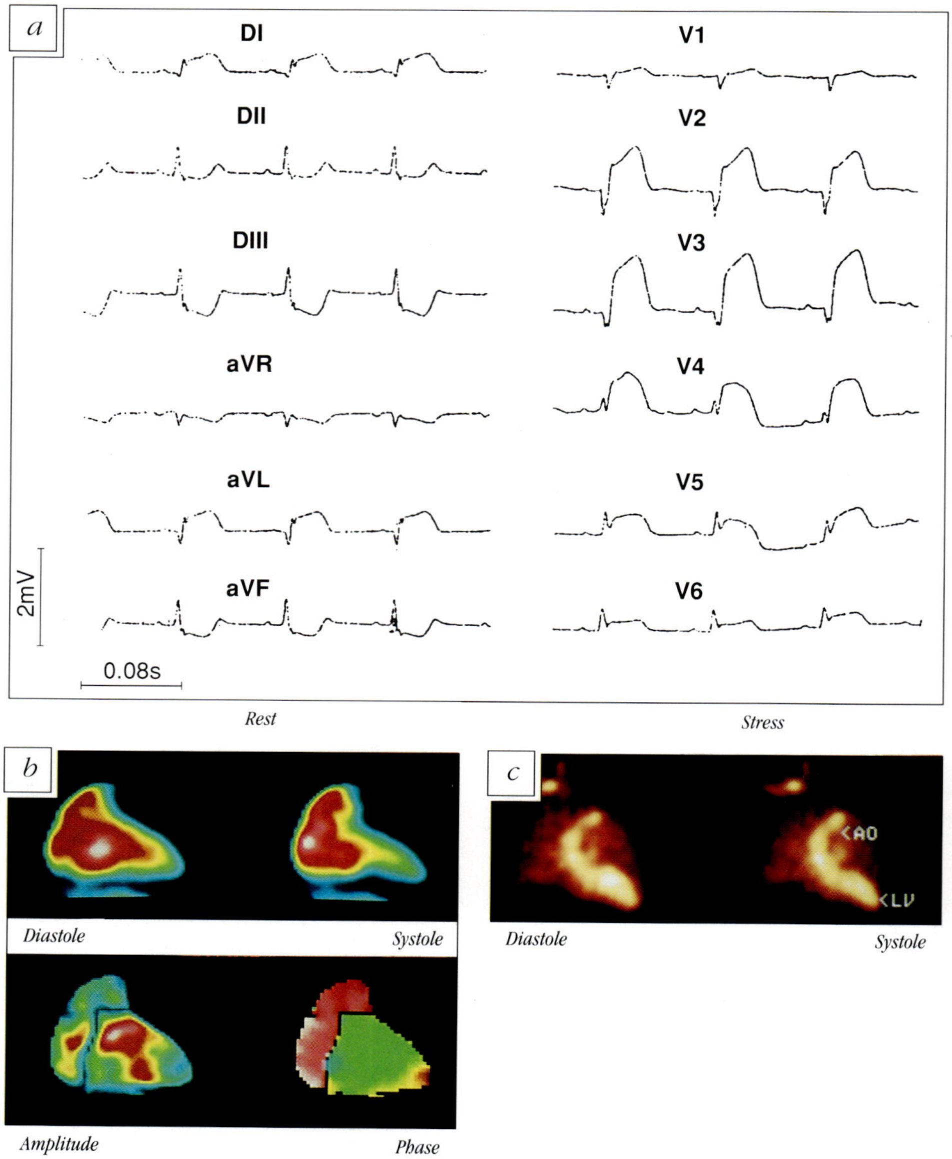

Myocardial perfusion imaging demonstrated fixed large perfusion defects corresponding to a large anteroseptal MI without residual ischaemia (Figs. IV.5d,e, arrows).

Angiography confirmed the presence of an LAD occlusion proximal to the origin of the diagonal branch (Fig. IV.5f, arrow) while the LCx and RCA were normal (Fig. IV.5g). The patient was then maintained on medical therapy.

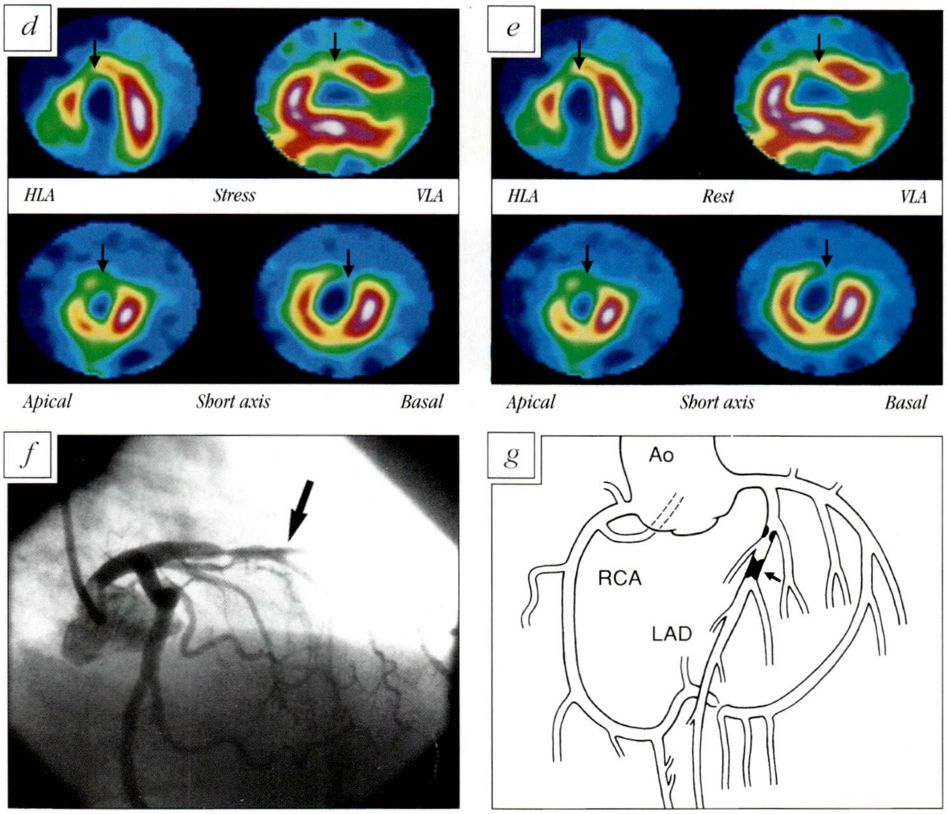

RAO view LAO view

Case Study IV.6

Assessment of residual ischaemia after myocardial infarction with perfusion imaging

Mr AD (48 years old) was admitted to the intensive care unit 2 h after inaugural left precordial chest pain, radiated to his left upper limb and not relieved by nitrates.

The rest ECG showed an acute anteroseptal MI and the patient received thrombolytic therapy. The hospital course was event free and the patient was evaluated before discharge.

Sestamibi demonstrated larger perfusion defects at stress than at rest in the anteroseptal and in the apical walls of the LV corresponding to residual ischaemia in the infarcted area (Figs. IV.6a,b, arrows).

Angiography showed a residual LAD stenosis that was successfully dilated (Fig. IV.6c, arrow).

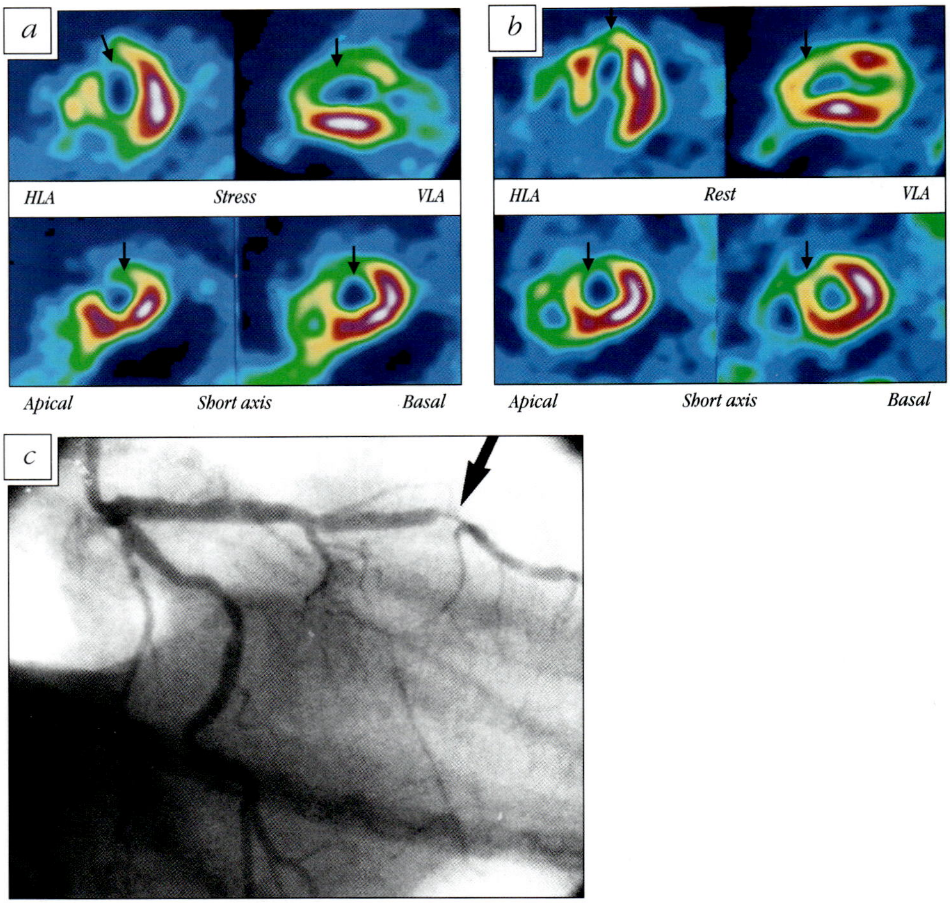

Case Study IV.7

Assessment of myocardial ischaemia in a patient with previous myocardial infarction

Mr WF, a 56-year-old patient with a previous MI, complained of recurrent episodes of anginal pain. The exercise test was interrupted for angina pectoris and dyspnoea.

Tomography performed at stress and at rest demonstrated fixed perfusion defects in the inferior wall corresponding to a myocardial scar and reversible perfusion defects in the anteroseptal wall suggesting myocardial ischaemia at a distance, in the LAD territory (Figs. IV.7a,b, arrows).

The angiogram showed an occlusion of the RCA and a lesion on the LAD (Figs. IV.7c,d, arrows) and the patient underwent revascularization.

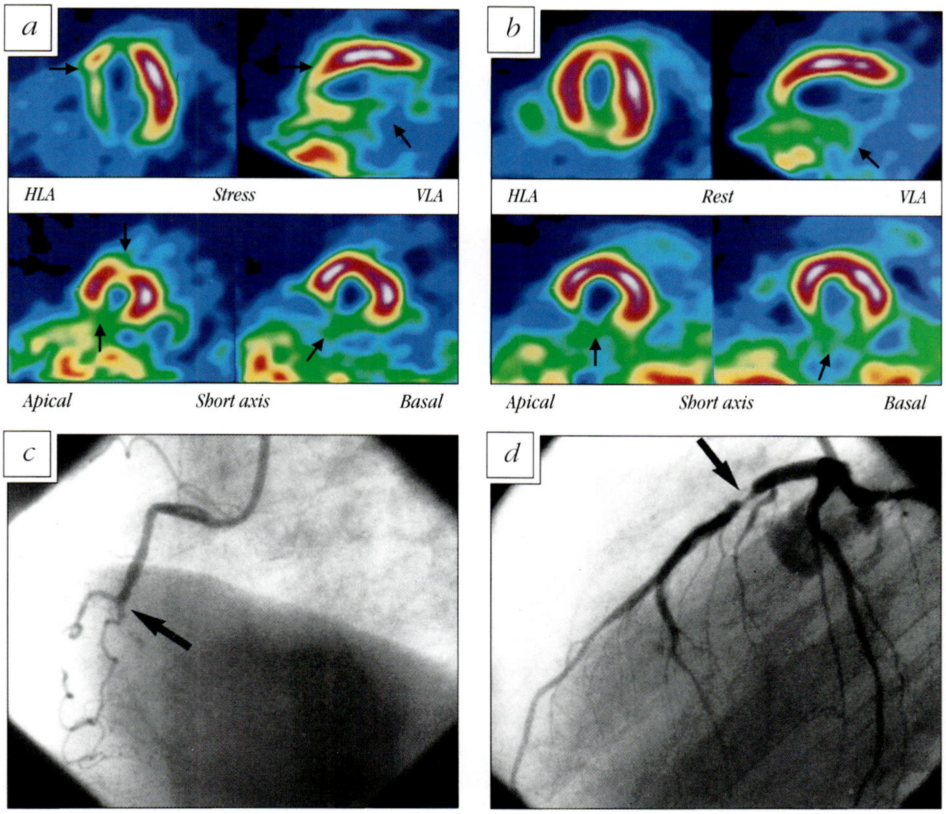

Case Study IV.8

Assessment of CAD in a patient with vascular disease using dipyridamole stress test combined with perfusion imaging

Mr GJ is a 72-year-old man suffering from hypertension and polyvascular disease. In December 1991, he was found to have an abdominal aortic bruit and a renal scan performed with captopril showed evidence of a left renal artery stenosis. Surgery was planned but as the patient had a previous inferolateral MI and atypical chest pain, a dipyridamole scan was performed to rule out ischaemia.

The sestamibi dipyridamole scan revealed posterolateral and inferoposterior defects, with a smaller resting defect (Figs. IV.8a,b, arrows), demonstrating an inferoposterior MI with lateral ischaemia.

Renal surgery was delayed pending coronary angiography.

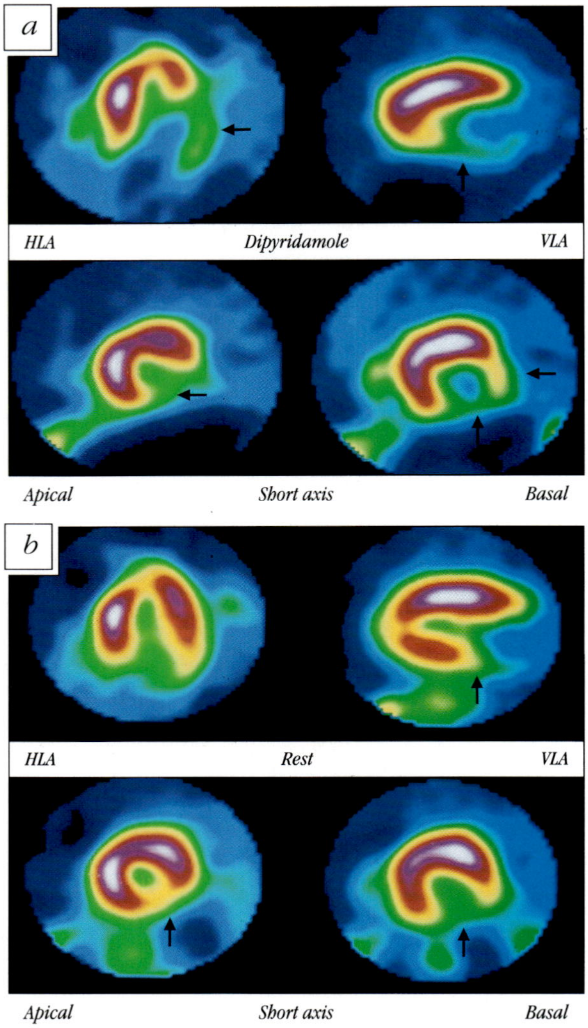

5 ASSESSMENT OF THE FUNCTIONAL SIGNIFICANCE OF CORONARY LESIONS

Clinical Background

Coronary angiography is the standard technique used to assess morphological changes of the vessels and to evaluate the severity of coronary stenoses. Limitations in the subjective qualitative assessment of coronary angiograms have been clearly demonstrated by studies showing the rather poor reproducibility, both between observers and in the same observer, under blind controlled conditions, as well as by studies comparing in vivo and post-mortem angiographic data with pathological assessment of the severity of stenosis.[1–3]

Quantitative assessment of coronary lesions using computer analysis of processed coronary outlines or videodensitometric techniques provide more reproducible results, but discrepancies with pathology or with measurement of coronary flow reserve (either by Doppler or angiography) remain.[4–7]

The need therefore exists for techniques to assess the significance of lesions depicted by angiography and myocardial perfusion imaging can do this non-invasively.[8,9]

Clinical Problems

A number of clinical situations can be described in which one would wish to assess the myocardial perfusion pattern with the angiogram on hand.

Defining the significance of a given coronary artery lesion

Demonstration of a lesion of borderline significance frequently leaves the cardiologist in doubt as to whether that lesion is responsible for the patient's symptoms. It is therefore advisable to find out if the lesion can be demonstrated to produce perfusion abnormalities or objective signs of myocardial ischaemia. Myocardial perfusion imaging is increasingly used for that purpose, particularly now that single photon emission computed tomography (SPECT) has increased both the sensitivity and the localizing value of imaging.

The potential of myocardial imaging to assess the significance of a given lesion varies, however, with the extent of coronary artery disease (CAD). In patients with single vessel disease, perfusion imaging has a high sensitivity (± 90%) for detecting significant (> 70%) lesions. It has been shown that the detection sensitivity drops with the angiographic severity of the lesions, but this finding might simply reflect the increasing frequency of patients in whom the angiographic abnormality is in fact not functionally significant.

Patients with multiple vessel lesions present a more difficult evaluation problem. Indeed, these patients may develop angina and stop exercising when they develop ischaemia in the territory of the most significant lesion. The detection sensitivity for second and third lesions is therefore less than optimal. Recent tomographic studies have indicated a sensitivity value of around 70% in these situations and this should be kept in mind when requesting such a study.[10–13]

The situation is somewhat different, however, when the patient has prior myocardial infarction (MI) in the territory of the first coronary artery obstruction, and the significance of the second lesion is sought. The detection sensitivity for a left anterior descending (LAD) abnormality after a small inferior infarct is almost as high as that for a first lesion. The detection sensitivity for a right coronary artery (RCA) or a left circumflex (LCx) lesion after a first large anterior MI is somewhat lower, but much improved by tomography.[14–16]

Identifying the culprit lesion

Single vessel angioplasty

Patients with angina pectoris who are not candidates for coronary artery bypass graft (CABG) surgery may have multiple vessel disease. A strategy has been proposed to use perfusion imaging to identify the lesion responsible for the initial manifestations of ischaemia and symptoms, 'the culprit lesion', and first to selectively dilate this lesion rather than performing more risky multiple vessel angioplasty. Subsequent evaluation and scans are then needed to assess the results of the procedure and to detect the presence of residual ischaemia in the territory of the dilated artery or of another stenosed vessel and to assess the need for secondary procedures.

Multiple vessel angioplasty

In patients undergoing multiple vessel angioplasty, it is also indicated to assess the functional severity of the lesions to decide which stenosis needs to be dilated and in which order. It is not always possible or necessary to perform complete revascularization and therefore it is essential to establish a priority list before proceeding with dilatation.[17]

Assessing the effectiveness of collateral supply

Segments distal to a complete coronary occlusion may remain partially or completely viable through collateral supply. Effectiveness of collateral supply is, however, often difficult to assess by angiography.

Demonstration by myocardial imaging of a normal perfusion pattern at rest and exercise would be a rare finding, but indicative of adequate collateral supply.

Observation of an exercise-induced perfusion defect would indicate the presence of viable myocardium receiving adequate collateral supply at rest but the inability of the collateral bed to supply the increased demand of exercise.[18,19]

Finally, the presence of an abnormal perfusion pattern at rest would indicate partial or total necrosis (depending on the intensity of the defect) and the inadequacy of collateral supply.

Aims of Sestamibi Studies

Sestamibi SPECT studies at rest and exercise are well suited to detecting myocardial ischaemia on a regional basis and relating it to the results of coronary angiography. The sensitivity is adequate for this purpose with the possible exception of patients with multiple vessel disease in the absence of previous MI. Quantitative evaluation of tracer uptake in relation to normal areas allows stratification of the severity of the defect and assessment of the level of collateralization in patients with complete occlusion. Concomitant evaluation of function and perfusion provides another way to define more precisely the significance of coronary lesions and their effects on the myocardium.

Clinical Points

- Functional criteria provide more precise definition of stenosis severity than angiographic criteria.
- Presence of an angiographic lesion does not necessarily imply that that lesion is responsible for the patient's symptoms.
- Recognition and dilatation of 'the culprit lesion' may provide in some patients an alternative to complete revascularization procedures.
- Myocardial perfusion imaging allows assessment of the effectiveness and the limitations of the collateral supply.

References

1 ZIR LM, MILLER SW, DINSMORE RE et al, Interobserver variability in coronary angiography, *Circulation* (1976) **53**:627.

2 BEAUMAN GJ, VOGEL RA, Accuracy of individual and panel visual interpretations of coronary arteriograms: implications for clinical decisions, *J Am Coll Cardiol* (1990) **16**:108.

3 ARNET EN, ISNER JM, REDWOOD DR et al, Coronary artery narrowing in coronary heart disease: comparison of cineangiographic and necropsy findings, *Ann Intern Med* (1979) **91**:350.

4 GOULD KL, KELLEY KO, BOLSON EL, Experimental validation of quantitative coronary arteriography for determining pressure flow characteristics of coronary stenosis, *Circulation* (1982) **66**:930.

5 REIBER JHC, Morphologic and densitometric quantitation of coronary stenoses: an overview of existing quantitative techniques. In: Reiber JHC, Serruys PW, eds, *New developments in quantitative coronary arteriography* (Kluwer Academic Publishers: Dordrecht 1988) 34.

6 WHITE CW, WRIGHT CB, DOTY DB et al, Does visual interpretation of the coronary arteriogram predict the physiologic importance of a coronary stenosis? *N Engl J Med* (1984) **310**:819.

7 LEGRAND V, MANCINI GBJ, BATES ER et al, A comparative study of coronary anatomy and the results of radionuclide exercise tests in patients with coronary artery disease, *J Am Coll Cardiol* (1986) **9**:1022.

8 BATESMAN T, RAYMOND M, IZER L et al, Stenosis severity. Analysis using Tl-201 scintigraphy and intracoronary pressure gradients, *J Am Coll Cardiol* (1984) **3**:606.

9 BROWN KA, OSBAKKEN M, BOUCHER C et al, Positive exercise thallium-201 test response in patients with less than 50% maximal coronary stenosis: angiographic and clinical predictors, *Am J Cardiol* (1985) **55**:54.

10 RIGO P, BAILEY IK, GRIFFITH LSC et al, Value and limitations of segmental analysis of stress thallium myocardial imaging for localization of coronary artery disease, *Circulation* (1980) **61**:973.

11 DEPACE NL, ISKANDRIAN AS, HAKKI AH, Relation between the extent of coronary artery disease and exercise-induced thallium-201 perfusion abnormalities, *J Cardiac Rehabil* (1983) **3**:611.

12 LAROCK MP, CANTINEAU R, LEGRAND V et al, 99mTc-MIBI (RP-30) to define the extent of myocardial ischemia and evaluate ventricular function, *Eur J Nucl Med* (1990) **16**:223.

13 MAHMARIAN JJ, BOYCE TM, GOLDBERG RK et al, Quantitative exercise thallium-201 single photon emission computed tomography for the enhanced diagnosis of ischemic heart disease, *J Am Coll Cardiol* (1990) **15**:318.

14 RIGO P, BAILEY IK, GRIFFITH LSC et al, Stress thallium-201 myocardial scintigraphy for the detection of individual coronary artery lesions in patients with and without previous myocardial infarction, *Am J Cardiol* (1981) **48**:209.

15 GIBBONS R, VERANI MS, BEHRENBECK T et al, Feasibility of tomographic 99mTc-hexakis-2-methoxy-2-methylpropyl-isonitrile imaging for the assessment of myocardial area at risk and the effect of treatment in acute myocardial infarction, *Circulation* (1989) **80**:1277.

16 LEPPO JA, O'BRIEN J, ROTHENDLER JA et al, Dipyridamole thallium-201 scintigraphy in the prediction of future cardiac events after acute myocardial infarction, *N Engl J Med* (1984) **310**:1014.

17 MYLER RK et al, Multiple vessel coronary angioplasty: classification, results and patterns of restenosis in 494 consecutive patients, *Cathet Cardiov Diagn* (1987) **13**:1.

18 RIGO P et al, Influence of coronary collateral vessels on the results of thallium-201 myocardial stress imaging, *Am J Cardiol* (1979) **44**:452.

19 KOLIBASH AJ, BUSH CA, WEPSIC RA et al, Coronary collateral vessels: spectrum of physiologic capabilities with respect to providing rest and stress myocardial perfusion, maintenance of left ventricular function and protection against infarction, *Am J Cardiol* (1982) **50**:230.

Case Study V.1

Assessment of borderline significant coronary lesion (1)

This young male patient (38 years old) developed prolonged precordial chest pain at rest, radiated to his back. He was referred to the coronary care unit for further investigations.

The ECG at rest and the myocardial enzymes were normal. Because of his age and the presence of cardiovascular risk factors (heredity, lipid disorders and hypertension), an angiogram was performed and revealed the presence of an isolated 50% LAD stenosis (Fig. V.1a, arrow).

A tomographic study was performed at stress to assess the functional significance of the LAD lesion. The patient exercised on a bicycle up to a load of 210 W, his heart rate rose from 80 beats/min to 150 beats/min with a normal blood pressure response. The ECG at stress did not show any significant ST–T changes (Fig. V.1b) and myocardial perfusion imaging demonstrated a normal perfusion pattern (Fig. V.1c).

According to the scintigraphic results, the patient was not considered for angioplasty. Further diagnostic work-up revealed the presence of a hiatus hernia.

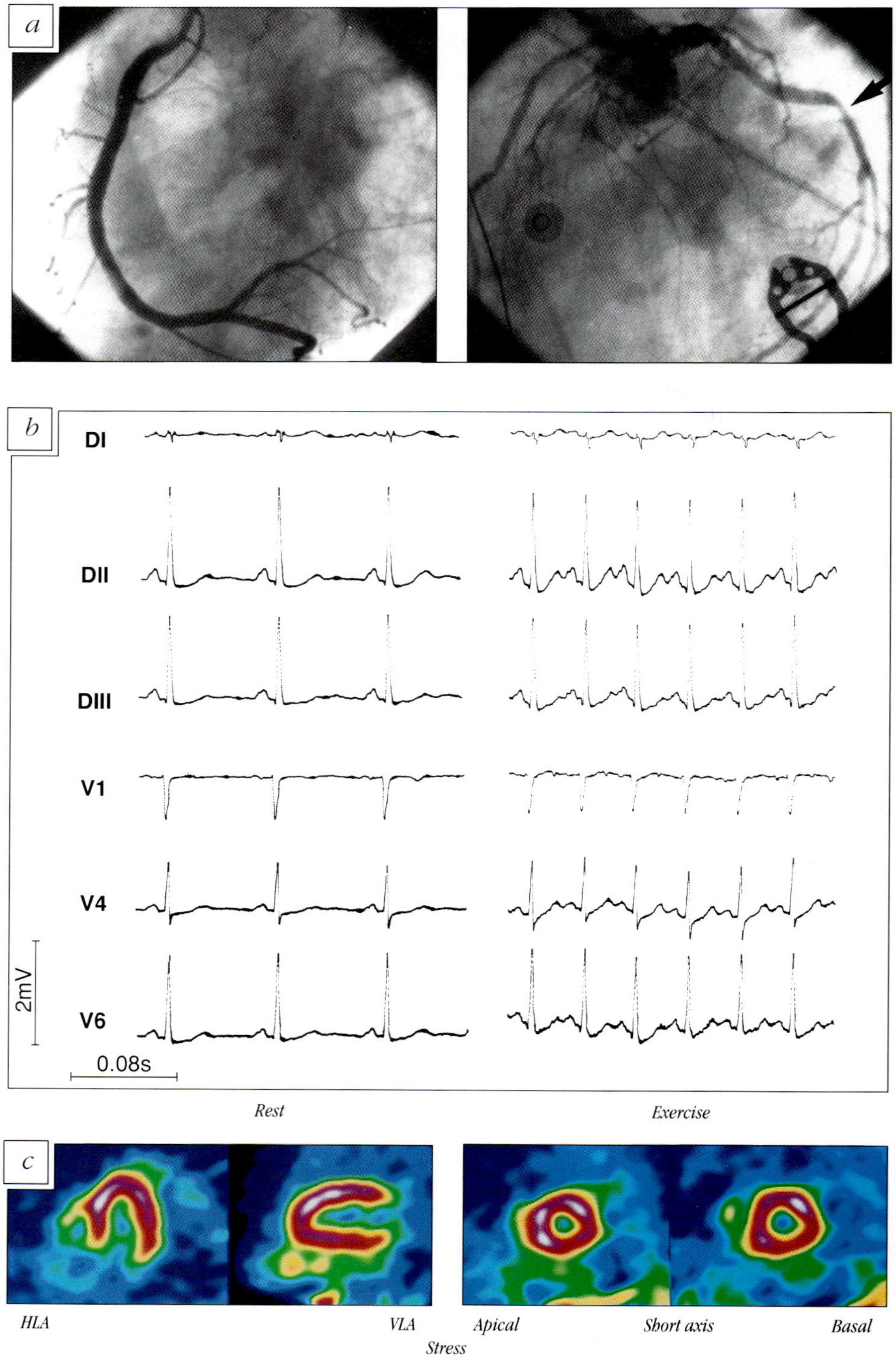

Case Study V.2

Assessment of borderline significant coronary lesion (2)

Mr KG, 42 years old with previous inferior myocardial infarction, was admitted to the coronary care unit for recurrent angina pectoris.

Thrombolysis had not been performed for his previous inferior myocardial infarction because the delay between the onset of pain and hospital admission was more than 12 h.

An angiographic control performed to assess the extent of CAD revealed the presence of a distal LCx occlusion and a 50% stenosis of the marginal branch (Fig. V.2a, arrows). A comparative rest and stress tomographic study was then realized, to evaluate the functional repercussion of the marginal stenosis.

Scintigraphic results demonstrated at rest small perfusion defects in the inferolateral wall of the LV on the short axis views (Fig. V.2b, arrows) and at stress larger perfusion defects involving the lateral and inferoposterior walls of the LV on the horizontal (HLA) and on the vertical long axis (VLA) views (Fig. V.2c, arrows) corresponding to MI with residual ischaemia. The patient was therefore referred for angioplasty of his marginal branch.

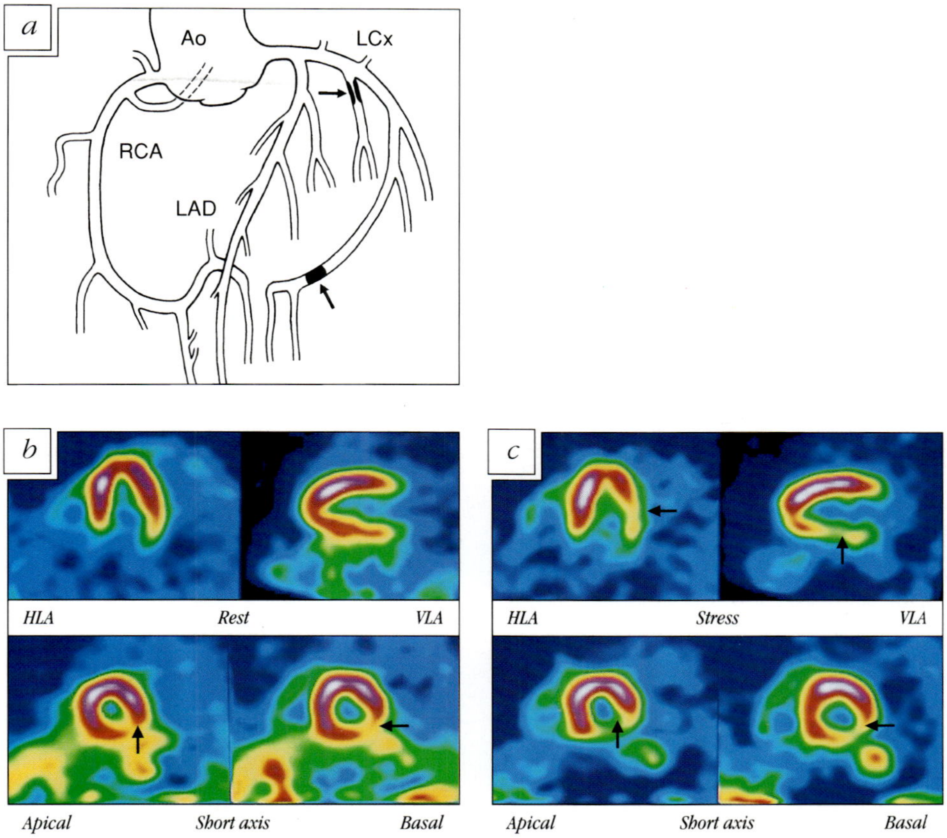

Case Study V.3

Assessment of functional significance of borderline coronary lesion

Mr L (40 years old) was admitted to the coronary care unit for an inaugural anteroseptal myocardial infarction.

The ECG on admission showed the presence of Q-wave and ST–T-wave changes (Fig. V.3a).

As he was admitted within 3 h of the onset of chest pain, he was treated by intravenous thrombolysis.

An angiographic control performed a few days later to assess the extent of CAD revealed a patent LAD and a 50% stenosis in the RCA (Fig. V.3b, arrow).

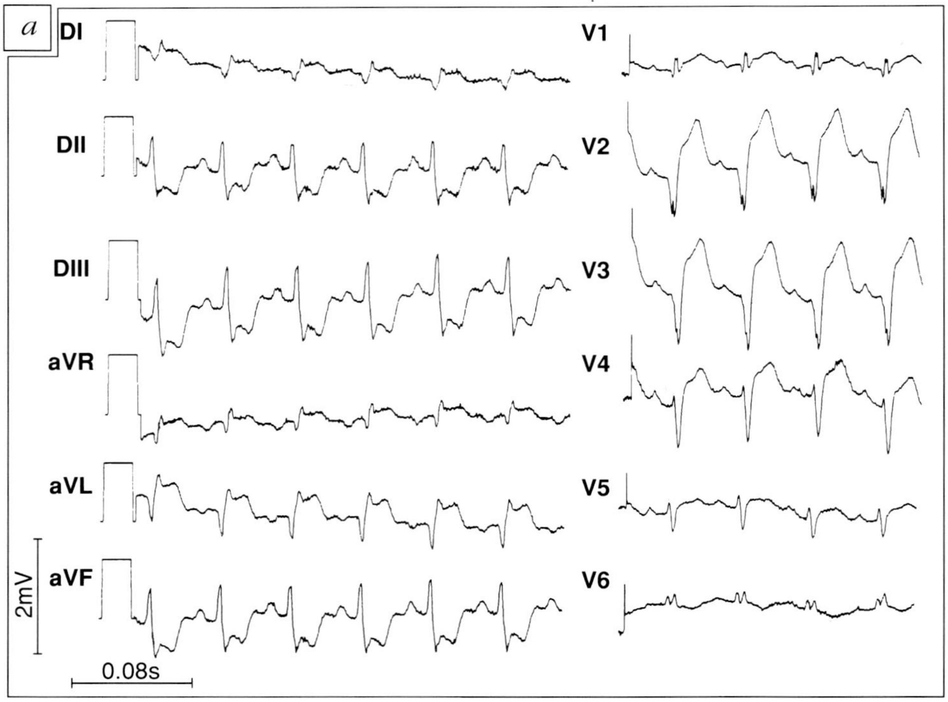

ECG at admission

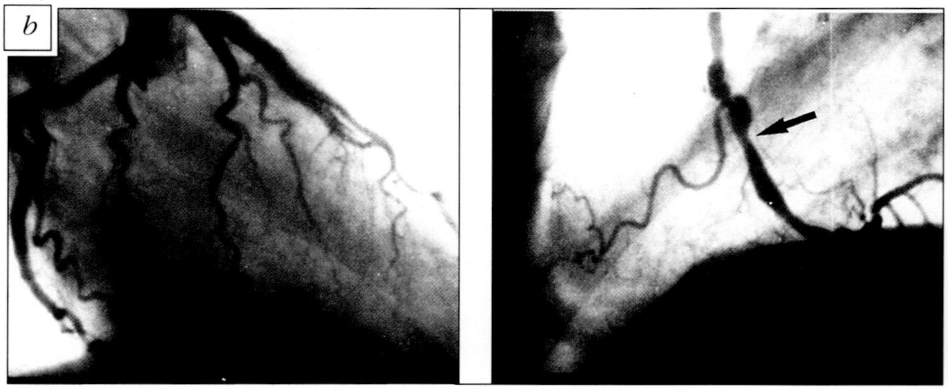

A rest and stress tomographic study was performed to evaluate the repercussion of the RCA stenosis on regional myocardial perfusion. Results indicated the presence of fixed perfusion defects in the anteroseptal walls of the LV corresponding to a small anteroseptal MI. The perfusion pattern was normal in the RCA vessel territory (Figs. V.3c,d, arrows). Accordingly, the patient was not considered for angioplasty of his RCA but was treated medically.

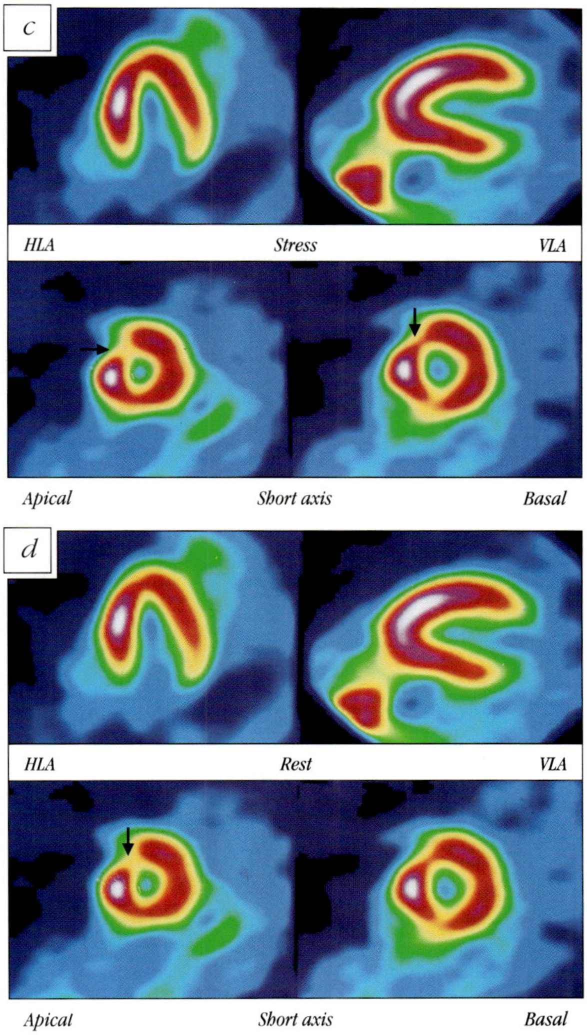

Case Study V.4

Assessment of the functional significance of angiographic lesions in a patient with multiple vessel disease

When Mr SE first came to the out-patient clinic he complained of left precordial chest pain radiated to his arms which was induced by physical exercise such as walking. He was a heavy smoker and suffered from hypertension.

The patient was evaluated at stress and described angina pectoris for a load of 90 W with significant ST–T changes (Fig. V.4a).

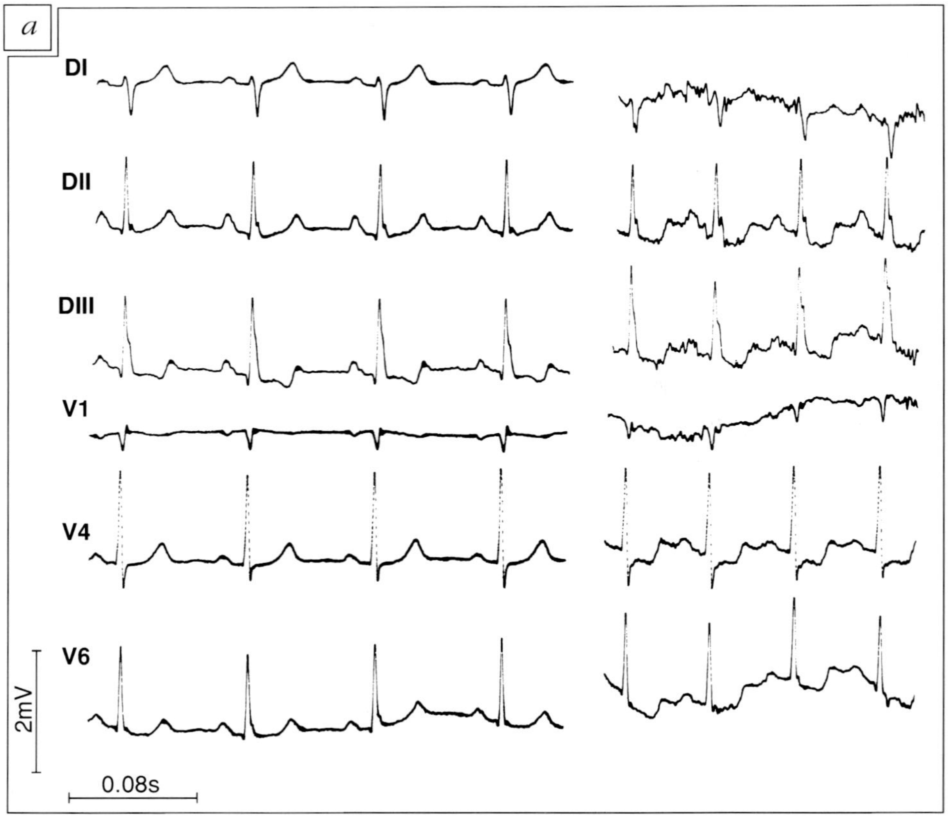

Rest *Stress*

Sestamibi was injected at peak exercise to assess the extent of perfusion abnormalities. Tomography showed perfusion defects only at stress in the anteroseptal, apical and inferior walls of the LV (Figs. V.4b,c, arrows) corresponding to myocardial ischaemia in two vessel territories.

Coronary angiography realized 3 days later demonstrated severe lesions on the LAD and RCA (> 90%) and one less severe lesion ±70%) in the LCx not detected by tomography (Figs. V.4d,e, arrows).

This case illustrates the lack of sensitivity of tomography to assess all the lesions in patients with triple vessel disease as the patient stopped exercising as a result of angina pectoris induced by the most severe stenosis (in this case, the LAD and RCA lesions but not the LCx lesion).

According to the angiographic and scintigraphic results the patient was considered for revascularization. As angioplasty was considered for this patient, the priority list was set as: (1) LAD, (2) RCA, (3) LCx.

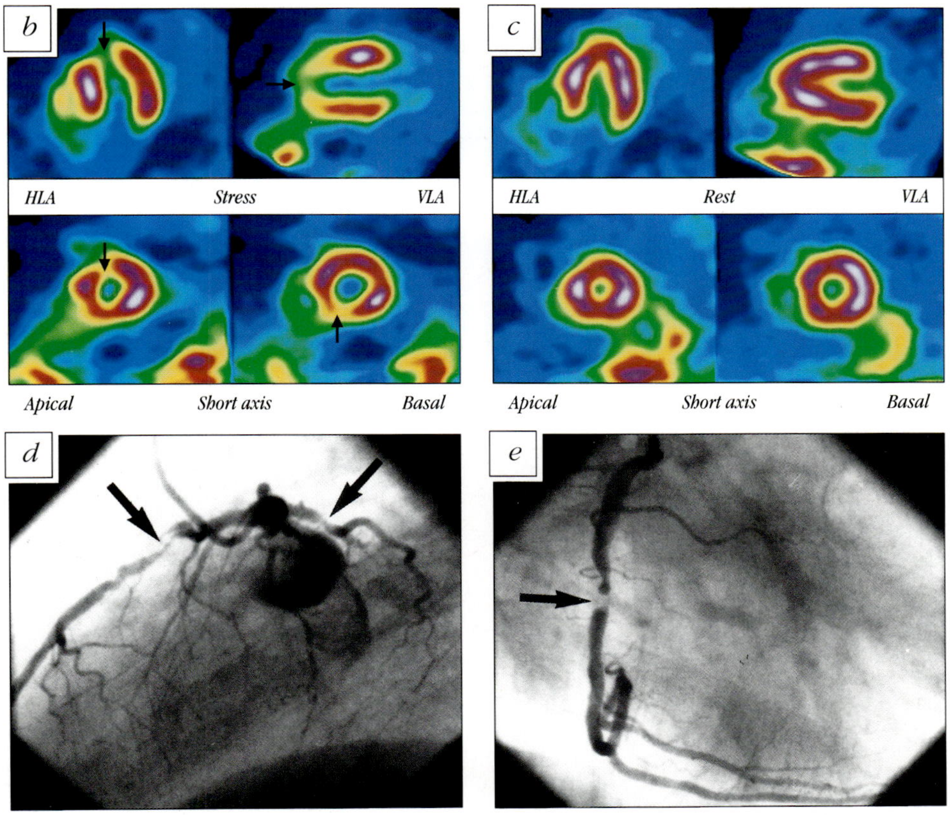

Case Study V.5

Assessment of functional coronary lesion after previous anteroseptal myocardial infarction

This case study concerns a 51-year-old patient who complained of angina pectoris and dyspnoea at stress. Recurrent chest pain occurred 16 months after an inaugural transmural anteroseptal MI.

A comparative rest and stress planar scintigraphy was performed to detect residual ischaemia and showed left ventricular dilatation and large perfusion defects in the anteroseptal and in the apical walls of the LV, both on rest and stress, corresponding to MI without residual ischaemia (Figs. V.5a,b, arrows).

As symptoms persisted, an angiographic control was performed and demonstrated an LAD occlusion and a significant RCA lesion subsequently treated by a revascularization procedure (Fig. V.5c, arrows).

This case illustrates the inadequate sensitivity of planar imaging to detect residual lesions after a large anterior MI.

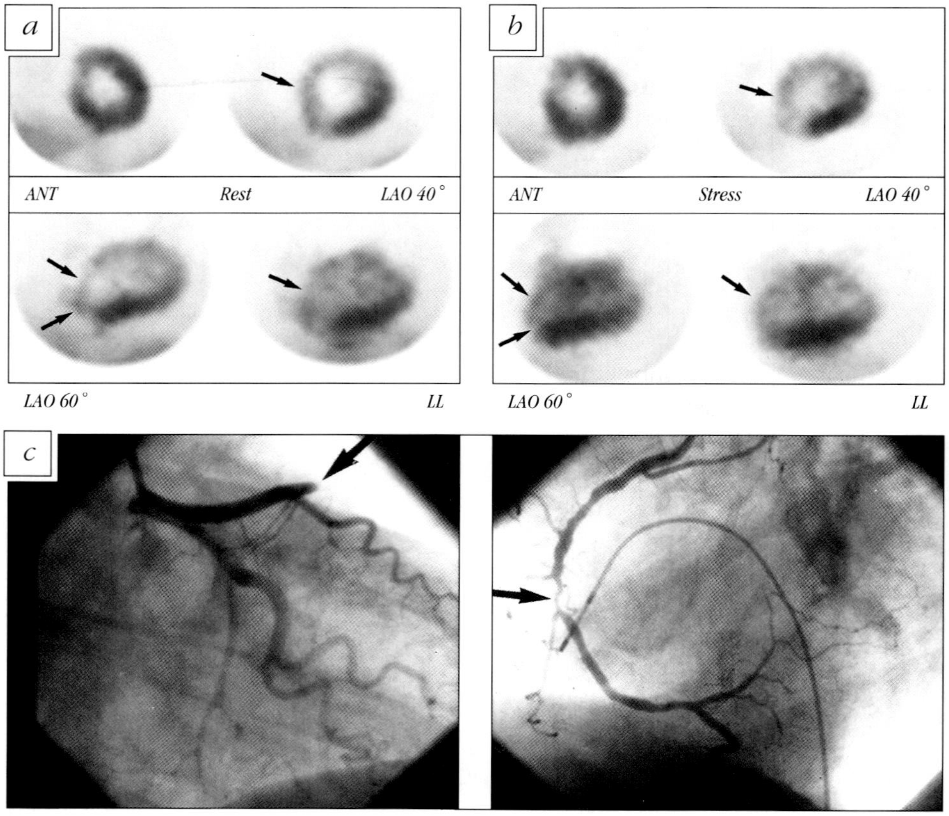

Case Study V.6

Functional assessment of a lesion after previous anteroseptal myocardial infarction using sestamibi tomography

Mr WG was admitted at the end of February 1992 to the coronary care unit for an acute anteroseptal myocardial infarction. Thrombolytic therapy was unsuccessful. Myocardial enzymes (CK) rose up to 1200 units/litre.

During the subacute phase, the patient complained several times of recurrent chest pain accompanied by significant ECG changes and a stress test was performed on day 10.

Tomography at stress demonstrated perfusion abnormalities in the anteroseptal and in the inferoposterior walls of the LV (Fig. V.6a, arrows) while at rest perfusion defects involved only the anteroseptal wall and were slightly less marked (Fig. V.6b, arrows), suggesting MI with residual ischaemia in the infarcted area and ischaemia at a distance in the RCA vessel territory.

The angiogram realized 48 h later confirmed the presence of an LAD occlusion and of a RCA stenosis (Fig. V.6c) and the patient underwent revascularization.

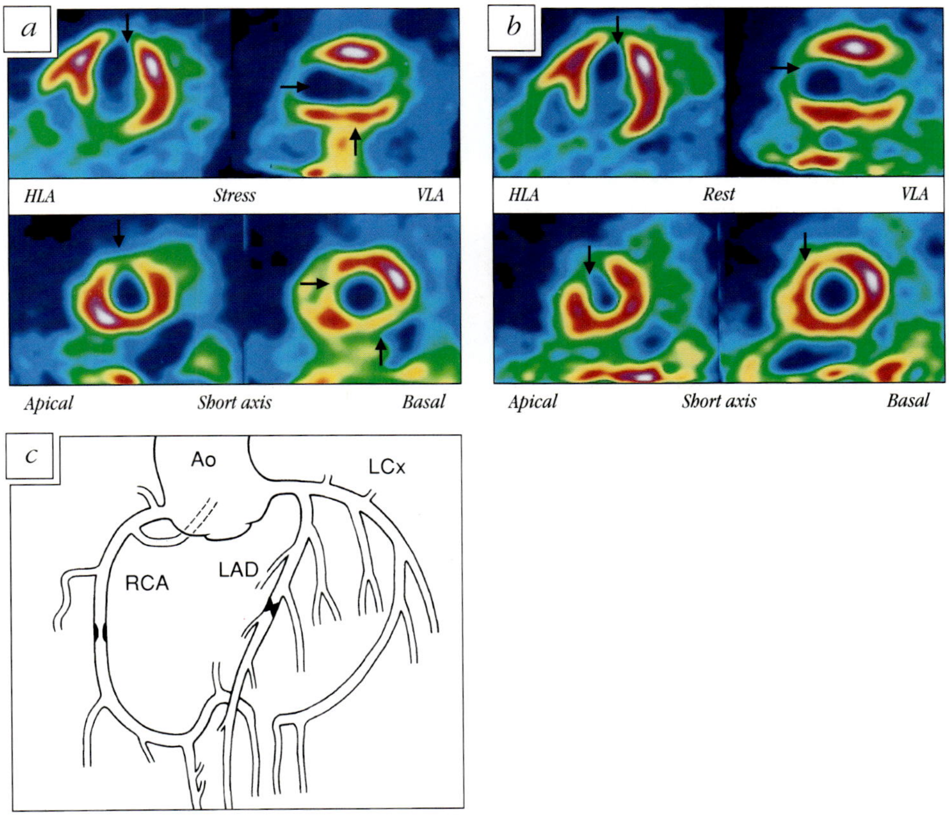

Case Study V.7

Myocardial perfusion imaging to define the optimal strategy for revascularization in the presence of multiple vessel disease (1)

Mr OR, 62 years old, first came to the out-patient clinic for left precordial chest pain radiated to his throat and left arm and induced by physical exercise such as gardening. A blood sample revealed lipid disorders and hyperglycaemia. The ECG recorded at rest was normal. He exercised on a bicycle up to a load of 120 W and described typical chest pain persisting during recovery and associated with significant ST changes. Perfusion defects in the anteroseptal wall of the LV were visualized with sestamibi at stress (Fig. V.7a, arrows), while the perfusion pattern was normal at rest (Fig. V.7b).

Coronary angiography performed 1 week later demonstrated the presence of an 80% stenosis on the LAD after the origin of the diagonal branch and a 60–70% stenosis on the LCx (Fig. V.7c, arrows).

The patient was first submitted for an angioplasty of the LAD, the vessel corresponding to the site of the myocardial ischaemia. The control 1 month later confirmed successful dilatation of the LAD but indicated the occurrence of perfusion defects in the lateral and inferoposterior walls of the LV, well visualized on the HLA and VLA views and on the short axis views (Fig. V.7d,e, arrows) corresponding to ischaemia in the LCx territory. A second angioplasty was performed successfully on the LCx coronary artery.

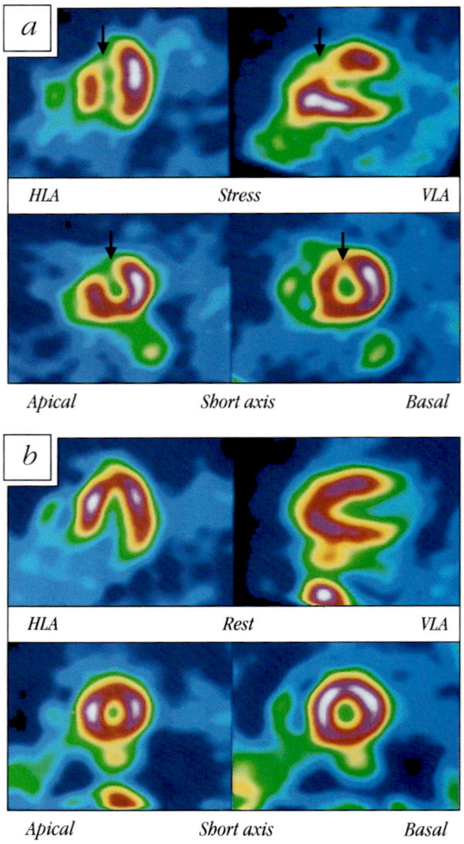

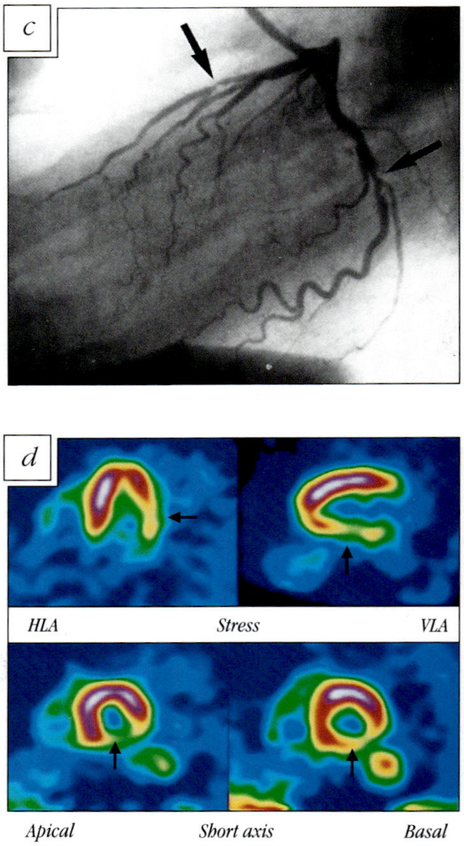

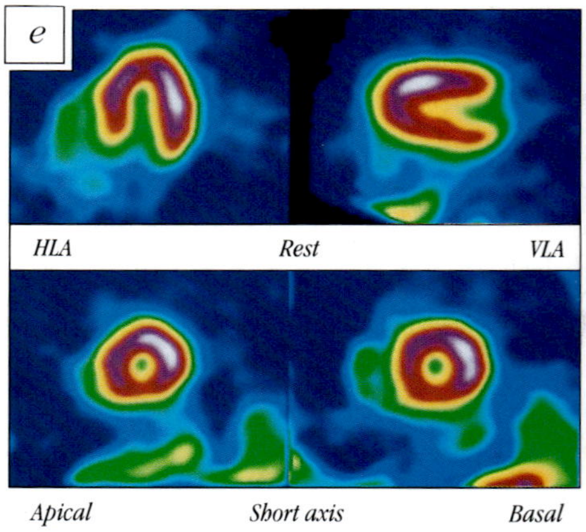

Case Study V.8

Myocardial perfusion imaging to define the optimal strategy for revascularization in the presence of multiple vessel disease (2)

Mr GA was admitted to the coronary care unit for unstable angina pectoris in September 1991. He had complained of chest pain induced by physical stress for 3 months and suffered from hypertension and renal dysfunction. Myocardial enzyme serum levels remained normal.

Myocardial perfusion imaging was performed after stabilization and showed stress perfusion defects in the anteroseptal and apical walls of the LV as well as left ventricular dilatation, suggesting severe myocardial ischaemia in the LAD vessel territory. Perfusion in the inferoseptal wall was slightly altered (Fig. V.8a,b, arrows).

The angiogram revealed the presence of 95% stenosis of the LAD and a less severe lesion (±60%) in the RCA (Fig. V.8c, arrows). The patient was referred for an LAD angioplasty. The scintigraphic control realized 3 months later indicated a normal perfusion pattern in the anteroseptal wall of the LV but the presence of perfusion abnormalities in the inferior walls (Fig. V.8d,e, arrows), requiring an angioplasty of the RCA.

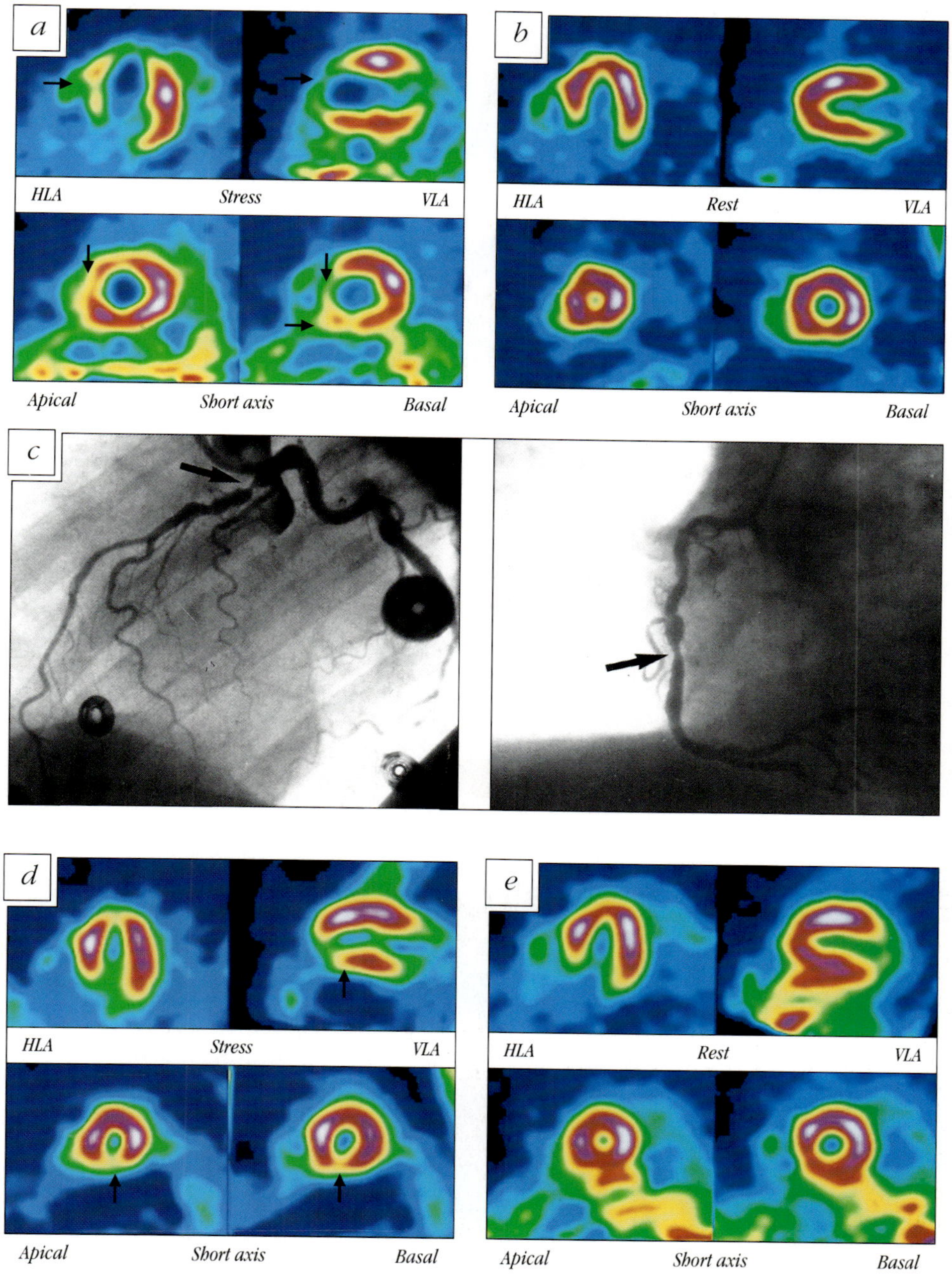

Case Study V.9

Assessment of the functional significance of a coronary lesion in a patient with collaterals

Mr DP is a 64-year-old male patient with predisposing factors for coronary artery disease. Three months ago, he experienced an episode of nocturnal chest discomfort, but did not consult his doctor as the pain finally went away. Subsequently, he complained of angina with exercise but the pain did not occur frequently.

When he came to the out-patient clinic, his resting ECG was normal but the exercise ECG was abnormal (ST segment depression in lead V6) at 125 W (Fig. V.9a).

Sestamibi scintigraphy at stress showed an anteroseptal defect while the resting images were normal (Fig. V.9b,c, arrows).

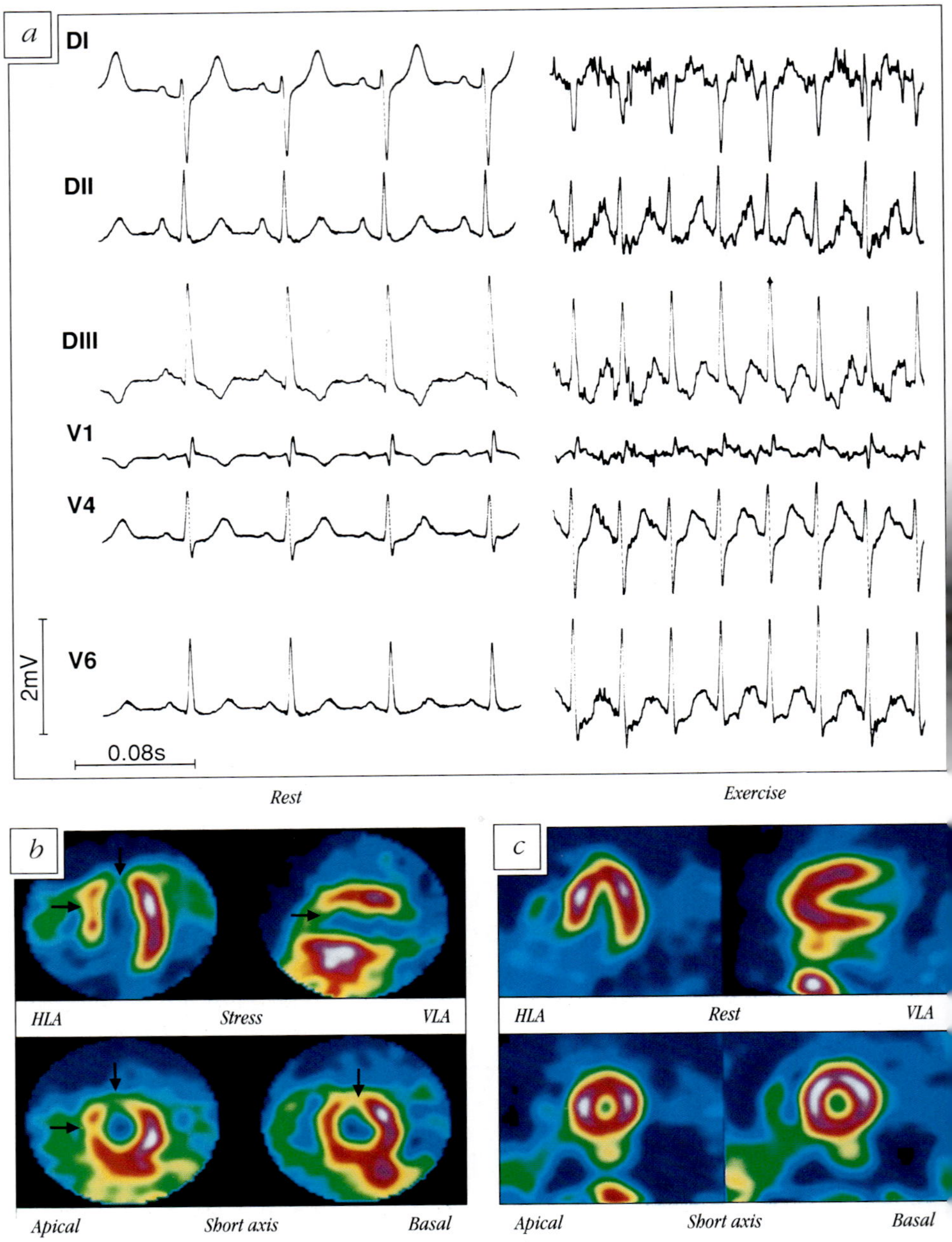

The angiogram revealed the presence of an LAD occlusion after the origin of the diagonal branch. The distal LAD vessel was revascularized by collaterals. The RCA and LCx were normal (Fig. V.9d, arrows).

Contrast ventriculography showed a normal systolic function and a good regional contractility (Fig. V.9e).

This case illustrates the protective effect of collaterals at rest.

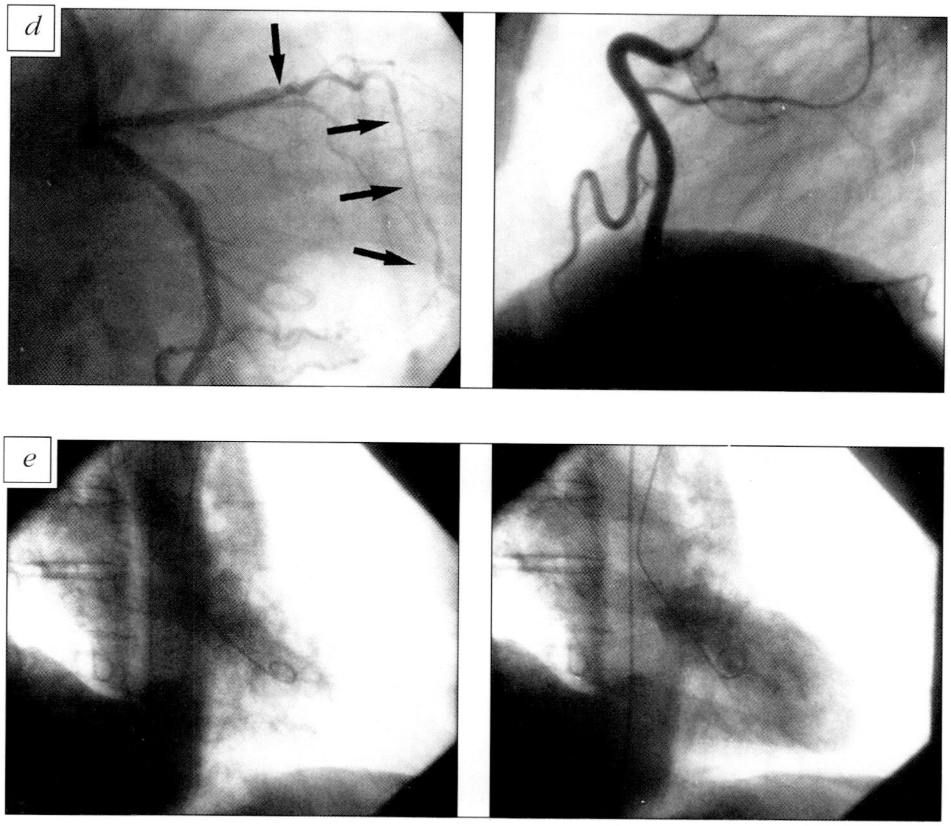

Case Study V.10

Functional assessment of coronary lesions in a patient with a high risk for bypass surgery

Mr SG, 65 years old, suffered from chronic obstructive pulmonary disease for several years when he developed precordial chest pain induced by stress and radiated to his back and to his shoulders. Pain was quickly relieved by nitrates.

He came to the clinic for further investigations. The stress ECG combined with sestamibi tomography at stress and at rest demonstrated the presence of small perfusion defects in the anteroapical wall and larger perfusion defects in the inferoposterior wall of the LV (Fig. V.10a,b, arrows). The angiogram, 4 days later, revealed the presence of a borderline significant stenosis on the LAD and the presence of an 80% stenosis on the RCA (Fig. V.10c, arrows).

As the risk area corresponding to the RCA stenosis was larger than the risk area corresponding to the LAD stenosis, the patient was considered for dilatation with priority being given to the RCA lesion.

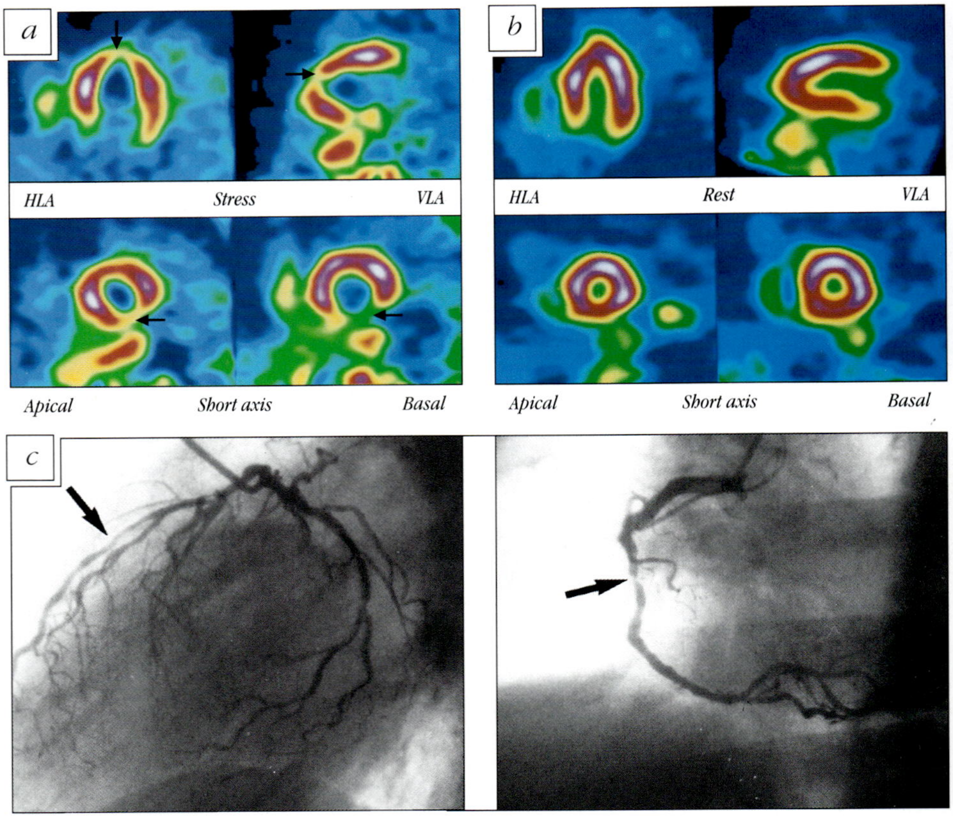

6 DIFFERENTIAL DIAGNOSIS OF ACUTE CHEST PAIN AND DIAGNOSIS OF UNSTABLE ANGINA PECTORIS

Clinical Importance of the Syndrome and Principles of Patient Management

The recognition of unstable angina pectoris (UAP) is one of the most important clinical diagnoses in modern cardiology as it has been shown that patients presenting with a syndrome of 'crescendo' type of chest pain or pain with increasing frequency and/or intensity as well as patients with de novo angina are an important subset of patients with coronary artery disease (CAD) with an unfavourable prognosis if not managed aggressively.[1,2] Key issues in unstable angina are given in Table 6.1.

In general, angina is characterized by the classical symptom of anginal pain, which typically is retrosternal, induced by effort and/or stress, and relieved by rest and/or nitroglycerin. This classical triad, when present, allows a diagnosis of CAD with a very high reliability, especially in male patients in the second half of their lives. Diamond and Forrester have characterized the pre- and post-test likelihood for such a clinical and purely intuitive approach (Fig. 6.1) which is valuable in many patients to make the initial diagnosis even before exercise testing may be warranted.[3]

While stable angina, especially when it has already been present for some time, does not indicate higher risk per se, the described syndrome of new onset of angina or the development of an unstable character of the clinical syndrome encompasses a completely different pathophysiological scenario.[4] With the information that can now be obtained from angioscopy and extensive previous experience with early angiography, it

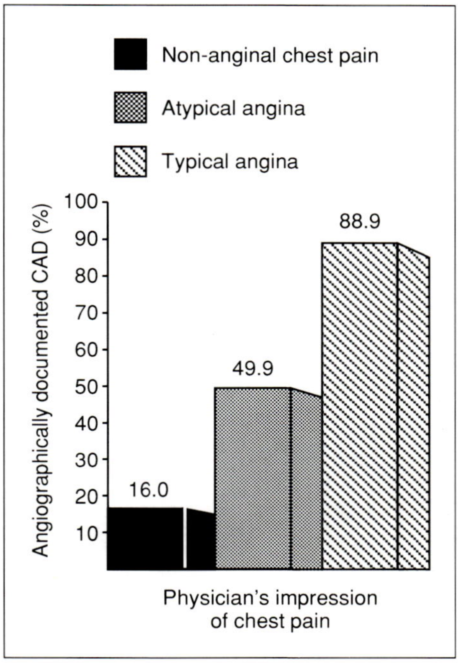

Figure 6.1
Prevalence of coronary artery disease in various chest pain syndromes. (Adapted from Diamond and Forrester.[3])

Table 6.1
Background: key issues in unstable angina.

- Increased incidence of acute myocardial infarction and death
- Treatment is efficient in reducing incidence of acute myocardial infarction and mortality
- Diagnosis sometimes difficult (atypical chest pain, no ECG changes)
- Hospital observation and coronary angiogram often necessary
- Non-invasive test to detect or rule out myocardial ischaemia during chest pain would be helpful

appears that the most important factor in the pathogenesis of myocardial infarction is thrombus formation and the 'complicated plaque' (Fig. 6.2).[5] In stable angina a fixed lesion usually leads to a well-defined effort-related threshold of the occurrence of ischaemia, mainly caused by demand/supply imbalance. The basis of instability, however, is the complicated, frequently ulcerated plaque, causing a vicious cycle of increased vasomotor tone, platelet deposition, thrombus formation, increased neurohumoral drive and possible progression to embolization (potential source of arrhythmias and electrical instability), coronary occlusion or healing with increase of stenosis degree and severity. This close relationship between clinical syndromes and morphological correlates is illustrated in Fig. 6.3.

However, similar to the area-at-risk concept for the assessment of myocardial salvage (i.e. reduction of the initial territory in jeopardy by early, aggressive treatment), this clinical entity usually requires dedicated assessment of the patient by the treating cardiologist leading to angiography to establish the morphological basis for further management. Most frequently, the diagnosis of UAP is a purely clinical one, supported by 12-lead electrocardiography. On the other hand, it is well known that in patients with left ventricular hypertrophy, bundle branch block, pacemakers, etc., ECG diagnosis has significant limitations. Additionally, a large number of patients with chest pain syndromes admitted to coronary care units (CCU) in the 1990s will be admitted to 'rule out myocardial infarction and UAP'.

A number of other disease entities such as aortic aneurysm, pericarditis, non-cardiac pain (e.g. gastric origin), etc. have to be considered and need to be integrated in order to make decisions about further aggressive diagnostic work-up or discharge.

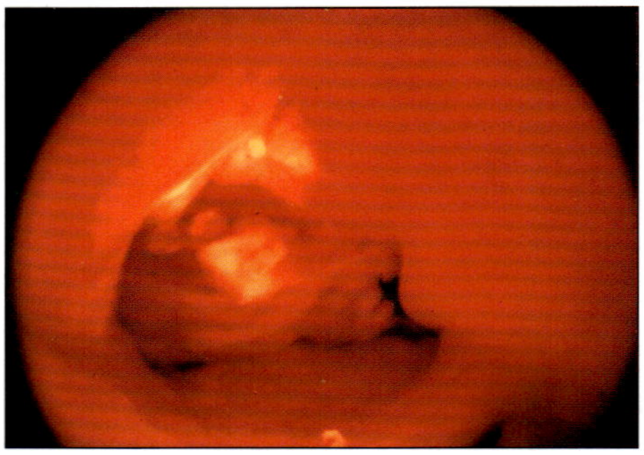

Figure 6.2
Angioscopic view through a human coronary artery. The highlighted area (upper part) shows an atheromatous plaque, and in the inner parts of the lumen, thrombus formation can be seen which leaves only a small area through which the blood can pass.

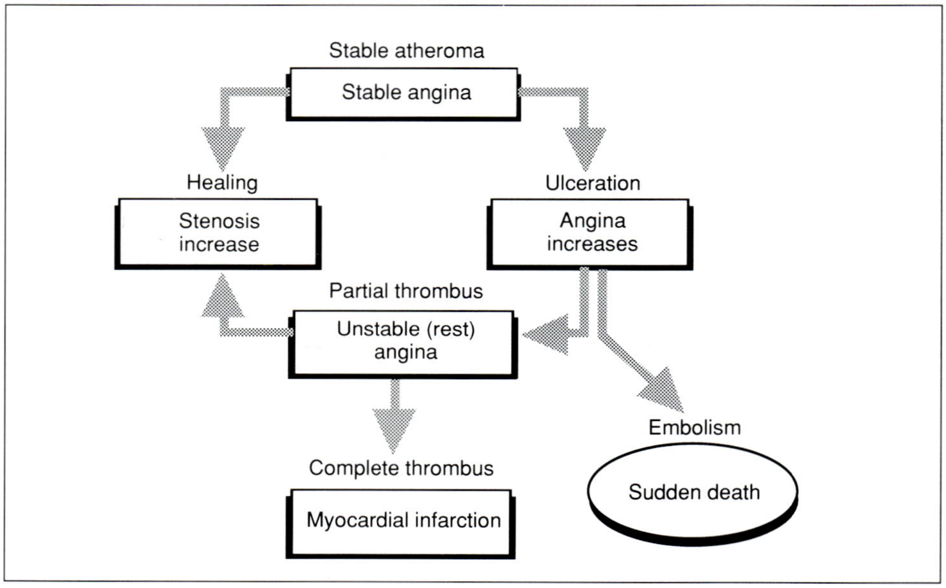

Figure 6.3
Schematic representation of relationship between clinical syndromes and morphological correlates.

Problem of silent ischaemia

It has been shown convincingly that during the chain of events of ischaemia in the myocardium, angina per se is a late symptom, preceded by reduction of flow, followed by increase of filling pressure, disturbed diastolic, then systolic function and ECG changes. Thus, the clinical syndrome of pain is a late but not an obligatory hallmark of ischaemia and the majority of ischaemic events may indeed be 'silent'; this is especially important in patients with previous myocardial infarction. In fact, studies with 24-h Holter monitoring and investigations using ^{82}Rb as a flow tracer have shown that the majority of events in a given patient may actually be silent. Therefore, the 'total ischaemic burden' will consist of episodes that are symptomatic as well as of episodes that may not be apparent clinically at all.[6,7]

Rationale for Perfusion Imaging for Differentiation of Acute Ischaemia

Any non-invasive test that could accurately identify myocardial ischaemia would be useful to aid diagnosis, to focus on 'culprit' vascular lesions (especially in known coronary disease) and may guide and optimize treatment regimens. Perfusion imaging with ^{201}Tl or with ^{99m}Tc sestamibi, which due to its favourable kinetic properties offers a unique approach, can be used.[8–11] While after injection of ^{201}Tl redistribution begins rapidly and may hide transient phenomena of ischaemia, sestamibi offers the major advantage of 'freezing' the perfusion distribution.[12] This tracer can be used to obtain an 'ischaemic fingerprint', allowing imaging at a time when ischaemia itself has already vanished. However, a single study often cannot differentiate ischaemia from infarct. By repeated injection of this new radiotracer and demonstration of reduction of the territory of decreased perfusion it can be deduced that transient ischaemia has been the cause of the clinical syndrome.

Initial experience with detection and assessment of UAP by sestamibi

Grégoire and Théroux[11] have evaluated the diagnostic value of this technique in patients with spontaneous chest pain (Fig. 6.4) and a presumable diagnosis of UAP in comparison with standard 12-lead ECG: sestamibi imaging with SPECT had a higher sensitivity for the diagnosis of UAP and better accuracy than 12-lead ECG, obtained during as well as between episodes of pain. (ECG obtained simultaneously with the radiotracer injection at the time of pain yielded a sensitivity of 35% and a specificity of 68%, whereas the presence of a perfusion abnormality during pain showed a sensitivity of 96% and specificity of 79% (Fig. 6.5).) It is interesting to note that in this early study, taking full advantage of the trace properties of sestamibi and relating this to a standard clinical signal, a few patients without any significant coronary stenosis also showed a perfusion defect.

It was found that the specificity when injecting during pain was 79%; when the presence of a reversible defect was taken as an end point specificity was 84%. Whether these false-positive judgements in relation to coronary anatomy do not in fact reflect the true pathophysiology of myocardial perfusion remains speculative, but alterations such as coronary vasospasm or spontaneous recanalization are also possible. However, the influence of methodological limitations such as soft tissue attenuation or patient movement have also to be considered.

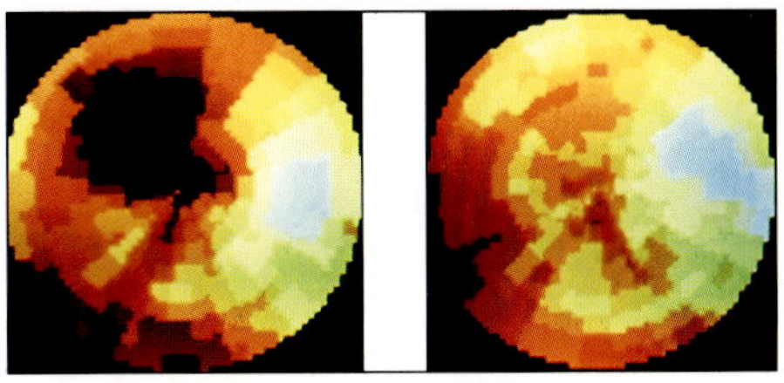

Figure 6.4 *^{99m}Tc sestamibi in spontaneous chest pain. (From Grégoire and Théroux[11], with permission)*

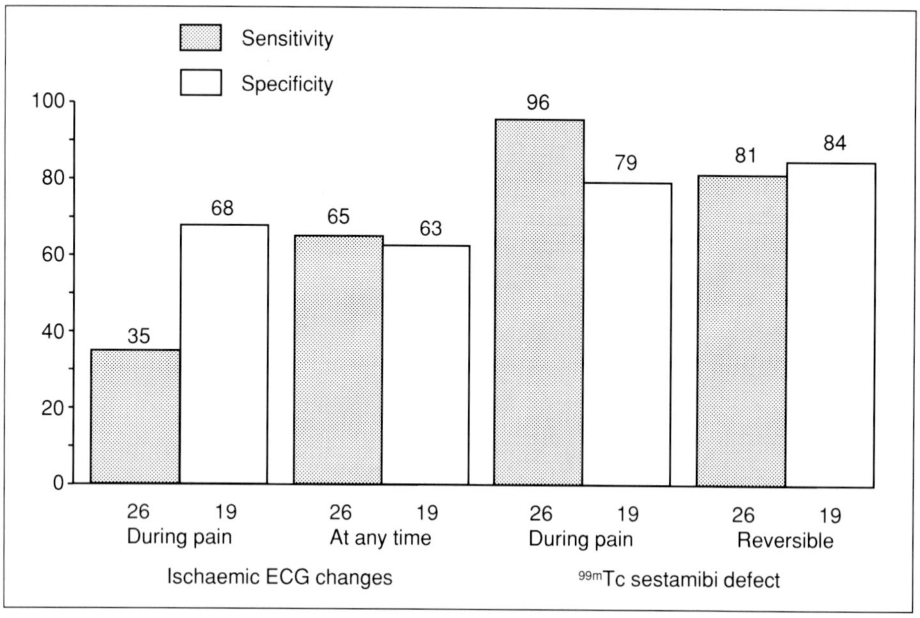

Figure 6.5
Sensitivity and specificity of ^{99m}Tc sestamibi vs ECGs in unstable angina. (From Grégoire and Théroux[11], with permission)

Aim of the Sestamibi Study in Unstable Angina

Initial experience in selected patients indicates an additive value to 12-lead electrocardiography for the recognition, localization and assessment of severity of ischaemia. This potential approach could be envisaged for the following applications:

- to offer improved possibilities to rule out ischaemia in borderline cases;
- to aid selection of patients for coronary angiography;
- to identify the culprit vessel and pinpoint the involved territory; and
- to provide insights into the phenomena of ischaemia when other markers are not necessarily positive.

In the clinical scenario, a negative sestamibi study, when injected during chest pain, suggests that ischaemia and significant coronary stenosis can be ruled out, while an abnormal study suggests significant coronary disease, especially when a reversible defect is evident on repeated injection.

Limitations

Despite its promise and conceptual novelty, the use of sestamibi imposes a number of logistical demands in a clinical setting: the tracer will have to be ready on a 24-h basis (as the time when pain occurs is not known), and facilities for imaging will also have to be available at all times.

Whether such an approach can aid in risk stratification and help in making management decisions in routine clinical practice remains to be determined from a larger series; trials and comparisons must be made with standard clinical and angiographically oriented management guidelines.

Clinical Points

- A negative study during chest pain rules out significant coronary stenosis with a high level of confidence.
- A positive study predicts significant coronary stenosis with high accuracy.
- A decrease in size of defect between pain and pain-free images supports a diagnosis of ischaemia.

References

1 Maseri A, Parodi O, Severi S, Pesola A, Transient transmural reduction of myocardial blood flow, demonstrated by Tl-201 scintigraphy, as a cause of variant angina, *Circulation* (1976) **54**:280.

2 Parodi O, Uthurralt N, Severi S et al, Transient reduction of regional myocardial perfusion during angina at rest with ST-segment depression or normalization of negative T wave, *Circulation* (1981) **63**:1238.

3 Diamond GA, Forrester JS, Analysis of probability as an aid in the clinical diagnosis of coronary artery disease, *N Engl J Med* (1979) **300**:1350.

4 Singh R, Progression of coronary arterosclerosis: clues to pathogenesis from serial coronary arteriography, *Br Heart J* (1984) **52**:451.

5 TIMI Research Group T, Immediate vs delayed catheterization and angioplasty following thrombolytic therapy for acute myocardial infarction, *JAMA* (1988) **260**:2849.

6 Tzivoni D, Gavish A, Zin D et al, Prognostic significance of ischemic episodes in patients with previous myocardial infarction, *Am J Cardiol* (1988) **62**:661.

7 Stern S, Tzivoni D, Early detection of silent ischaemic heart disease by 24 hour electrocardiographic monitoring of active subjects, *Br Heart J* (1974) **36**:481.

8 Wackers F, Lie K, Liem K et al, Thallium-scintigraphy in unstable angina pectoris, *Circulation* (1978) **57**:738.

9 Brown K, Okada R, Boucher C et al, Serial thallium-201 imaging at rest in patients with unstable and stable angina pectoris: relationship of myocardial perfusion at rest to presenting clinical syndrome, *Am Heart J* (1983) **106**:70.

10 Freeman M, Williams A, Chisholm R et al, Role of resting thallium-201 perfusion in predicting coronary anatomy, left ventricular wall motion and hospital outcome in unstable angina pectoris, *Am Heart J* (1989) **117**:306.

11 Grégoire J, Théroux P, Detection and assessment of unstable angina using myocardial perfusion imaging: comparison between technetium-99m Sestamibi SPECT and 12-lead electrocardiogram, *Am J Cardiol* (1990) **66**:42E.

12 Okada R, Glover D, Gaffney T, Williams S, Myocardial kinetics of Tc-99m-hexakis-2-methoxy-2-methyl propylisonitrile, *Circulation* (1988) **77**:491.

Case Study VI.1

Interest of sestamibi myocardial imaging in UAP

A 62-year-old woman with type 2 diabetes and with low lipid levels was admitted to the CCU with chest pain that increased when she did her housework. In addition, she suffered from osteoporosis and frequent back pain.

Admission ECG showed unspecific ST changes in leads DI, DII and aVL as possible signs of ischaemia with a small Q-wave in lead DIII. On several occasions during the first 24 h the patient experienced back pain and chest pain. However, ECGs did not reveal ischaemia. Therefore, it was decided to try to correlate her ischaemic syndrome with a stage of myocardial perfusion. When she re-experienced pain the ECG showed clear ST elevation in the inferior wall (Fig. VI.1a).

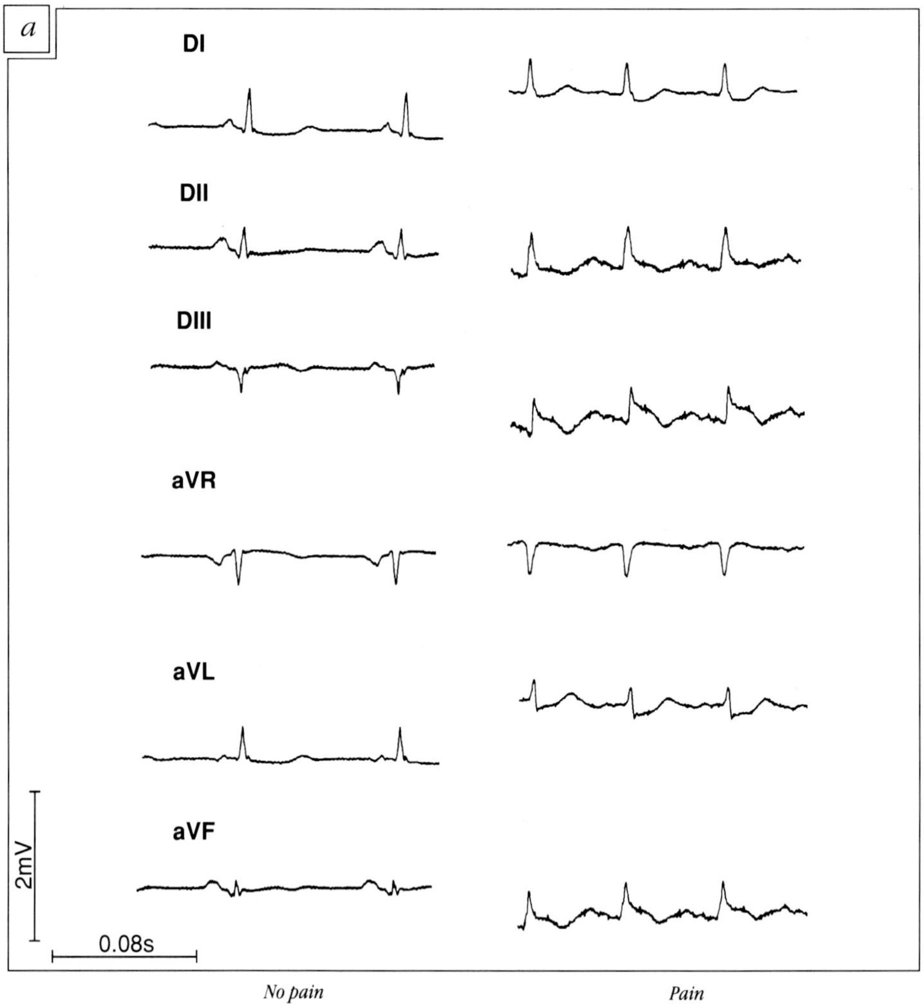

Tomographic imaging performed after sestamibi injection during an episode of pain demonstrated perfusion defects involving the inferoposterior and the inferior wall of the left ventricle on the sagittal long axis and on the short axis views (Fig. VI.1b).

Subsequently, because of the proof of significant ischaemia, coronary angiography was performed. The baseline angiogram showed one proximal and one mid- to high-grade right coronary artery (RCA) stenosis (Fig. VI.1c) and the patient underwent successful percutaneous transluminal coronary angioplasty (PTCA) of both lesions (Figs. VI.1d,e).

This study shows the correlation of the clinical syndrome of chest pain with ECG abnormality, significant abnormalities in myocardial perfusion and severe coronary disease.

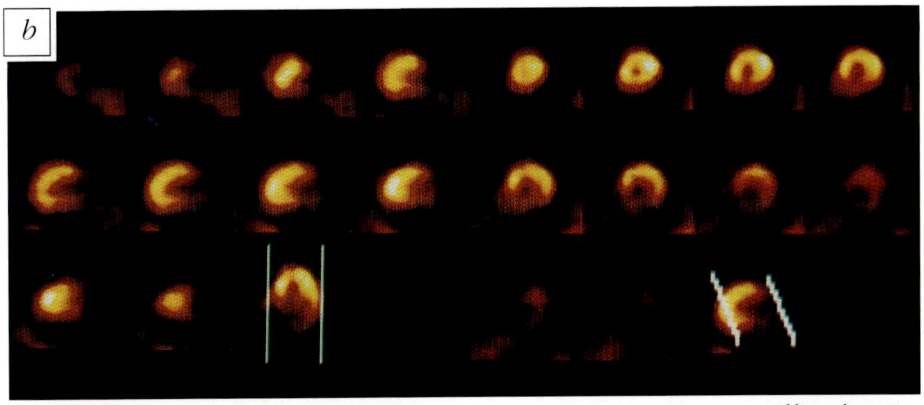

Sagittal long axis *Oblique short axis*

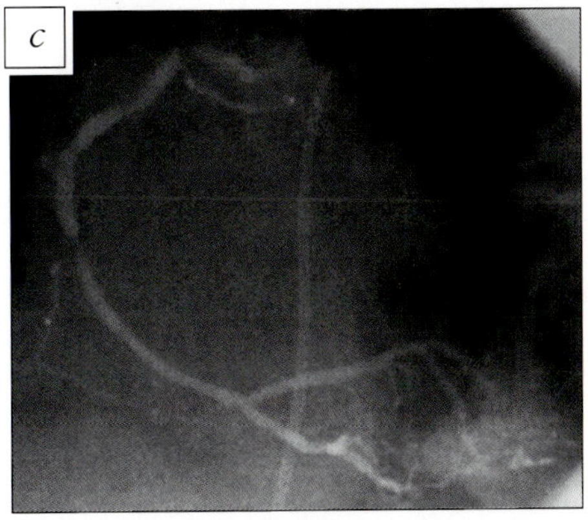

Before PTCA

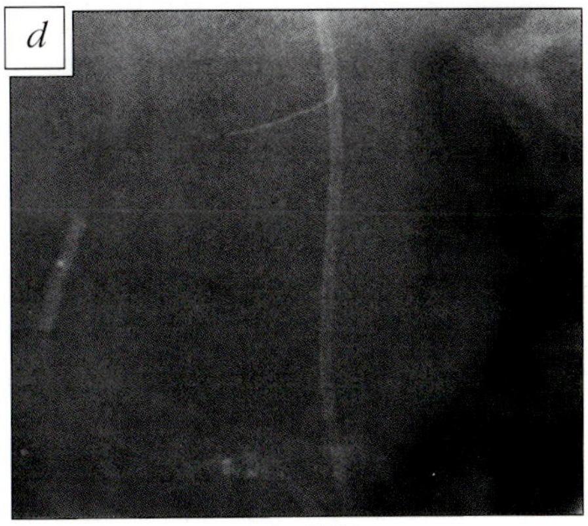

During PTCA

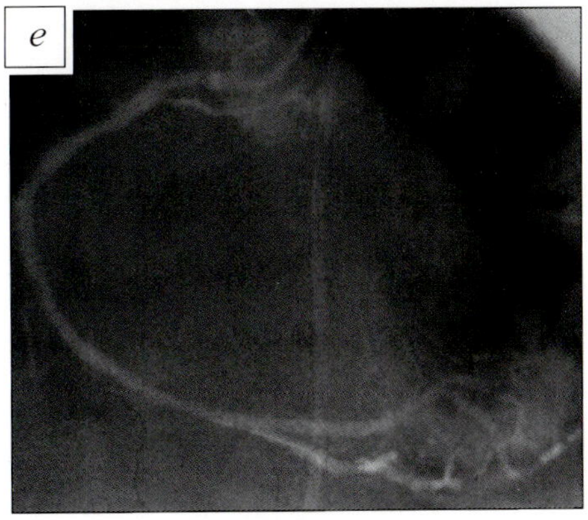

After PTCA

Case Study VI.2

Interest of gated SPECT imaging after injection during acute chest pain

A 75-year-old man was admitted to hospital following a period of partly typical, partly atypical chest pain radiating from between his shoulders towards the left side of the thorax and extending to his left arm. He experienced this when walking in the park with his dog and also to some degree at rest. He had hypertension and a history of a rib fracture of the left fourth and fifth ribs as a result of a tram accident.

The ECG at admission showed non-specific ST changes in the precordial leads (V1 to V6) (Fig. VI.2a). A second ECG immediately following anginal symptoms was again found not to be significantly different from that at admission and therefore sestamibi was injected (Fig. VI.2b). One hour later, a third ECG was recorded and showed significant ST–T changes and loss of R amplitude in the precordial leads V2 and V3 (Fig. VI.2c).

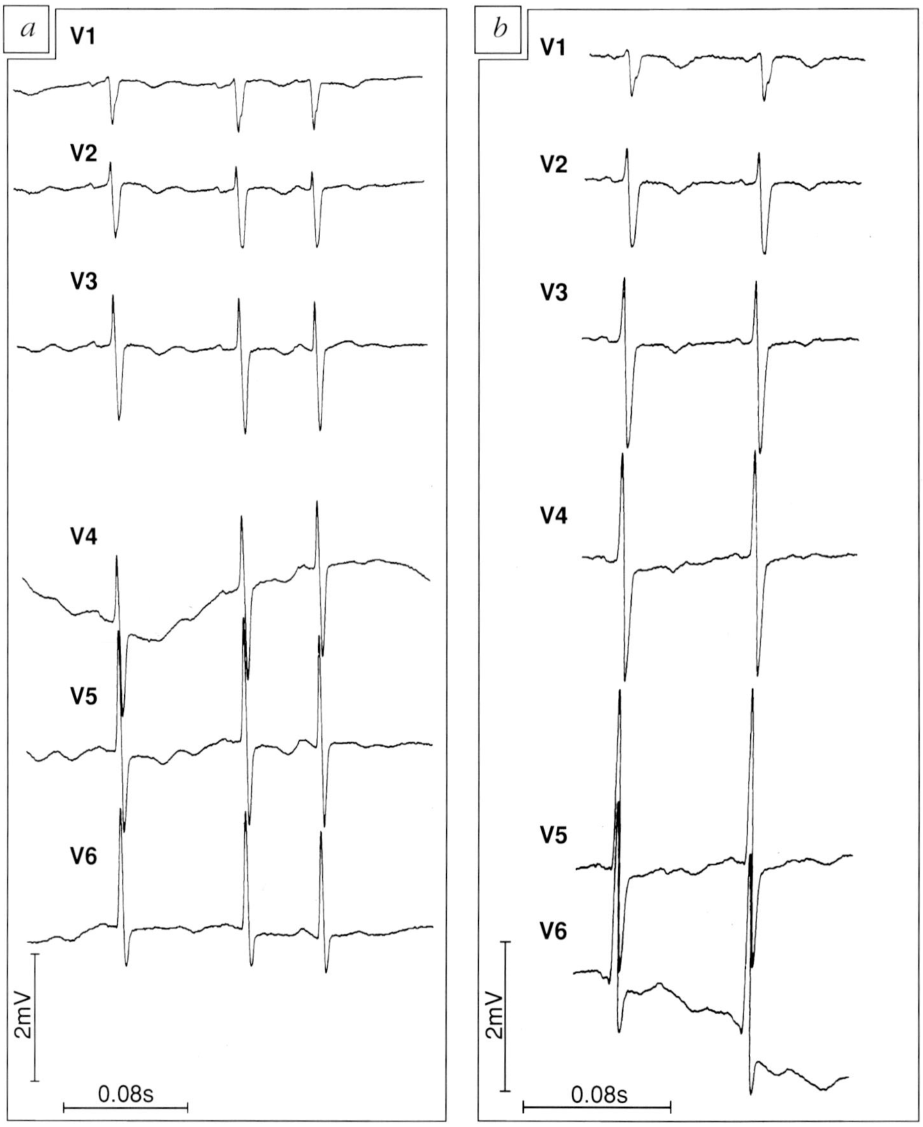

Admission

Pain *Sestamibi injection*

To analyse myocardial perfusion and myocardial wall thickening, we decided to perform a gated tomographic acquisition study (Fig. VI.2d). The eight frames represent an average cardiac cycle. The perfusion defect visualized in the apical, in the anterolateral and in the posterolateral walls of the left ventricle (LV), and in the left circumflex (LCx) vessel territory on diastolic frame disappeared on systolic frame, indicating well-preserved myocardial wall thickening. The physical and biological characteristics of sestamibi are such that in gated studies the perfusion distribution reflects the status at the time of injection (in this case myocardial ischaemia), while regional wall thickening reflects the status at the time of imaging (in this case, 1 h after pain). Thus, a gated study may aid in identifying transient and ischaemic events in perfusion but preserve regional left ventricular function suggesting reversibility.

Subsequent angiography revealed a 95% mid-stenosis and a subtotal occlusion of the LCx coronary artery immediately before the marginal branches. There was also discrete distant filling of the circumflex bed by bridging collaterals (Fig. VI.2e).

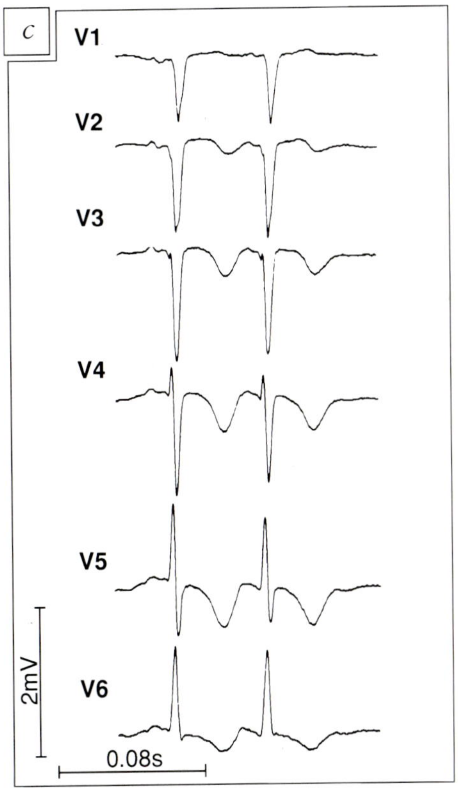

ECG 1 hour after pain

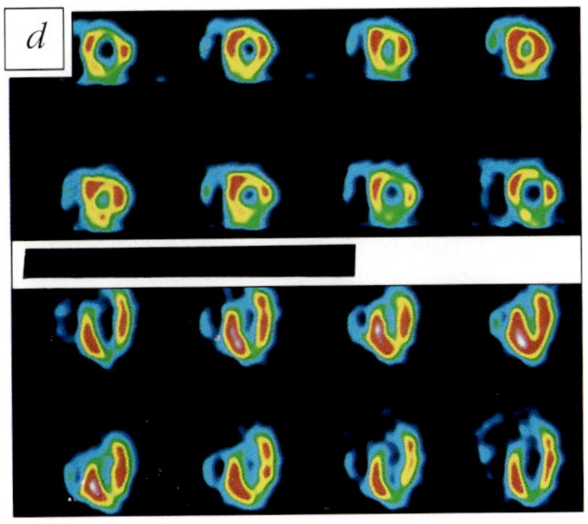

HLA

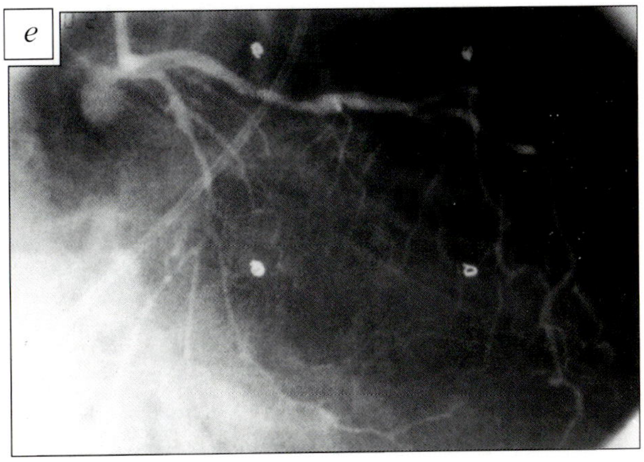

Case Study VI.3

Assessment of myocardial perfusion and myocardial wall thickening during acute chest pain with sestamibi gated planar imaging

A 60-year-old man with a DDD pacemaker, fitted as a result of recurrent syncopy one year ago caused by a reconduction abnormality in combination with a left interior block, was admitted with a history of short episodes of atypical chest pain, mainly occurring during exposure to cold weather.

The admission ECG showed normal pacemaker function of a DDD pacemaker (Fig. VI.3a). Because of the pacemaker, ECG diagnosis of ischaemia could not be based on the ECG alone. Therefore, it was decided to perform a perfusion study with sestamibi.

During one of the next brief episodes, the tracer was injected and 60 min later a planar gated study was performed in the anterior, in the LAO 40° and in the LAO 70° views. Scintigraphic results demonstrated clearly a perfusion defect in the septal, apical and inferior wall of the LV. However, myocardial thickening was preserved, particularly on the inferior wall in the anterior view (Fig. VI.3b). Judgement of thickening was not easily obtainable for the septum area but the suggestion of significant CAD was made.

An angiogram was therefore performed, highlighting the tight proximal/mid-stenosis of the LAD and irregularities in the LCx (Fig. VI.3c, arrows). Subsequently, the patient underwent coronary angioplasty. The post-intervention scan (not shown) showed normal perfusion both at stress and at rest.

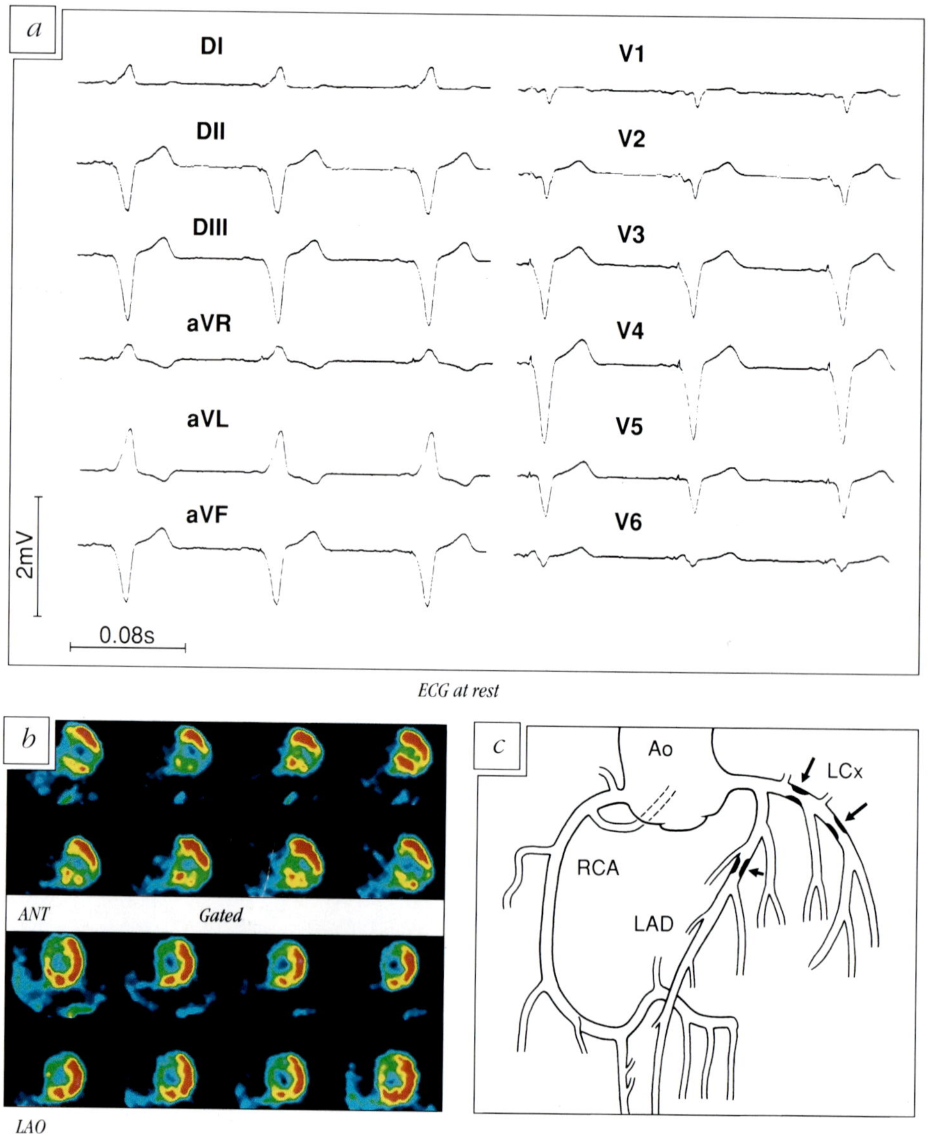

7 ASSESSMENT OF PTCA INTERVENTIONS

Clinical Background

Since the performance of the first coronary angioplasty by Gruentzig (1977), percutaneous transluminal coronary angioplasty (PTCA) has become an important method of myocardial reperfusion. More than 100 000 PTCA interventions are performed every year in Europe and more than 200 000 in the United States.[1,2]

The indications for PTCA have widened significantly over the last few years. They were in the beginning limited to cases of single proximal stenosis. Advances in the material used (balloon and guide wire), and the increased experience of the interventional cardiology teams, have resulted in changes in the clinical indications; more complex lesions as well as older patients are being approached, and dilatation is more frequently performed on multiple and more distal sites.[3,4]

PTCA is a highly attractive technique in that it is less aggressive, carries less risk of morbidity and implies significant reduction in cost as compared to coronary artery bypass (CABG) graft surgery. However, its major inconvenience remains a high rate of restenosis estimated at around 30–40% by most recent studies.[5]

Restenosis appears predominantly in the first 6 months following PTCA with the majority developing as early as 2 or 3 months later. At least initially, however, a large number of these restenoses remain asymptomatic. The causes of restenosis are not yet fully understood but might be related to intimal and medial tear, thrombus formation and proliferation of smooth muscular cells.[6] There is at present no known effective preventive treatment.

Clinical Problem

Clinical decision to perform angioplasty requires knowledge not only of the detailed coronary anatomy, but also of the functional significance of the lesions. Indeed, only stenosis responsible for myocardial ischaemia should be dilated, but in practice the question of whether or not to dilate a mild stenosis, or one for which the access is difficult, is frequently asked.

While, in many cases, coronary angiography will accurately identify significant lesions, the relationship between anatomy and functional significance remains complex and documentation of myocardial ischaemia in the distal perfusion bed of the stenosis is preferred.[7]

It is also important to assess the extent of myocardial ischaemia to evaluate the need for intervention on several vessels. In particular, in patients after myocardial infarction (MI), it is fundamental to assess both the presence of residual peri-infarcted ischaemia and of ischaemia at a distance. The enhanced ability of sestamibi tomography to detect the presence and extent of myocardial ischaemia in these patients should be of significant help in decision making.[8,9]

Recently, strategies have been presented in patients with multiple vessel stenosis of varying severity or in high-risk patients with complex lesions to subdivide revascularization in several sessions and use myocardial imaging as a guide after each session to assess the need to proceed. These strategies, designed to minimize the risk, require knowledge of the most severe (culprit) lesion(s) to decide on the dilatation sequence.[10]

Assessment of the completeness of revascularization after PTCA is the subsequent role of myocardial perfusion imaging. Residual myocardial ischaemia after PTCA may result from inadequate or incomplete dilatation of the treated artery, complications of the dilatation, or residual stenosis elsewhere, whether or not these were evident before the first PTCA.

Shortly after PTCA, however, perfusion imaging abnormalities have been described reflecting the presence of transient coronary flow abnormalities but non-predictive of the long-term results. These perfusion abnormalities may reflect factors such as arterial disruption and platelet deposition and can also be demonstrated by other techniques measuring the coronary flow reserve, such as intracoronary Doppler and digital angiography. It may therefore be necessary to delay routine exercise myocardial imaging after PTCA for 1–2 months after the procedure at a time when these transient problems have resolved and the incidence of restenosis increases.[11–13] Residual myocardial ischaemia reflecting incomplete revascularization will also be evident at that time. Myocardial scintigraphy is superior to clinical and ECG signs of residual ischaemia as, in addition to better sensitivity, it has the ability to localize the area of ischaemia and relate it to the known anatomy.[14]

Clinical signs of restenosis are also not very reliable. The recurrence of typical anginal symptoms is specific but not sensitive, whereas persistence, or increase, of atypical chest pain has a low specificity. Furthermore, the stress ECG alone has not proved to be a very adequate test for detecting a restenosis with a low sensitivity (30–65%) and specificity (60–80%).

To best assess the occurrence of restenosis and differentiate it from complications, residual ischaemia or disease progression elsewhere, myocardial imaging should be systematic and performed serially at 4–6 weeks, then 3–6 months and possibly at 6-monthly intervals thereafter. Tomography should be preferred to maximize the localizing value of the scan and differentiate among the various potential causes of ischaemia.[15,16]

As demonstrated by Breisblatt et al,[11] scintigraphic signs of restenosis may precede clinical evidence for restenosis by several months. However, the accuracy of the scintigraphic early 'prediction' of restenosis has been confirmed in almost all patients.

Aims of Sestamibi Studies

Before PTCA, information from perfusion scintigraphy is complementary to angiography and establishes the presence, extent and location of the myocardial ischaemia. This is particularly important in patients with previous MI. Comparison of scintigraphic or angiographic information is essential to establish a priority list of the stenoses to be dilated and to determine a treatment strategy.

After PTCA, especially when only partial revascularization has been attempted or achieved, myocardial scintigraphy is extremely useful in demonstrating the existence and the site of residual ischaemia and in deciding on the usefulness of a second procedure.

The most important contribution made by myocardial scintigraphy in the early months following PTCA is in the detection of restenosis. Myocardial scintigraphy is the best non-invasive test in the diagnosis of restenosis. It avoids the need for systematic angiographic control in the absence of typical chest pain or of positive ECG changes.

In addition, information on the site and size of myocardial ischaemia is frequently determinant in higher risk patients to decide on the desirability of a second PTCA.

Conclusion

Given the frequency of post-PTCA restenosis and the low reliability of clinical and ECG information after PTCA, myocardial scintigraphy is an excellent alternative to systemic coronary angiography in the detection of restenosis in the 6 months following PTCA.

In addition, myocardial scintigraphy enables the location and extent of a myocardial ischaemia to be determined and this improves the treatment strategy before and after PTCA.[17–19]

Clinical Points

- Only stenosis responsible for documented myocardial ischaemia should be dilated.
- The enhanced ability of tomography to define the extent of coronary artery disease (CAD) should be of significant help in decision making.
- One key role of scintigraphy may be to identify the culprit lesion and to define a priority list in patients with multiple vessel disease.
- Restenosis occurs in 30–40% of cases but may remain asymptomatic for long periods.
- Perfusion imaging is superior to clinical and other non-invasive tests for detecting restenosis.
- Serial imaging at 6 weeks, 3–6 months, and then according to the clinical situation may be necessary for optimal monitoring of PTCA.

References

1 GRUENTZIG AR, SENNING AK, SIEGENTHALER WE, Nonoperative dilatation of coronary artery stenosis: percutaneous transluminal coronary angioplasty, *N Engl J Med* (1979) **301**:61.

2 BOURASSA MG, ALDERMAN EL, BERTRAND M et al, Report of the Joint ISFC/WHO Task Force on coronary angioplasty, *Circulation* (1988) **78**:780.

3 VANDORMAEL MG, DELIGONUL U, KERN MJ et al, Multilesion coronary angioplasty: clinical and angiographic follow-up, *J Am Coll Cardiol* (1987) **10**:246.

4 LAMBERT M, BONAN R, COTE G et al, Early results, complications and restenosis rates after multilesion and multivessel percutaneous transluminal coronary angioplasty, *Am J Cardiol* (1987) **60**:788.

5 SERRUYS PW, LUIJTEN K, BEATT KJ et al, Incidence of restenosis after successful coronary angioplasty: a time-related phenomenon. A quantitative angiographic study in 242 consecutive patients at 1, 2, 3 and 4 months, *Circulation* (1988) **77**:361.

6 WILCOX JN, Thrombin and other potential mechanisms underlying restenosis, *Circulation* (1991) **84**:432.

7 LEGRAND V, AUERON FM, BATES ER et al, Value of exercise radionuclide ventriculography and thallium-201 scintigraphy in evaluating successful coronary angioplasty. Comparison with coronary flow reserve, transaxial gradient and percent stenosis. *Eur Heart J* (1987) **8**:329.

8 Hartzler GO, RUTHERFORD BD, McCONAHAY DR et al, Percutaneous transluminal coronary angioplasty with and without thrombolytic therapy for treatment of acute myocardial infarction, *Am Heart J* (1983) **106**:965.

9 TOPOL EJ, CALIFF RM, GEORGE BS et al, A randomized trial for immediate versus delayed elective angioplasty after intravenous tissue plasminogen activator in acute myocardial infarction, *N Engl J Med* (1987) **317**:518.

10 Breisblatt WM et al, Incomplete revascularization in multivessel percutaneous transluminal coronary angioplasty: the role for stress thallium-201 imaging, *J Am Coll Cardiol* (1988) **11**:1183.

11 Breisblatt WM, Weiland FL, Spaccavento LF, Stress thallium-201 imaging after coronary angioplasty predicts restenosis and recurrent symptoms, *J Am Coll Cardiol* (1988) **12**:1199.

12 Manyari DE, Knudtson M, Kloiber R et al, Sequential thallium-201 myocardial perfusion studies after successful percutaneous transluminal coronary artery angioplasty: delayed resolution of exercise-induced scintigraphic abnormalities, *Circulation* (1988) **77**:86.

13 Wilson RF, Johnson MR, Marcus ML et al, The effect of coronary angioplasty on coronary flow reserve, *Circulation* (1988) **77**:873.

14 DePuey EG, Myocardial perfusion imaging with thallium-201 to evaluate patients before and after percutaneous transluminal coronary angioplasty, *Circulation* (1991) **84** (Suppl. I):59.

15 Wijns W, Serruys PW, Reiber JHC et al, Early detection of restenosis after successful percutaneous transluminal coronary angioplasty by exercise-redistribution thallium scintigraphy, *Am J Cardiol* (1985) **55**:357.

16 Renkin J, Melin J, Robert A et al, Detection of restenosis after successful coronary angioplasty: improved clinical decision making with use of a logistic model combining procedural and follow-up variables, *J Am Coll Cardiol* (1990) **16**:1333.

17 Vandormael MG, Chaitman BR, Ischinger T et al, Immediate and short-term benefit of multilesion coronary angioplasty: influence of degree of revascularization, *J Am Coll Cardiol* (1985) **6**:983.

18 Bell MR, Bailey KR, Reed GS et al, Percutaneous transluminal angioplasty in patients with multivessel coronary disease: how important is complete revascularization for cardiac event-free survival? *J Am Coll Cardiol* (1990) **16**:553.

19 Nath A, Disciascio G, Kelly KM, Multivessel coronary angioplasty early after acute myocardial infarction, *J Am Coll Cardiol* (1990) **16**:545.

Case Study VII.1

Usefulness of myocardial perfusion imaging in the follow-up of PTCA interventions

Mr P is a 73-year-old male patient without previous cardiac disease who had suffered from right femoral artery occlusion several years before. In January 1989, he complained of an episode of nocturnal pain lasting around 35 min but resolving spontaneously.

An exercise test performed a few days later was abnormal with typical ECG changes and a sestamibi perfusion deficit in the anteroseptal region (Fig. VII.1a, arrows). A small septoapical abnormality persisted at rest (Fig. VII.1b, arrow).

Angioplasty was performed successfully but in February 1989 the post-PTCA scan revealed a persistent minimal apical abnormality as is commonly seen early after PTCA (Fig. VII.1c, arrow).

Two months later, this abnormality had spontaneously disappeared and the sestamibi scintigraphy was normal at stress (Fig. VII.1d).

In May 1989, symptomatic recurrence was observed and the presence of myocardial ischaemia was confirmed by perfusion scintigraphy (Fig. VII.1e, arrows). Angioplasty was repeated, this time with lasting success (Fig. VII.1f).

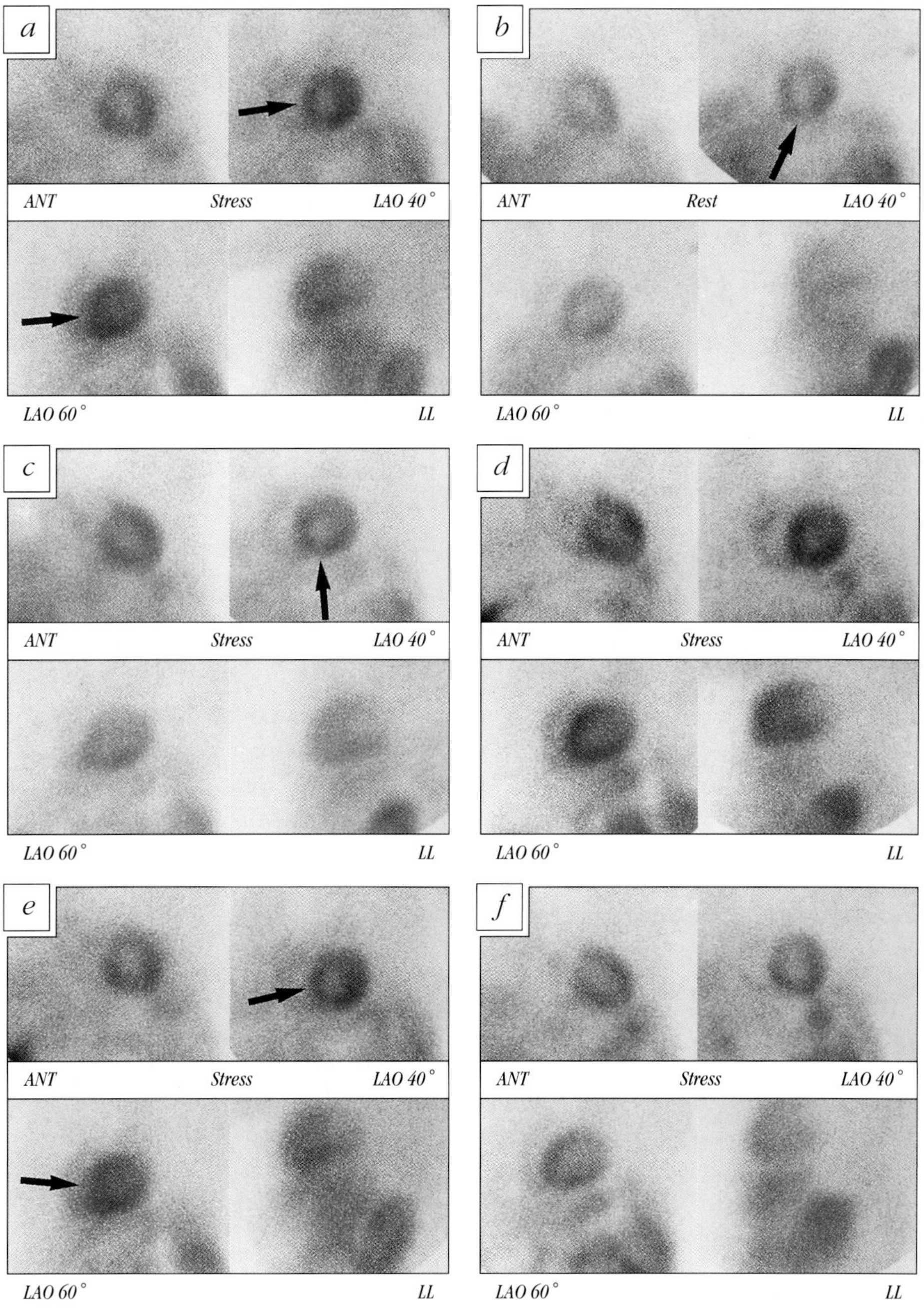

Case Study VII.2

Evaluation of the results of PTCA with myocardial perfusion imaging

Mr LM, a 59-year-old man, suffered for several years from occasional exercise chest pain well controlled by medical therapy. Recently the pain has become more severe and more frequent.

His exercise test was interrupted for angina pectoris and ST depression in the inferior leads (Fig. VII.2a).

Tomography at stress and at rest demonstrated partially reversible inferoposterior defects corresponding to a small inferior MI with residual ischaemia in the right coronary artery (RCA) territory (Figs. VII.2b,c, arrows).

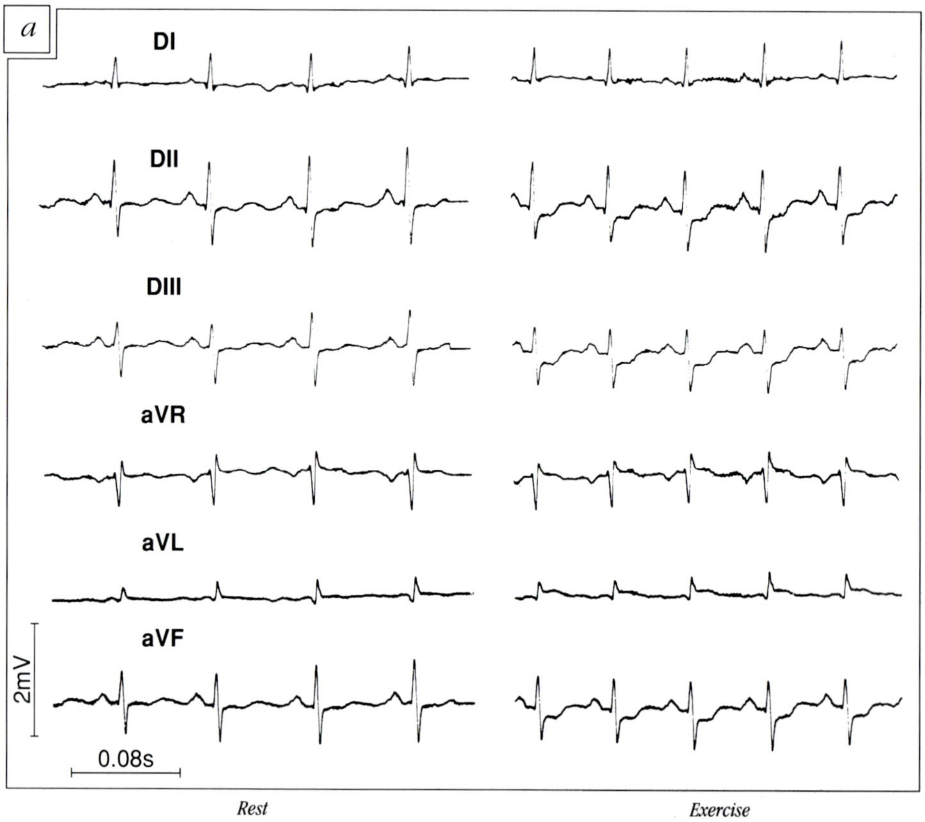

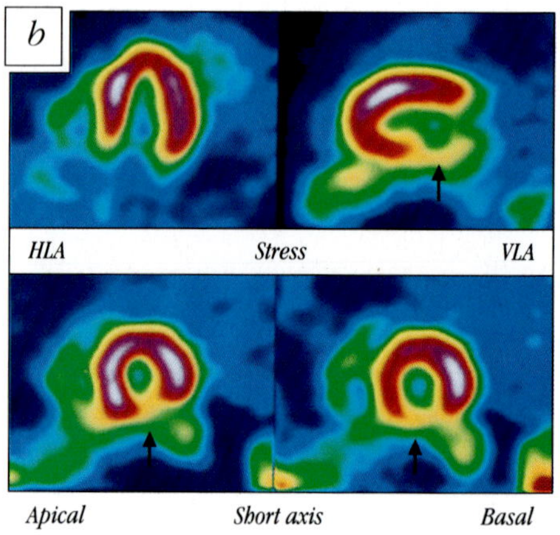

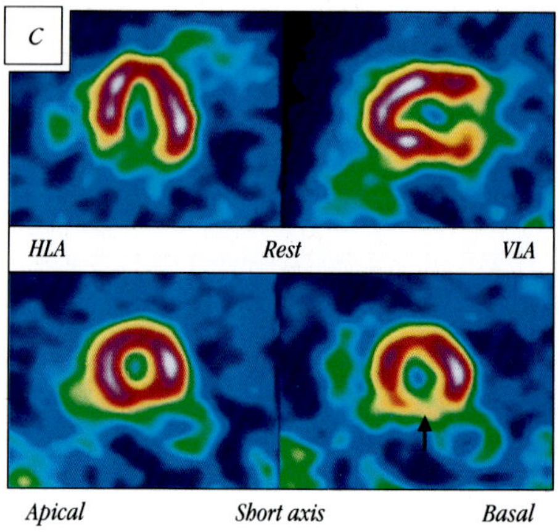

Angiography confirmed the presence of a significant RCA stenosis that was later dilated (Fig. VII.2d, arrow).

The angioplasty was successful, as confirmed by the angiographic control (Fig. VII.2e). The scintigraphic control performed 1 month later was completely normal (Fig. VII.2f).

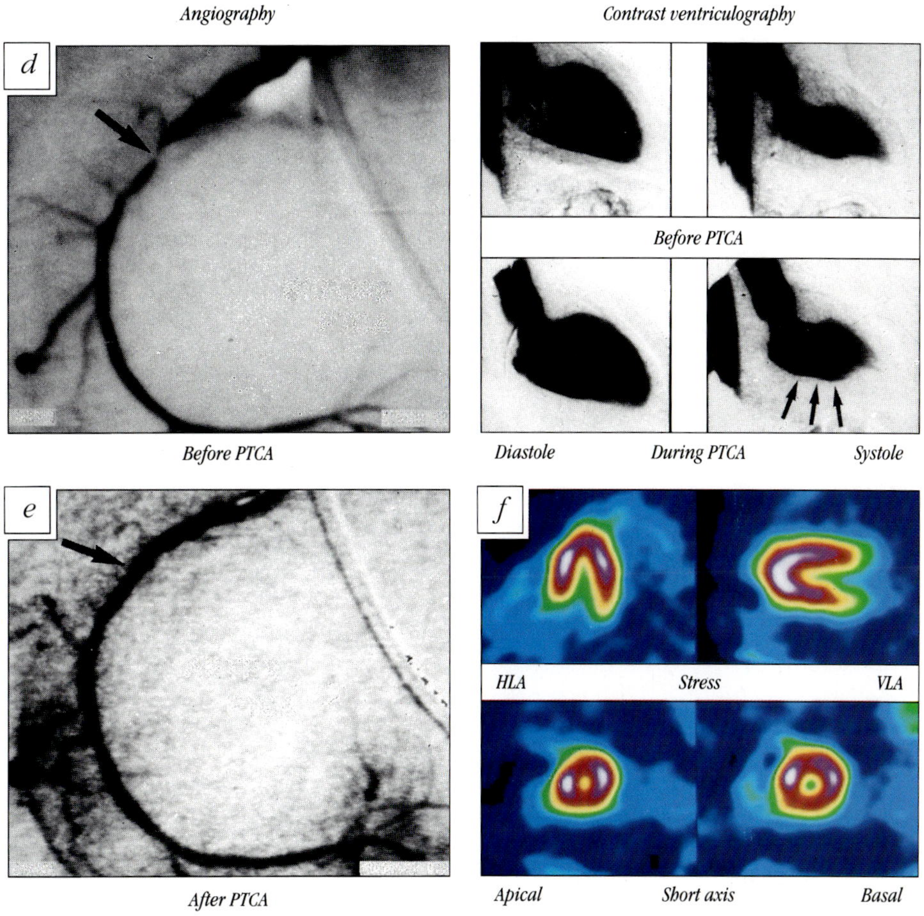

Case Study VII.3

Myocardial perfusion imaging to assess PTCA complications

Mrs ES, a 50-year-old female patient, was referred for investigations of anginal chest pain induced by activities such as shopping. Her cardiovascular risk factors were heredity and hypertension.

She exercised on a bicycle up to a load of 120 W and complained at peak exercise of left precordial pain persisting during recovery.

Sestamibi tomography at stress and at rest revealed reversible perfusion defects involving the anteroseptal wall of the left ventricle (LV), suggesting myocardial ischaemia (Figs. VII.3a,b, arrows).

The angiogram performed later demonstrated irregular and significant LAD lesions located after the origin of the diagonal branch (Fig. VII.3c, left upper, arrows).

An angioplasty was attempted but was not completely successful and led to a coronary dissection (Fig. VII.3c, right upper and bottom left, arrows).

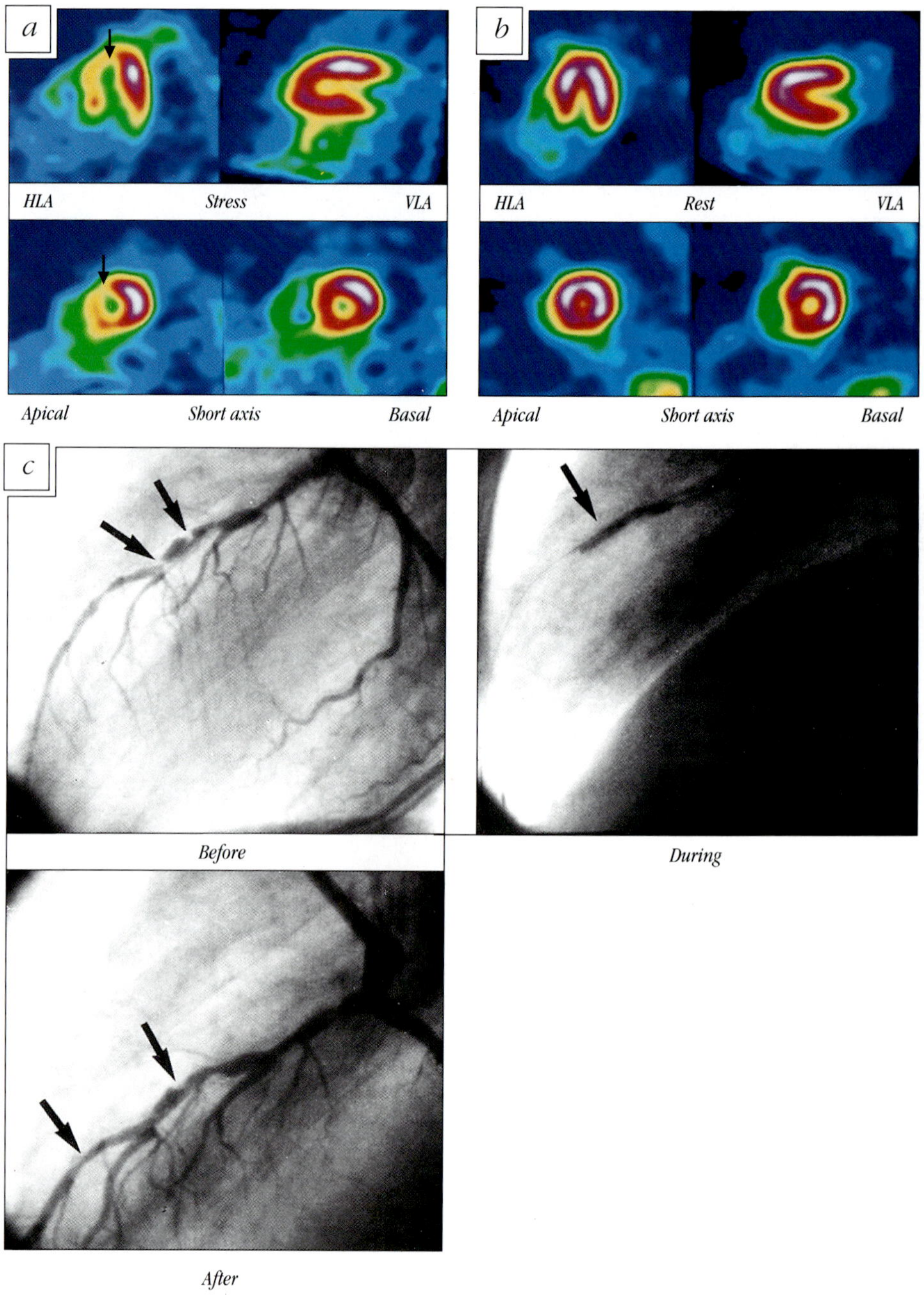

Two months later, the patient was referred for control. The scan at that time showed perfusion defects in the anteroapical wall corresponding to restenosis and requiring the angioplasty to be done again (Figs. VII.3d,e, arrows).

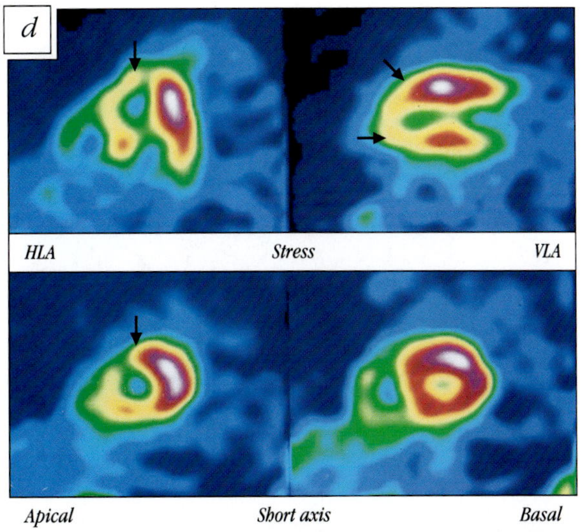

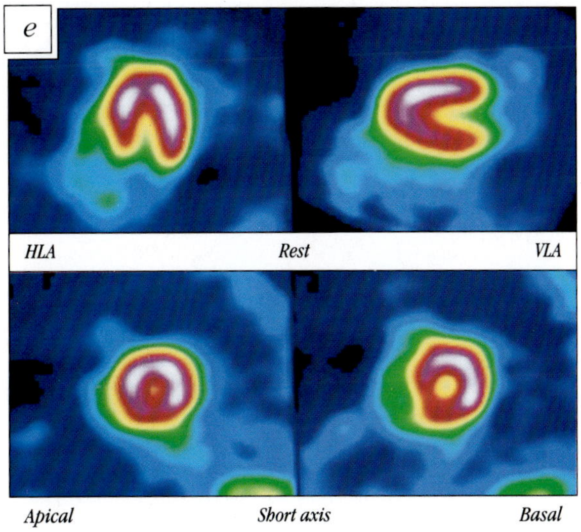

Case Study VII.4

Detection of restenosis and prevention of reocclusion with sestamibi tomography

This case concerns a 54-year-old male patient with angina pectoris of recent onset.

Scintigraphic evaluation 1 week later demonstrated anteroseptal reversible perfusion defects consistent with myocardial ischaemia (Figs. VII.4a,b, arrows).

Coronary angiography confirmed a severe stenosis in the LAD coronary artery before the origin of the diagonal branch; this was successfully dilated (Fig. VII.4c, arrow).

Three months later, the patient complained of atypical chest pain. He was re-evaluated at stress and tomography revealed recurrent perfusion abnormalities in the LAD territory indicative of restenosis (Figs. VII.4d,e, arrows) confirmed by angiography (Fig. VII.4f, arrow).

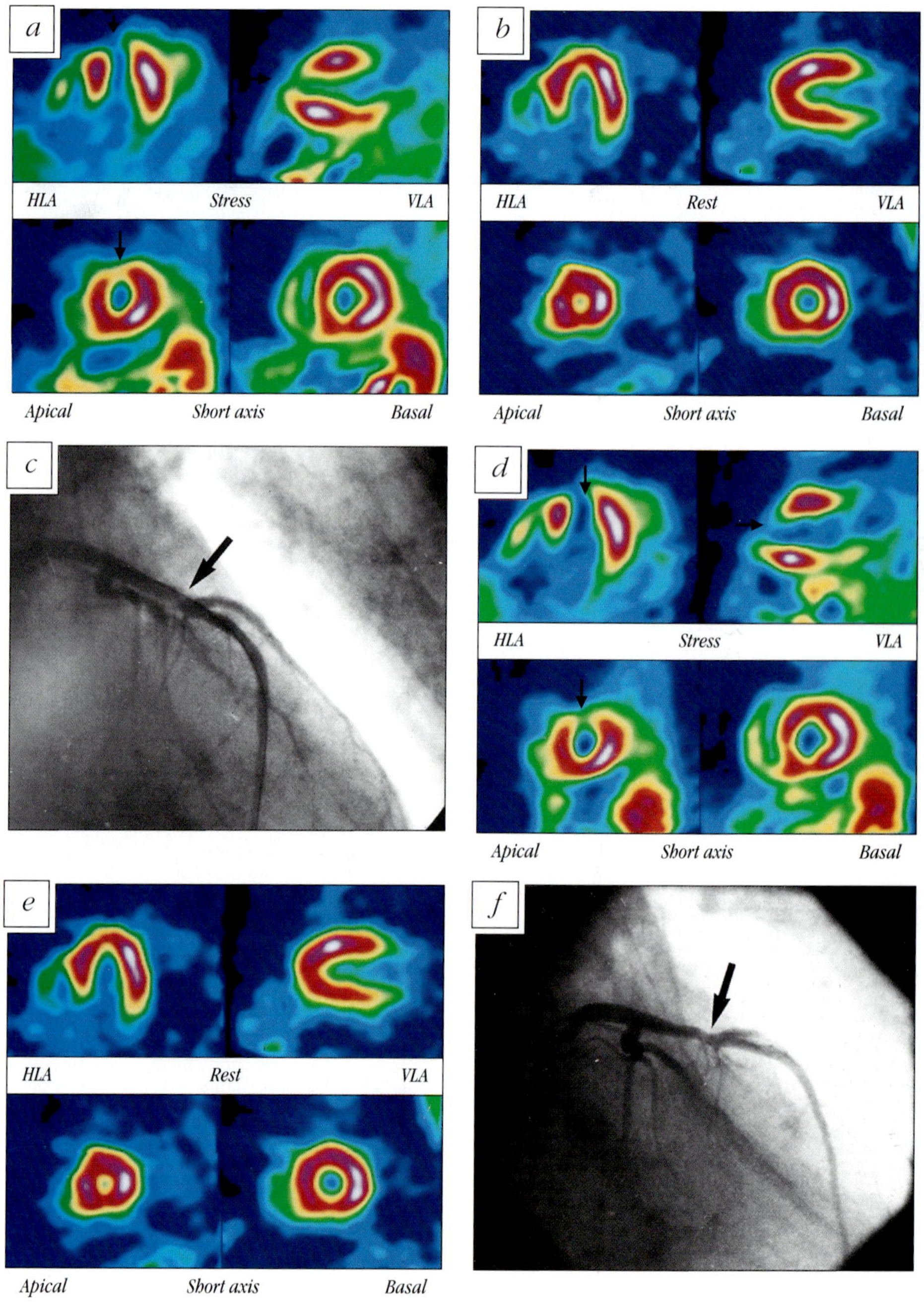

Case Study VII.5

Evaluation of restenosis and indication for a second dilatation

Mr TR (68 years old) was submitted in September 1991 to a coronary angioplasty for RCA disease.

The angiographic control performed after balloon dilatation indicated a good anatomical result (Figs. VII.5a,b, arrow). The patient was asymptomatic during the following weeks but the evaluation at stress realized 2 months later revealed a small perfusion defect in the inferoposterior wall on the vertical long axis (VLA) view (Fig. VII.5c, arrow).

The patient was maintained under modified medical therapy for 3 months until he complained of recurrent chest pain.

Tomography at stress demonstrated larger perfusion defects in the inferior and inferoposterior regions (Fig. VII.5d, arrows).

The patient was therefore re-evaluated by angiography and a repeated angioplasty was performed (Fig. VII.5e, arrow).

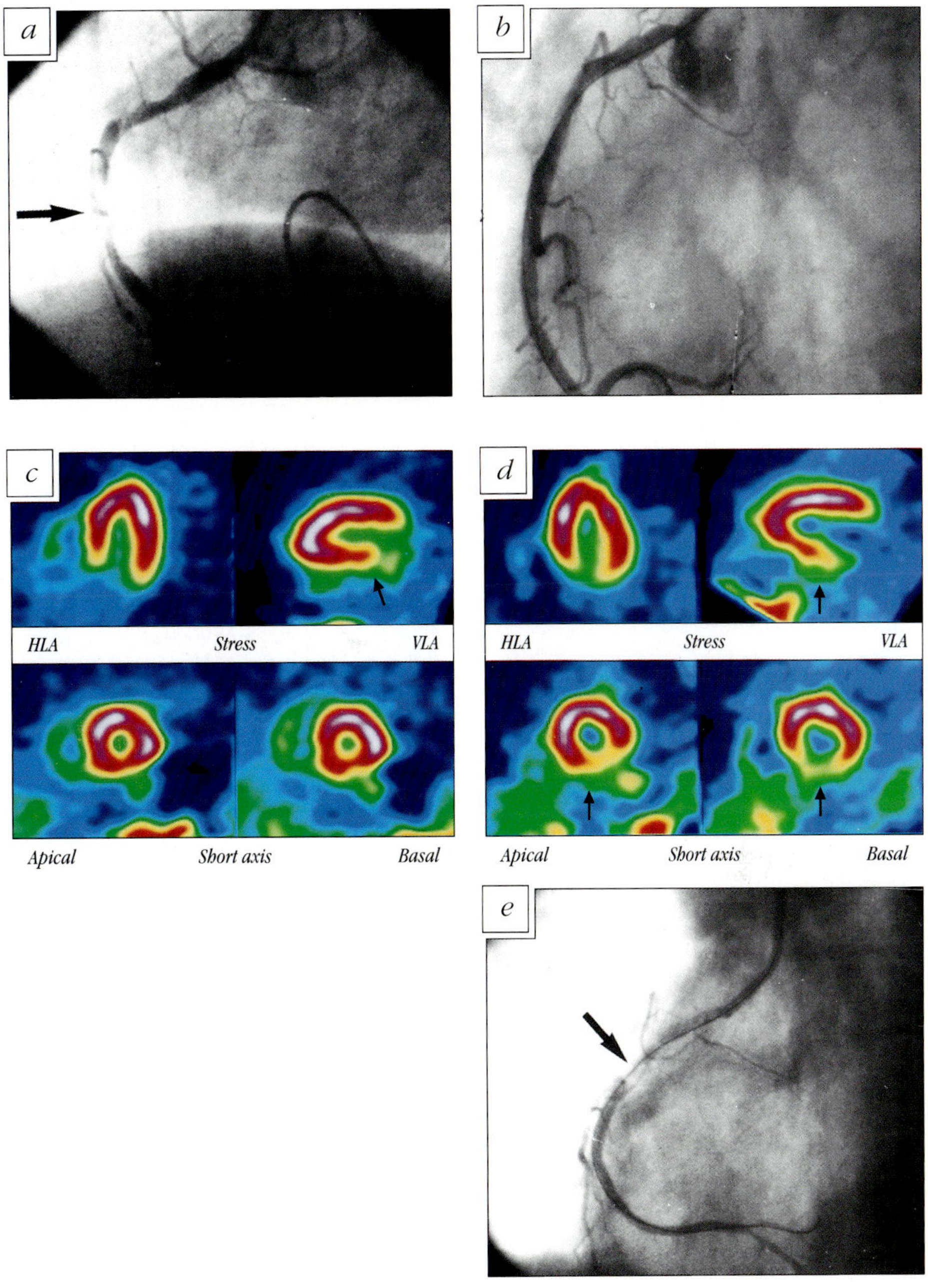

Case Study VII.6

Detection of progression of CAD in patients submitted for angioplasty

Mr KD, a 51-year-old man, complained 3 years ago of left precordial chest pain radiated to his back and to his throat and induced by physical exercise and mental stress.

As angiography and myocardial perfusion imaging demonstrated the presence of an RCA lesion inducing myocardial ischaemia, he was submitted for angioplasty which was successful (Figs. VII.6a,b,c, arrows).

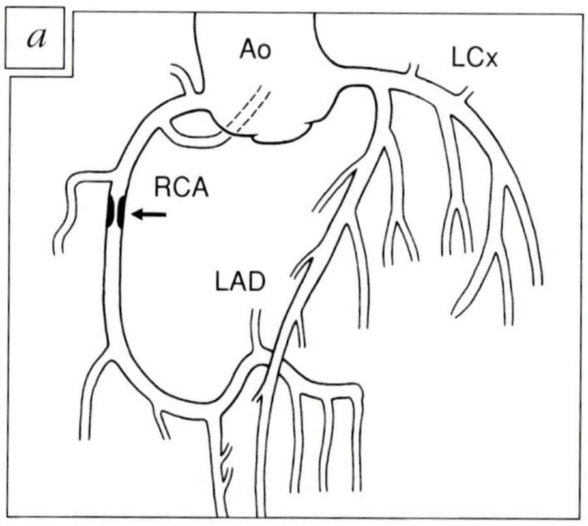

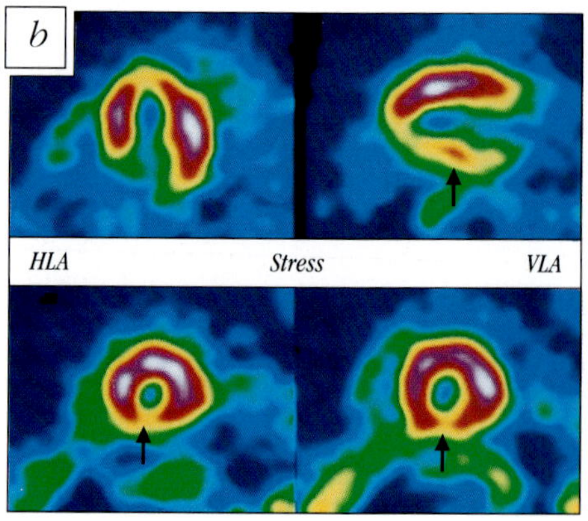

Apical Short axis Basal
Before PTCA

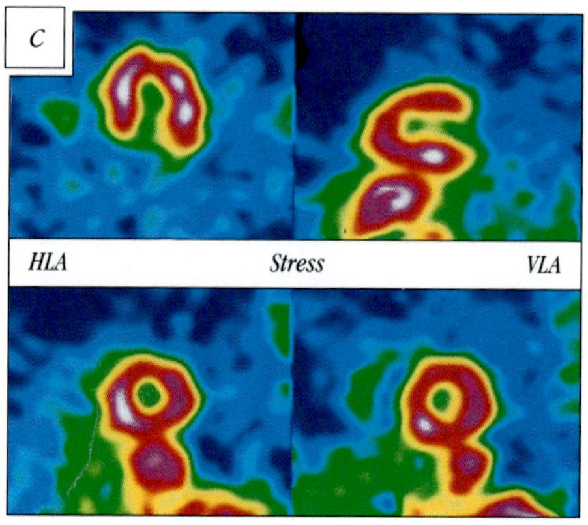

Apical Short axis Basal
After PTCA

He remained asymptomatic for 15 months, but then described recurrent anginal pain. The evaluation at stress revealed reversible perfusion abnormalities involving the inferoposterior and posterolateral walls of the LV, suggesting ischaemia in the left circumflex (LCx) territory (Figs. VII.6e,f, arrows).

Angiography confirmed the presence of an LCx stenosis, which was also treated successfully by angioplasty (Figs. VII.6g,h,i, arrow).

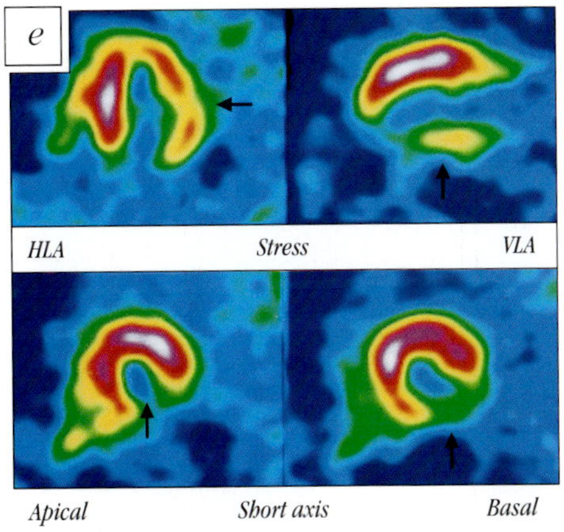

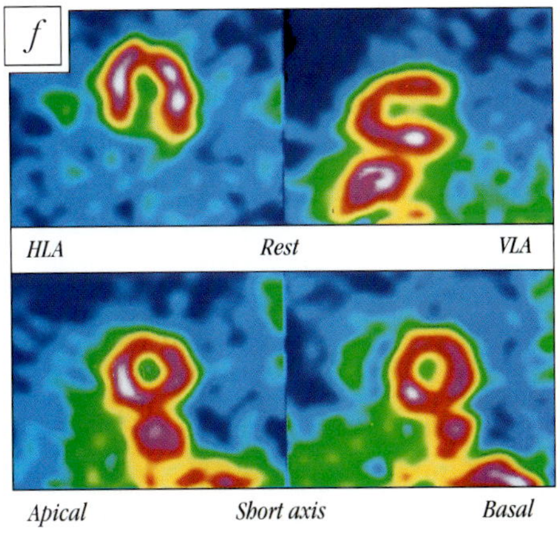

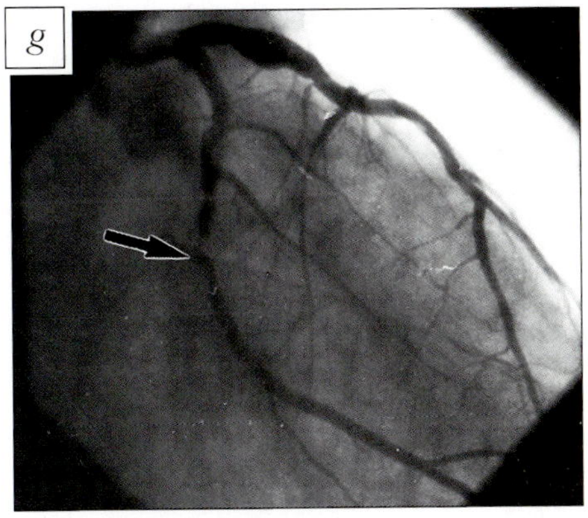

Before PTCA

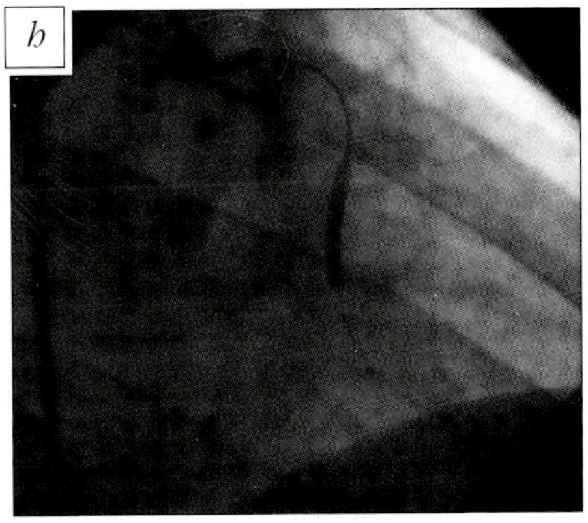

During PTCA

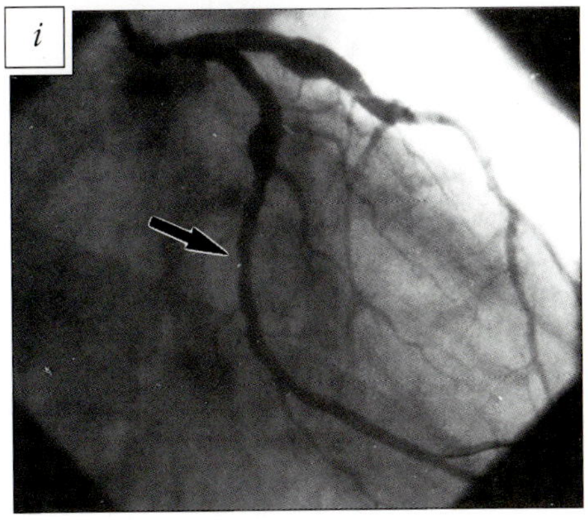

After PTCA

Case Study VII.7

Prognostic significance of early versus delayed scintigraphic controls after PTCA

Mr FCh, having cardiovascular risk factors, developed RCA stenosis which was treated by angioplasty.

His follow-up was uneventful. To assess the results of revascularization, sestamibi tomography was performed at stress 1 week later and demonstrated a small reversible perfusion defect in the inferoposterior and in the inferoseptal walls of the LV (Fig. VII.7a, arrows).

As this study was early, he was reevaluated 1 month later and this study showed normal myocardial uptake in the three orthogonal planes (Fig. VII.7b), indicating successful reperfusion in the RCA territory.

This example illustrates the occurrence of early scintigraphic abnormalities post-dilatation corresponding to remodelling of the arterial wall or to transient increased distal vascular tone with abnormal perfusion reserve.

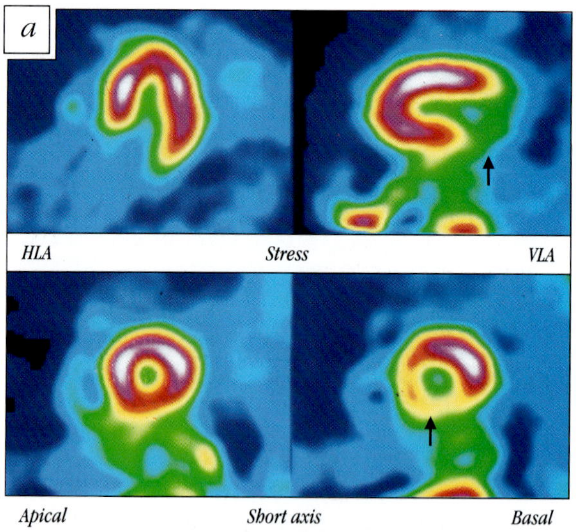

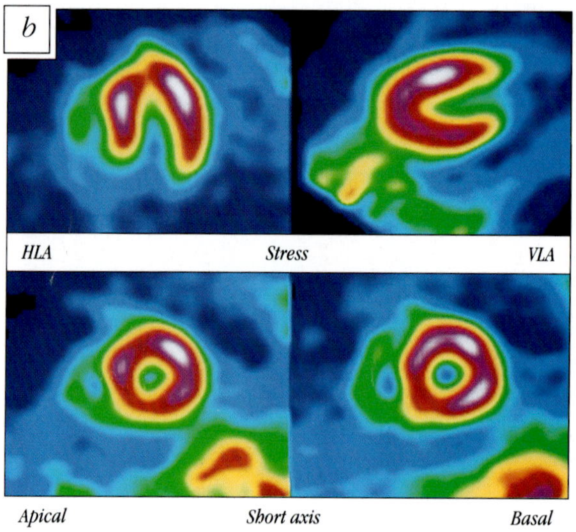

8 ASSESSMENT OF THE EFFECTIVENESS OF CORONARY ARTERY BYPASS GRAFT SURGERY

Clinical Background

Coronary artery bypass graft (CABG) surgery has for more than 20 years profoundly altered the fate of patients with coronary artery disease (CAD).[1] First performed primarily for symptomatic relief, it has been shown that CABG surgery can provide regional functional improvement at rest and more so during exercise, and can improve the prognosis. Patients with severe disease, such as left main stenosis or multiple vessel stenoses associated with an altered left ventricular function, have been shown to be the chief beneficiaries in terms of life expectancy.[2–4]

Optimal functional improvement is dependent upon complete revascularization and the absence of perioperative complications or postoperative reocclusion. To diminish the attrition rate of vein grafts and to perform more complete revascularization procedures, surgeons now extensively use arterial conduits such as the internal mammary arteries, or bypass several lesions using one graft and sequential anastomoses.[5] Using these techniques and antiaggregant therapy, the incidence of graft occlusion has been reduced from approximately 15–20% in the first year to less than 10%, or even as low as 5% for the internal mammary artery.[5–7] The incidence of perioperative complications, essentially perioperative myocardial infarction, has also diminished over the years. It now stands at approximately 5% but most infarcts are small. Although patients experiencing myocardial infarction have a higher perioperative mortality, no difference is observed in the 5-year survival rate.[8,9]

Although providing successful relief of coronary obstructions, bypass surgery does not alter the natural progression of the atherosclerotic disease and subsequent stenoses are likely to develop elsewhere. Furthermore, changes in the flow pattern resulting from bypass accelerate the progression of native vessel stenosis proximal to the point of anastomosis and complete obstruction of the native vessel frequently results from these situations of flow competition.

Clinical Problems

Less than optimal results from bypass surgery, whether persistence of anginal pain, lack of functional improvement or functional alterations, can result from a variety of causes often difficult to differentiate clinically.

Perioperative infarction

Diagnosis of perioperative infarction can be difficult as a result of the non-specific ECG changes and enzyme release consecutive to the intervention. It can be recognized early on using necrosis-specific tracers such as ^{99m}Tc pyrophosphate or ^{111}In-labelled antimyosin monoclonal antibodies.[10] Myocardial imaging at rest can recognize the presence of a new or of a larger perfusion defect in patients without previous myocardial infarction or in whom a preoperative scan is available for comparison. Myocardial perfusion imaging cannot, however, diagnose small perioperative infarcts.

Incomplete revascularization

Incomplete revascularization can be the result of an incomplete procedure for technical or other reasons, or can be due to the early obstruction of one of the grafts. Rest and stress perfusion imaging can document the site and extent of residual ischaemia and should be interpreted in the context of information about the preoperative angiographic results and details of the surgical procedure. Secondary obstruction of an initially patent graft can also lead to myocardial necrosis, especially if disease in the native coronary artery has progressed.[11] Progression of disease in non-grafted arteries will usually be the cause of later events.

Differentiation between these various complications cannot usually be done non-invasively unless one can, in favourable cases, rely on the full angiographic and operative reports as well as on preoperative, immediate postoperative and subsequent perfusion scans at the time of symptoms.[12] Although not routinely done in all institutions, serial imaging post-bypass surgery could be very helpful in complicated cases to assess the need for re-interventions despite the increased risk of redo procedures.

Prognostic Information

Valuable information about the patient's prognosis post-bypass can be provided by serial imaging. Measurements of both myocardial perfusion and left ventricular function have been shown to relate to prognosis in patients with CAD pre- and post-bypass surgery. The myocardial scintigraphy variables that provide the greatest prognostic information are those that reflect both the extent and severity of perfusion abnormalities and their functional correlates. Left ventricular ejection fraction at rest and especially after exercise, size of total perfusion defect at stress, presence and size of exercise-induced reversible perfusion defect indicating the presence of residual myocardial ischaemia post-bypass – all these carry important prognostic information.[13–16] A degree of redundancy of information is assured by the demonstrated correlation between perfusion and function, yet additive information might be expected from the simultaneous evaluation of these parameters considering the occasional discrepancies between the extent of perfusion and the functional abnormalities observed in individual patients. In these patients it is therefore advisable to combine first-pass or gated wall motion functional information with information gained from perfusion analysis using sestamibi.[17]

Aims of the Sestamibi Studies

Initial exercise myocardial imaging in clinically uncomplicated bypass cases are indicated 1–2 months after the procedure to document the absence of perioperative infarction and the functional results of the procedure. Availability of a preoperative scan is most useful for this purpose, especially in patients with previous myocardial infarction. Absence of residual ischaemia is evidence of a functionally complete revascularization and implies a good result and a good prognosis. Evidence for a new myocardial infarction or for residual ischaemia indicates the occurrence of complications or of an incomplete revascularization. The degree of impairment determines the prognosis.

This early scan can serve as the basis for follow-up to assess the occurrence of later complications (bypass occlusion) or of disease progression.

Conclusions

Myocardial imaging post-bypass is useful in assessing the functional results of surgery. Comparison with preoperative data or with early postoperative scan is preferred to differentiate pre- or perioperative abnormalities from later complications. The strength of the test is the elimination of ischaemia suggestive of patent graft, while demonstration of new abnormalities cannot always differentiate between complications and progression of the disease in the native vessels.

Clinical Points

- Monitoring CABG surgery implies detecting perioperative myocardial infarction, graft occlusion and the ischaemic consequences of incomplete revascularization or disease progression.
- Perioperative infarction is best recognized acutely using ^{99m}Tc pyrophosphate or ^{111}In antimyosin.
- Functional improvement is usually associated with perfusion scans demonstrating the absence of residual ischaemia.
- Availability of a preoperative scan is often necessary to differentiate among the various possible complications.
- Prognosis after bypass surgery remains closely related to the level of left ventricular function.

References

1 CASS PRINCIPAL INVESTIGATORS AND ASSOCIATES, CORONARY ARTERY SURGERY STUDY (CASS), A randomized trial of coronary artery bypass surgery. Survival data, *Circulation* (1983) **68**:939.

2 PASSAMANI E, DAVIS KB, GILLESPIE MJ et al, A randomized trial of coronary artery bypass surgery. Survival of patients with a low ejection fraction, *N Engl J Med* (1985) **312**:1665.

3 KRONENBERG MW, PEDERSON RW, HARSTON WE et al, Left ventricular performance after coronary artery bypass surgery, *Ann Intern Med* (1983) **99**:305.

4 DILZIZIAN V, BONOW RO, CANNON RO et al, The effect of coronary artery bypass grafting on left ventricular systolic function at rest: evidence for preoperative subclinical myocardial ischemia, *Am J Cardiol* (1988) **61**:1248.

5 LOOP FD, LYTLE DW, COSGROVE DM et al, Influence of the internal mammary artery graft on 10 year survival and other cardiac events, *N Engl J Med* (1986) **314**:1.

6 LIMET R, DAVID JL, MAGOTTEAUX P et al, Prevention of aortocoronary bypass occlusion. Beneficial effect of Ticlopidine on one year patency rate of coronary bypass grafts: a double-blind study, *J Thor Cardiovasc Surg* (1987) **94**:773.

7 CHESEBRO JH, FUSTER V, ELVEBACH LR et al, Effect of dipyridamole and aspirin on late vein graft patency after coronary bypass operation, *N Engl J Med* (1984) **310**:209.

8 GRAY RJ, MATLOFF JM, CONKLIN CM et al, Perioperative myocardial infarction: late clinical course after coronary artery bypass surgery, *Circulation* (1982) **66**:1185.

9 BURDINE JA, DEPUEY EG, ORZAN F et al, Scintigraphic, electrocardiographic, and enzymatic diagnosis of perioperative myocardial infarction in patients undergoing myocardial revascularization, *J Nucl Med* (1979) **20**:711.

10 Braat SH, de Zwaan C, Teule J et al, Value of Indium 111 monoclonal antimyosin antibody for imaging in acute myocardial infarction, *Am J Cardiol* (1987) **60**:725.

11 Campeau L, Enjalbert M, Lesperance J et al, The relation of risk factors to the development of atherosclerosis in saphenous vein bypass grafts and the progression of disease in the native circulation. A study 10 years after aortocoronary bypass surgery, *N Engl J Med* (1984) **311**:1329.

12 Pfisterer M, Emmenegger H, Schmitt HE et al, Accuracy of serial myocardial perfusion scintigraphy with thallium-201 for prediction of graft patency early and late after coronary artery bypass surgery: a controlled prospective study, *Circulation* (1982) **66**:1017.

13 Bates ER, Aueron FM, Legrand V et al, Comparative long term effects of coronary artery bypass graft surgery and percutaneous transluminal coronary angioplasty on regional coronary flow reserve, *Circulation* (1985) **72**:833.

14 Frick MH, Valle M, Harjola PT, Progression of coronary artery disease in randomized medical and surgical patients over a 5 year angiographic follow up, *Am J Cardiol* (1983) **52**:681.

15 Jones RA, Floyd RD, Austin EH et al, The role of radionuclide angiography in the preoperative prediction of pain relief and prolonged survival following coronary bypass grafting, *Ann Surg* (1983) **197**:743.

16 Wilson RF, White CW, Does coronary artery bypass surgery restore normal maximal coronary flow reserve? *Circulation* (1987) **76**:563.

17 Jones RH, Borges-Neto S, Potts JM, Simultaneous measurement of myocardial perfusion and ventricular function during exercise from a single injection of technetium 99m sestamibi in coronary artery disease, *Am J Cardiol* (1990) **66**:68E.

Case Study VIII.1

Successful revascularization associated with improvement of left ventricular function in a patient with multiple vessel disease

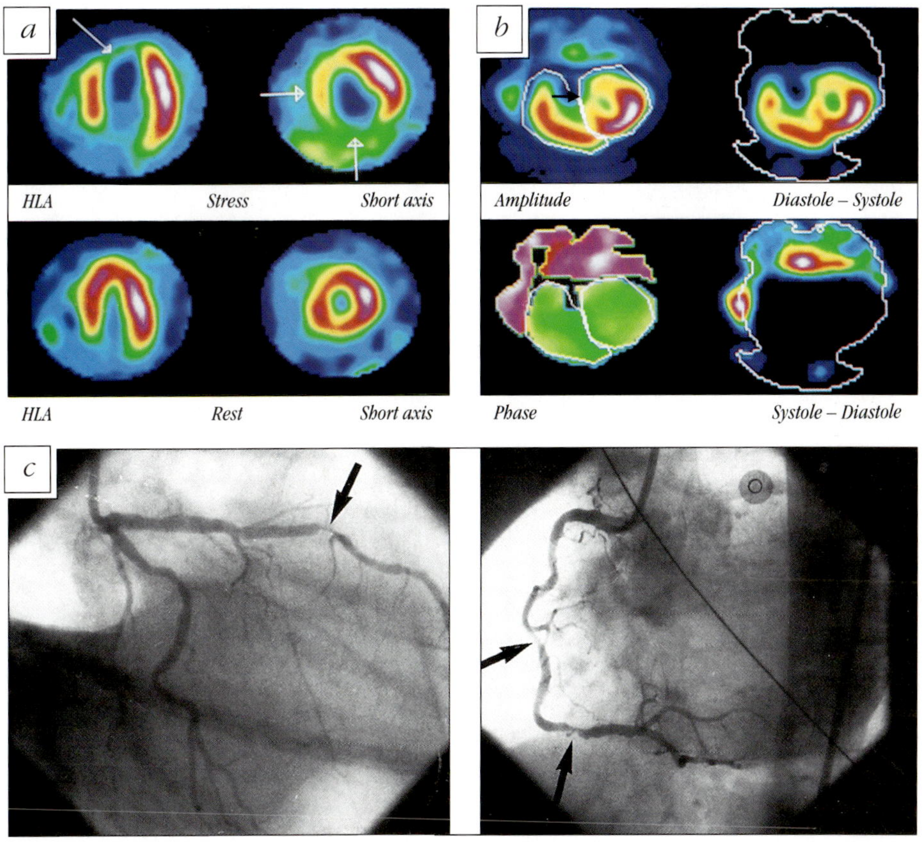

In September 1990 this patient visited the out-patient clinic with typical chest pain, as well as dyspnoea and fatigue induced by exercise.

He exercised on a bicycle for 5 min up to a load of 90 W and his heart rate increased from 85 to 130 beats/min. He stopped because of dyspnoea and pain while significant ECG changes were present.

The tomographic sestamibi stress study showed ventricular dilatation and sestamibi defects in the anteroseptal and the inferior walls of the LV suggesting multiple vessel disease (Fig. VIII.1a, upper panel, arrows).

Equilibrium radionuclide ventriculography at rest revealed a moderately decreased ejection fraction (48%) and an abnormal filling rate. Mild hypokinesia of the septum was also apparent on the amplitude image (Fig. VIII.1b, arrow).

The patient underwent bypass of the left anterior descending (LAD) and right coronary (RCA) arteries (Fig. VIII.1c).

Radionuclide ventriculography at rest 3 months later showed a normalization of the left ventricular ejection fraction (60%), while sestamibi demonstrated a normal perfusion pattern (Fig. VIII.1d).

In this case, the combined analysis of perfusion and function illustrates successful revascularization with improvement of left ventricular function.

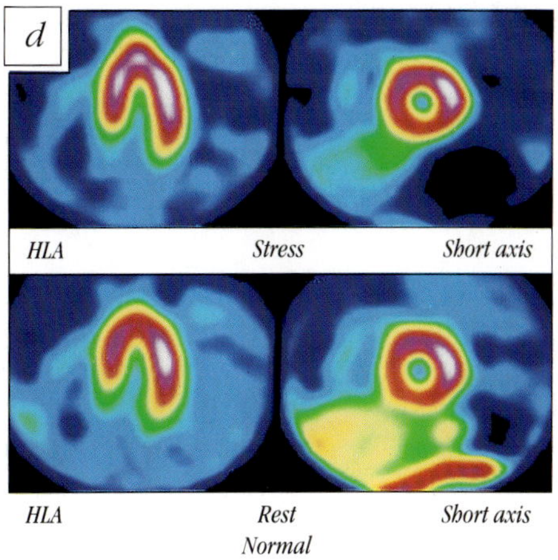

Case Study VIII.2

Incomplete revascularization after CABG in a patient with previous myocardial infarction

Mr B suffered an inferior myocardial infarction in 1989. He remained asymptomatic for 10 months. In November 1990 he began to complain of typical exercise chest pain, relieved by rest.

The resting ECG showed the presence of an inferoposterior myocardial infarction (Fig. VIII.2a).

Rest and stress tomography demonstrated the presence of sestamibi defects in the inferior wall of the LV accentuated during exercise, and sestamibi defects at stress only in the anterolateral, lateral and apical walls of the LV (Figs. VIII.2b,c, arrows).

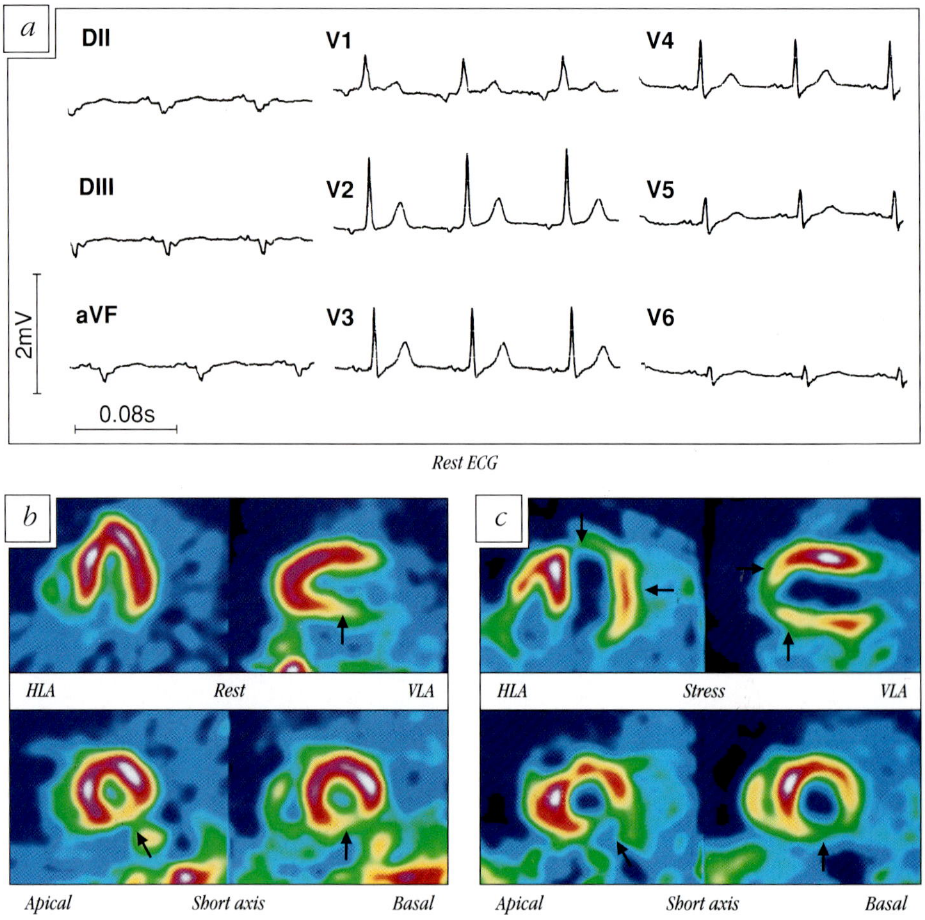

The angiogram confirmed the presence of an RCA occlusion corresponding to the previous myocardial infarction and also the presence of significant lesions on the LCx and the LAD coronary arteries (Fig. VIII.2d, arrows). The patient was referred for bypass surgery.

Six weeks later scintigraphic evaluation of the results at rest and at stress demonstrate improvement of the perfusion in the postlateral wall. However, there were still signs of residual ischaemia in this area, suggesting incomplete revascularization (Figs VIII. 2e,f, arrows).

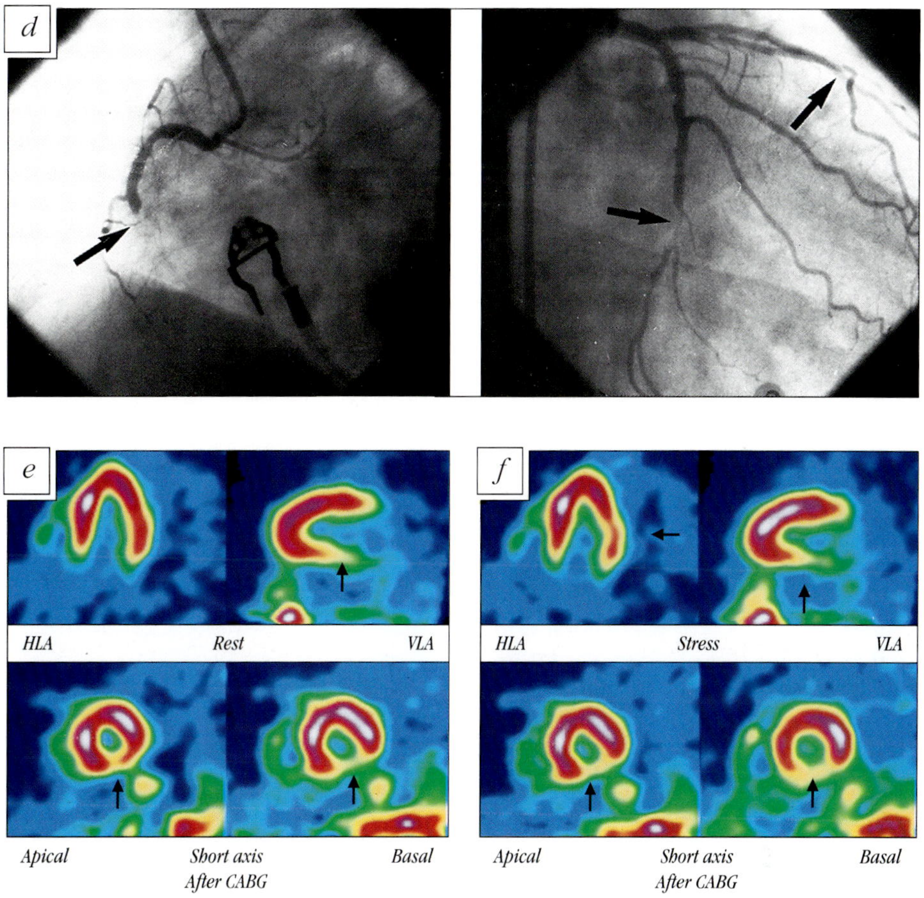

Case Study VIII.3

Successful myocardial reperfusion after coronary artery bypass grafting

Mr A was referred to the cardiology department for left precordial chest pain radiated to his throat and his left arm, induced by stress and by walking quickly.

The ECG performed at stress showed widening of the QRS complex at a workload of 120 W, associated with typical chest pain. Ischaemic abnormalities were present during recovery (Fig. VIII.3a).

Sestamibi tomography at stress demonstrated severe perfusion abnormalities involving the anterolateral, the lateral and the inferior walls of the LV, as well as important left ventricular dilatation (Fig. VIII.3b, arrows; upper panel).

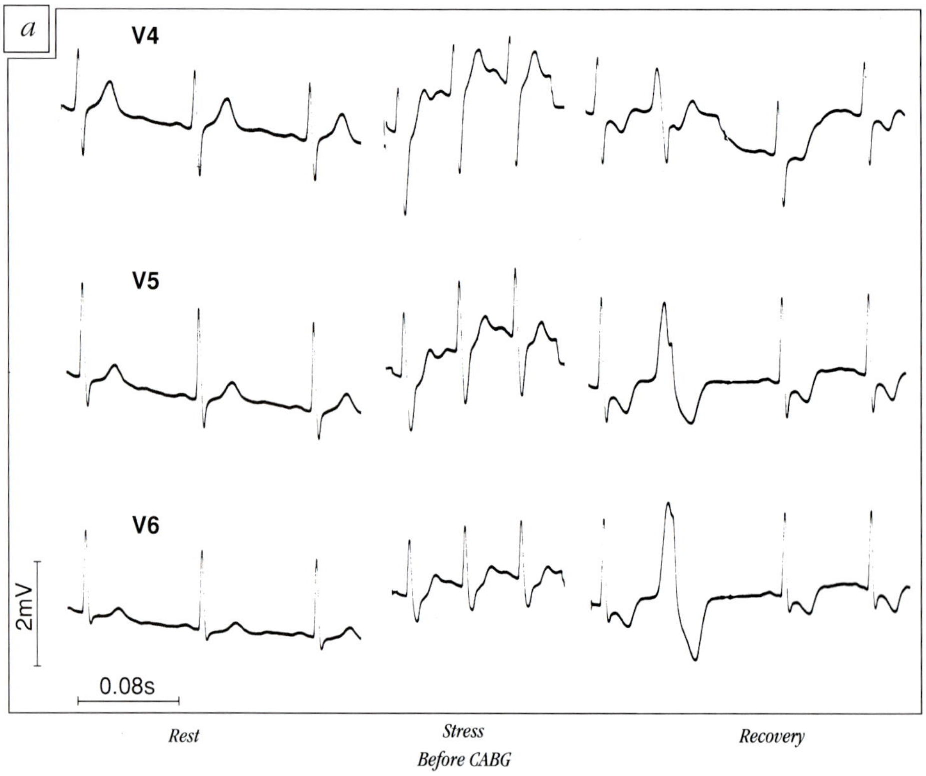

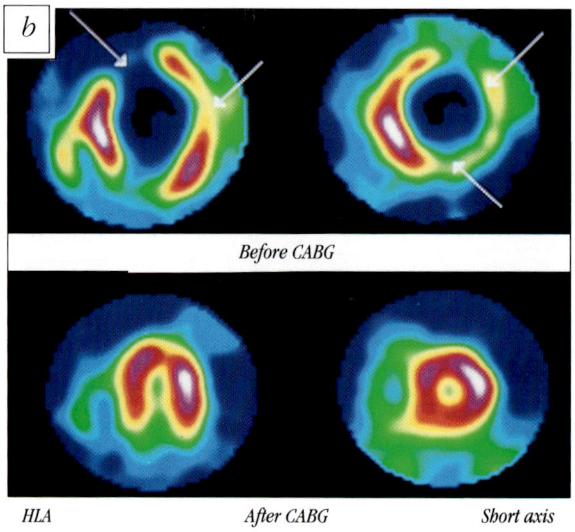

The diagnostic coronary angiogram confirmed the presence of significant stenoses in the proximal LAD, the left circumflex (LCx) arteries and the RCA arteries (Fig. VIII.3c, arrows).

Scintigraphic control performed at stress 2 months after CABG demonstrated successful revascularization (Fig. VIII.3b, lower panel). The ECG stress test was normalized (Fig. VIII.3d).

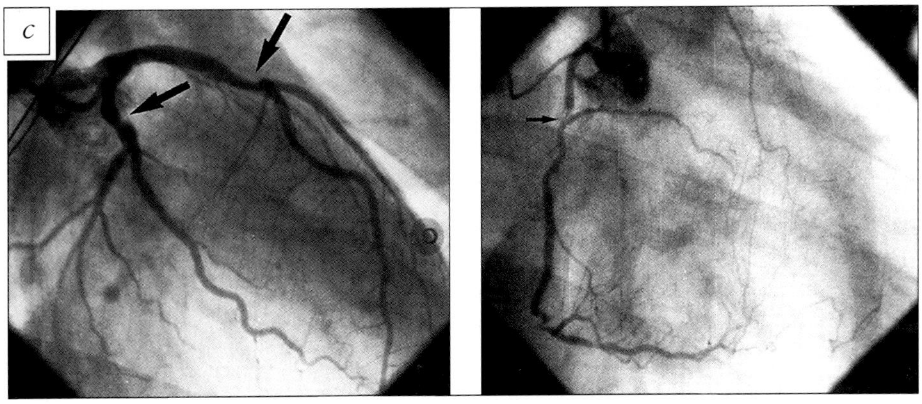

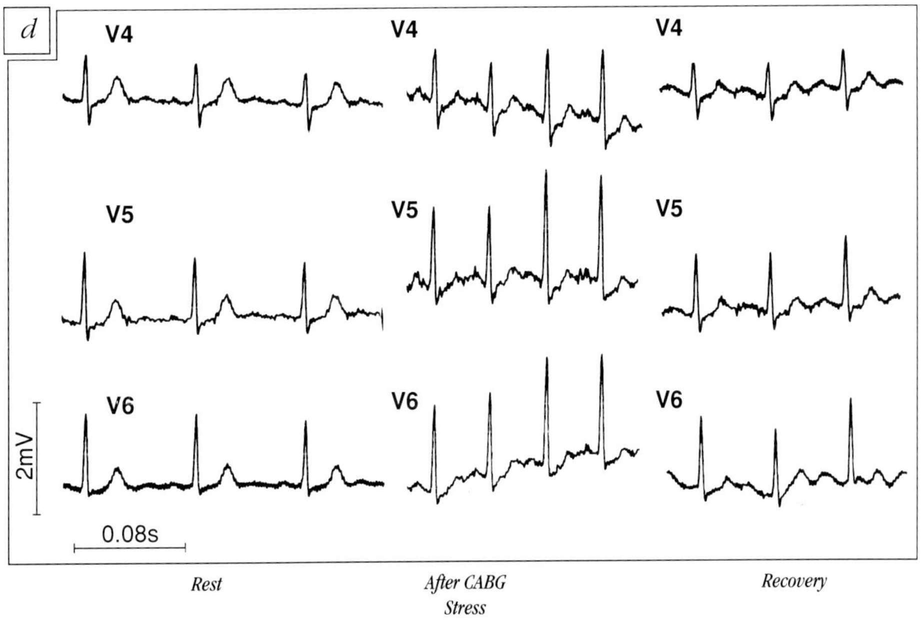

Case Study VIII.4

Perioperative myocardial infarction in a patient with a normal resting perfusion pattern before CABG

This patient underwent bypass surgery for triple vessel disease. The distal segment of the RCA was suboccluded (Fig. VIII.4a, arrow). The ECG at rest was normal (Fig. VIII.4b) and sestamibi at rest showed a normal perfusion pattern (Fig. VIII.4c, upper panel).

To allow bypass grafting of the distal RCA, the surgeon performed thromboendarterectomy on this artery. After the operation, the patient developed ST–T wave abnormalities in the inferior leads (Fig. VIII.4b) and a rise of the CK–MB isoenzyme serum level was noted.

Sestamibi tomography performed at rest before discharge revealed the presence of defects in the inferior wall of the LV (Fig. VIII.4c, lower panel, arrow) corresponding to the perioperative infarct.

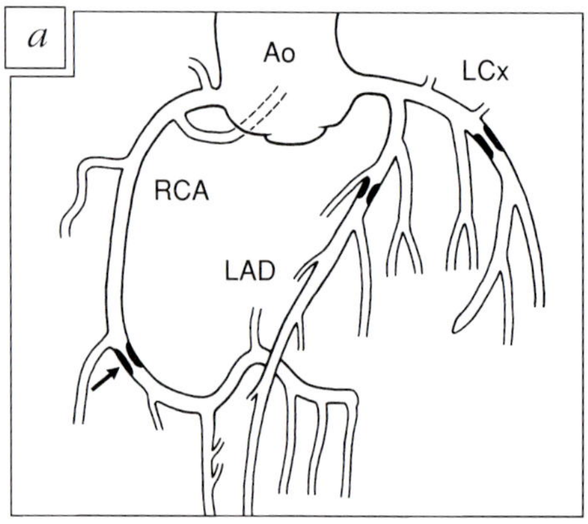

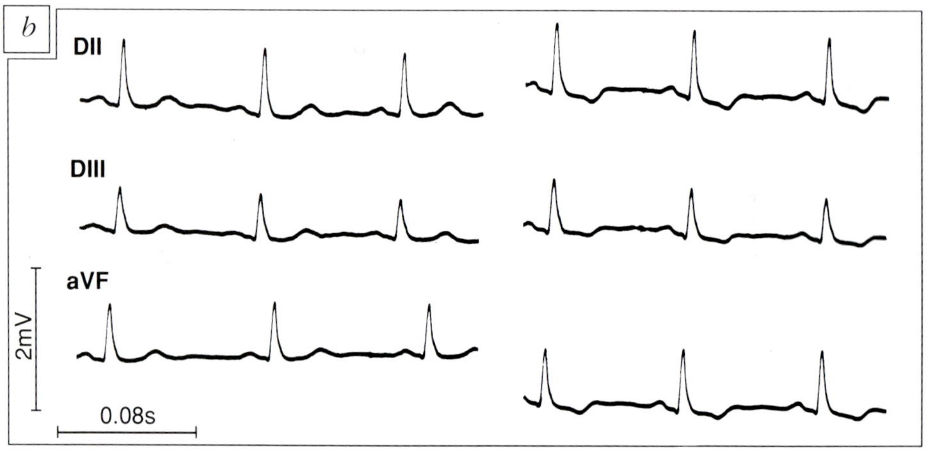

Before CABG *Rest* *After CABG*

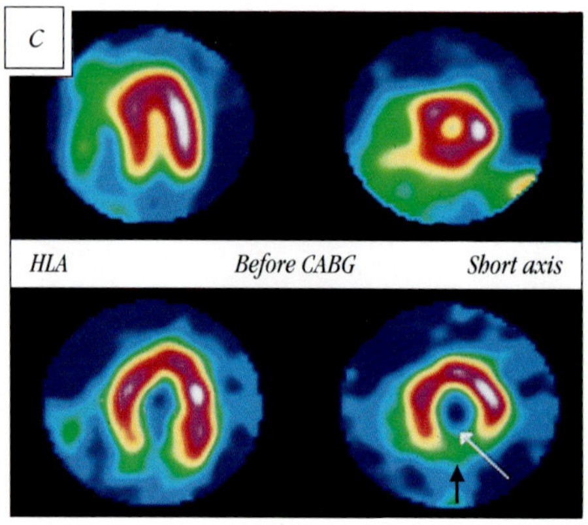

HLA *After CABG Rest* *Short axis*

Case Study VIII.5

Perioperative myocardial infarction in a patient with previous myocardial scar

The patient is a 55-year-old man who developed an inferior myocardial infarction 2 years ago treated by thrombolysis. The angiogram performed at that time revealed the persistence of a significant residual stenosis in the RCA, which was successfully dilated. The patient remained asymptomatic for 20 months. In July 1991, he complained again of typical angina. A second coronary angiogram demonstrated coronary lesions in the LAD and in the RCA (Fig. VIII.5a, arrows).

The patient underwent double bypass surgery. The CK–MB isoenzyme level rose significantly but the ECG showed only a slight axis shift as compared to those realized before surgery.

Comparison of the rest sestamibi planar scintigraphy before and after CABG showed a much larger defect in the inferior and inferoposterior area, demonstrating the extension of the inferior myocardial infarction (Fig. VIII.5b, arrow; Fig. VIII.5c, arrows).

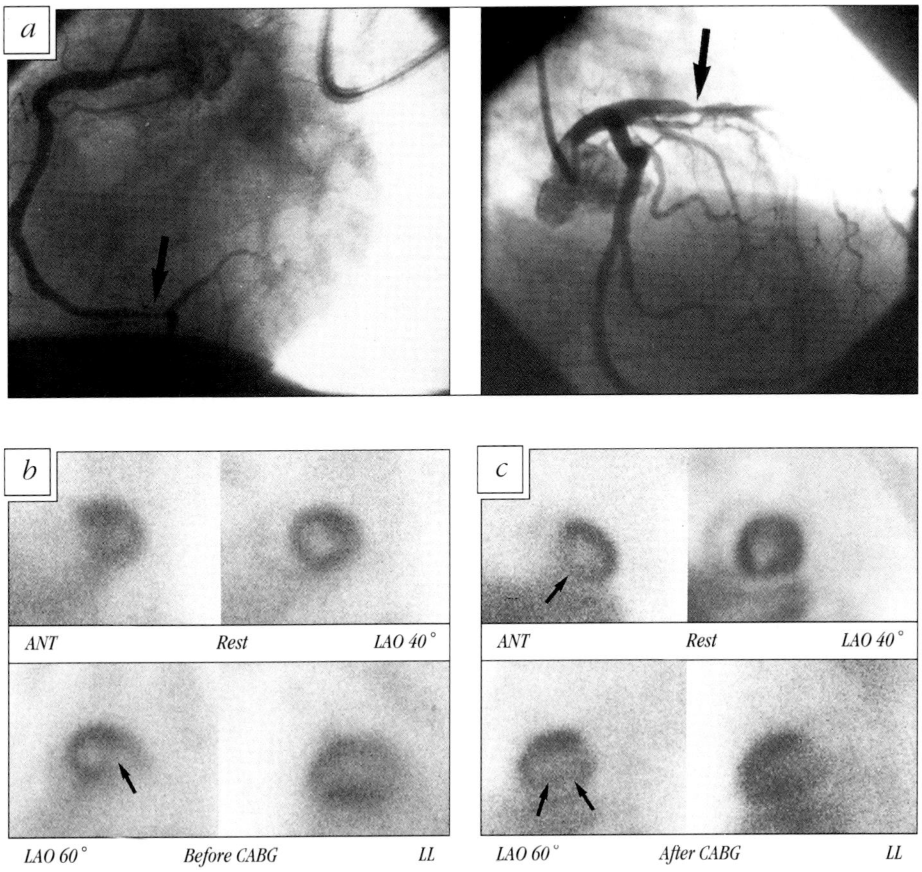

Case Study VIII.6

Graft stenosis with recurrent angina pectoris

This patient was referred to the cardiology department for angina pectoris. The exercise test showed marked ST–T segment changes in the precordial leads.

Stress tomography demonstrated extensive perfusion abnormalities in the lateral, inferoposterior and inferior walls of the LV associated with ventricular dilatation (Fig. VIII.6a, arrows).

Coronary angiography showed the presence of significant stenoses in the LCx and RCA requiring bypass surgery (Fig. VIII.6b).

Six months later, the patient developed a recurrence of chest pain. Sestamibi tomography again showed defects in the lateral wall of the LV (Fig. VIII.6c, arrows) suggesting recurrent myocardial ischaemia in the LCx vessel territory.

The angiographic control demonstrated the presence of stenosis in the LCx graft while the RCA graft remained patent (Fig. VIII.6d, arrows).

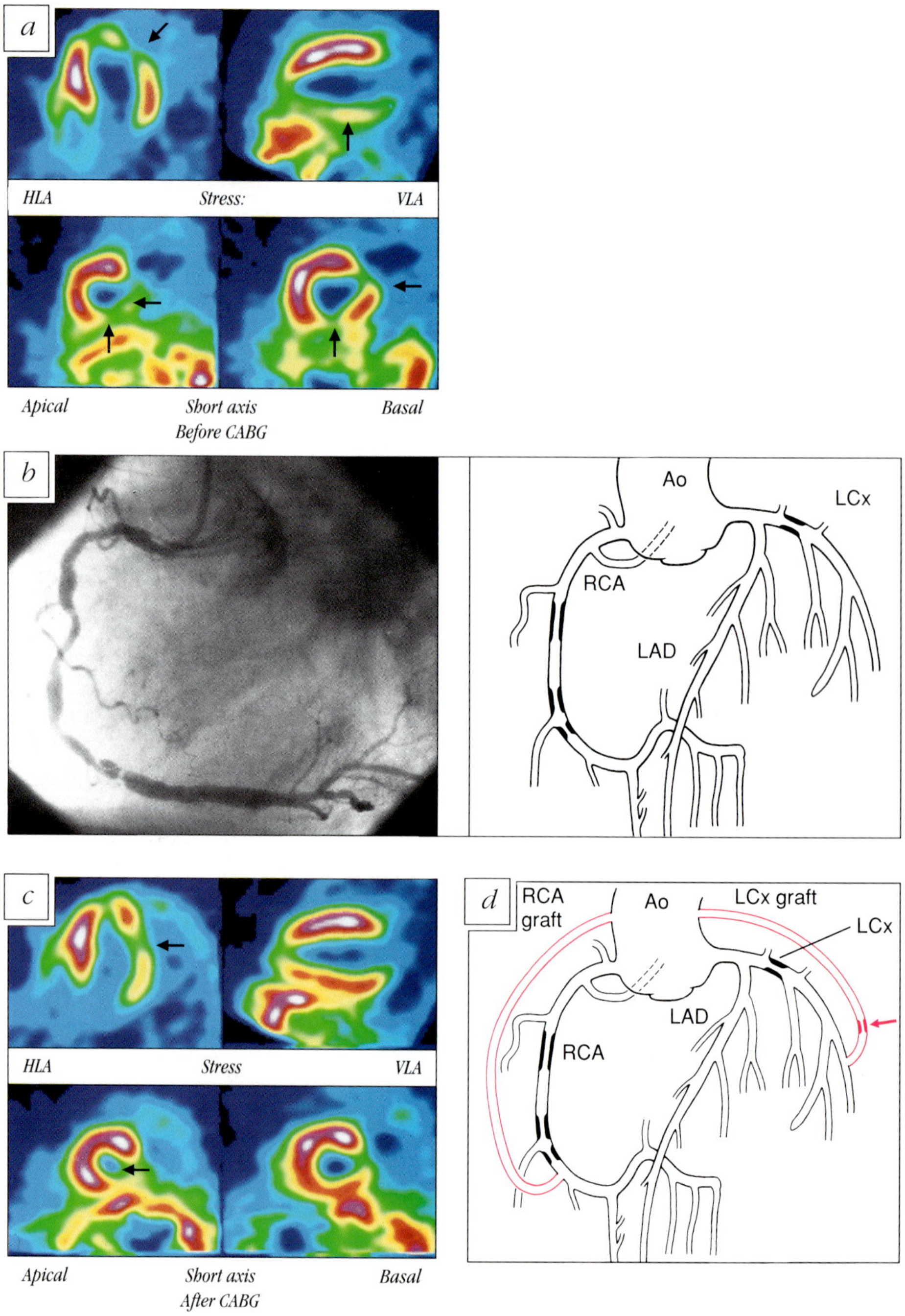

Case Study VIII.7

Incomplete revascularization after CABG

This case concerns a 51-year-old patient who underwent recent bypass surgery for double vessel disease.

His tomographic study performed at stress before CABG indicated perfusion abnormalities in the anteroseptal, inferoposterior and inferior walls of the LV corresponding to myocardial ischaemia in the LAD and in the RCA vessel territories (Fig. VIII.7a, arrows).

Coronary angiography realized 1 week later confirmed the presence of coronary lesions located in the LAD after the diagonal branch and in the distal segment of the RCA (Fig. VIII.7b, arrows).

The distal RCA lesion could not be bypassed, however, for technical reasons and the surgeon performed bypass only in the LAD coronary artery.

Tomographic evaluation at stress 6 weeks after CABG demonstrated reperfusion in the LAD vessel territory, but incomplete reperfusion of the territory corresponding to the distal RCA lesion (Fig. VIII.7c, arrows).

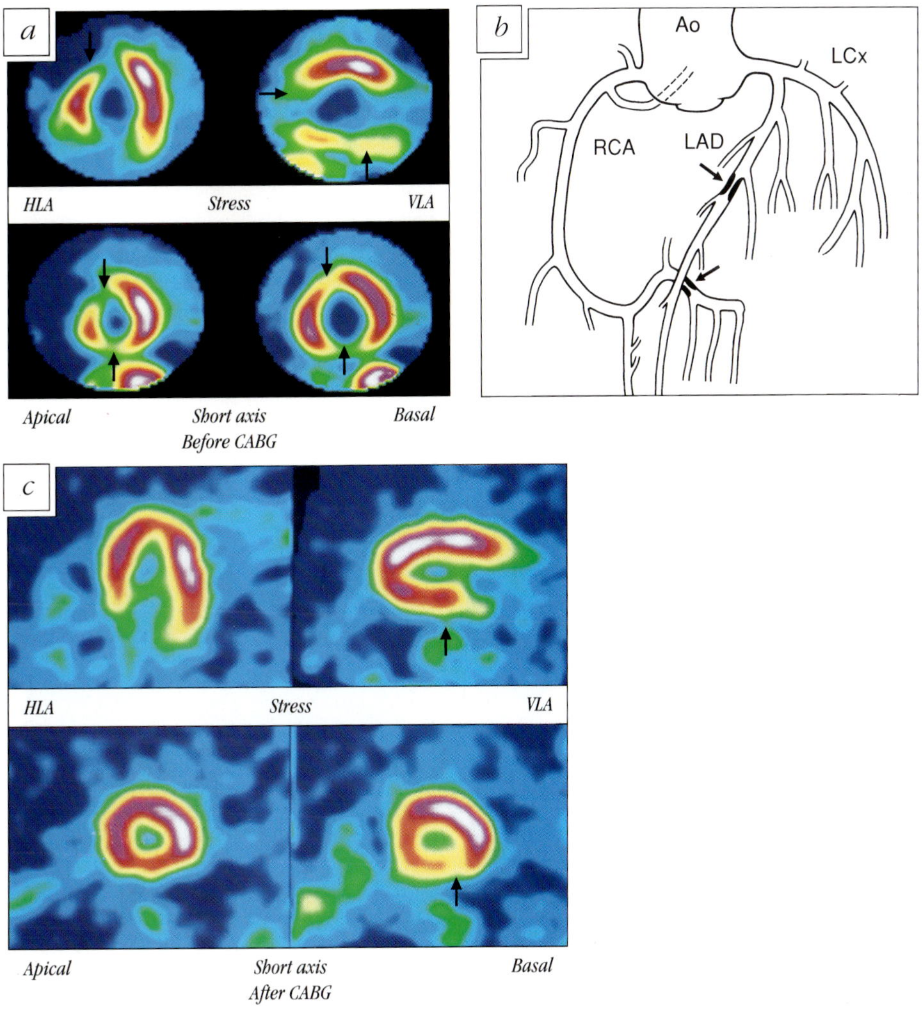

Case Study VIII.8

Progression of CAD

Mr AM, 61 years old, underwent 4 years ago a double coronary bypass on his LAD and RCA arteries.

The scintigraphic evaluation performed at stress with sestamibi showed severe defects in the anteroseptal and in the inferoposterior walls of the LV corresponding to myocardial ischaemia in the LAD and in the RCA vessel territories (Fig. VIII.8a, arrows).

These results were confirmed by coronary angiography (Fig. VIII.8b) and the patient was referred for CABG. A graft was placed on the LAD and another on the RCA.

A scintigraphic control 3 months after surgery demonstrated successful revascularization (Fig. VIII.8c).

The patient remained asymptomatic for 3 years, but in November 1991 he complained again of angina pectoris.

Tomography showed stress perfusion abnormalities in the lateral wall of the LV while the perfusion pattern was normal in the LAD and RCA vessel territories (Fig. VIII.8d, arrows).

The angiogram demonstrated graft patency of the LAD and RCA (Fig. VIII.e, arrows), but significant stenosis on the LCx coronary artery, as suggested by tomography, which was treated successfully by percutaneous transluminal coronary angioplasty (PTCA).

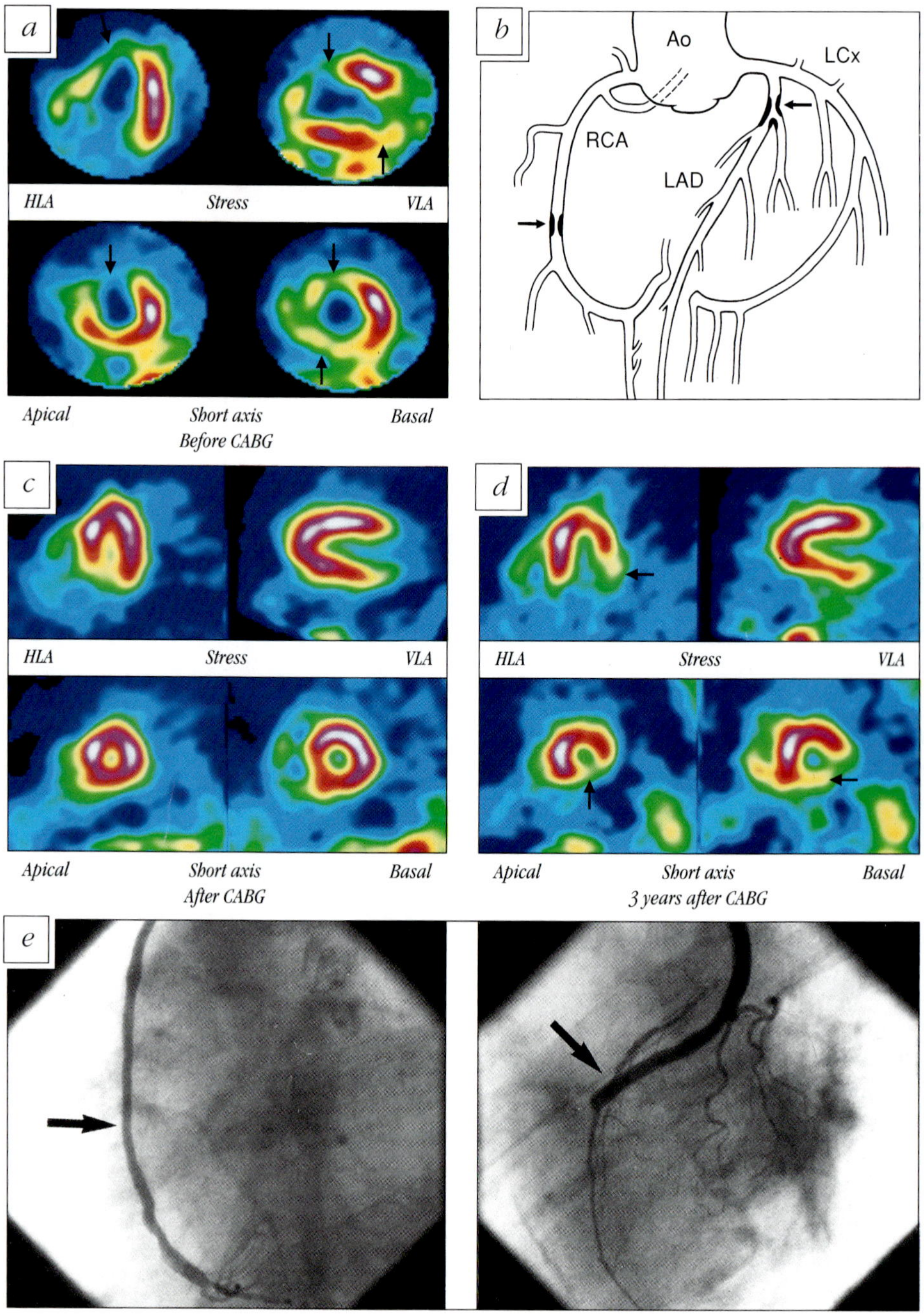

Case Study VIII.9

Late closure of bypass grafts requiring a redo operation

In 1990 this patient developed severe precordial chest pain which radiated to his left arm when he was walking and when he became anxious. The pain sometimes occurred even at rest. He was immediately referred to the cardiology department for further investigations.

The patient exercised on a bicycle and reached a load of 90 W. The pulse rose from 82 to 150 beats/min and his blood pressure from 150/95 to 190/100 mmHg. The stress ECG showed ST changes in leads V4, V5 and V6.

Sestamibi tomography demonstrated severe hypofixation in the lateral, in the anterior and in the inferior walls of the LV suggesting triple vessel disease (Fig. VIII.9a, arrows).

Coronary angiography confirmed these results (Fig. VIII.9b, arrows) and the patient underwent CABG.

The results seemed successful because the scintigraphic control performed 2 months after surgery showed a normal perfusion pattern at stress (Fig. VIII.9c).

Unfortunately, 10 months after the operation, the patient described recurrent angina pectoris. The scintigraphic control demonstrated myocardial ischaemia in the LCx and RCA vessel territories and the angiogram showed an occlusion of the LCx and RCA bypasses requiring the operation to be done again (Figs. VIII.9d,e, arrows).

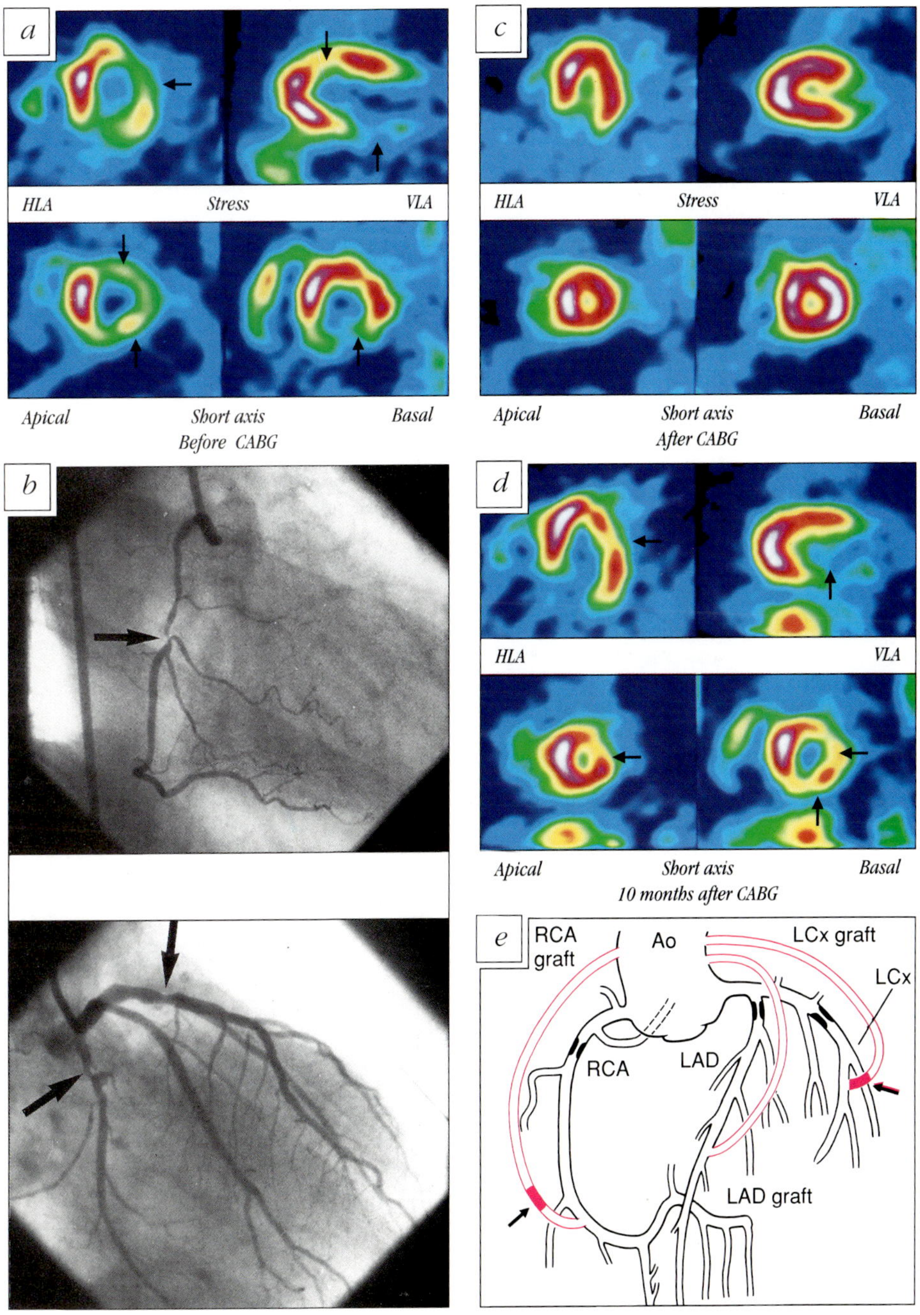

Case Study VIII.10

Indication of CABG in presence of unsuccessful angioplasty

This case study concerns a 54-year-old man who presented in September 1990 with unstable angina pectoris and ECG signs of ischaemia in leads V3, V4, V5 and V6. Sestamibi was injected at rest and tomography acquired 1 h later showed defects in the anteroseptal and inferoseptal walls of the LV (Fig. VIII.10a, arrows).

The angiogram performed the same day demonstrated the presence of 60% stenosis of the RCA and 90% stenosis of the LAD located after the origin of the diagonal branch (Fig. VIII.10b).

PTCA performed on the LAD coronary artery reduced the stenosis from 90% to 30%. Good anatomical and functional results were achieved and myocardial imaging returned to a normal perfusion pattern at stress (Figs. VIII.10b, lower right panel; c).

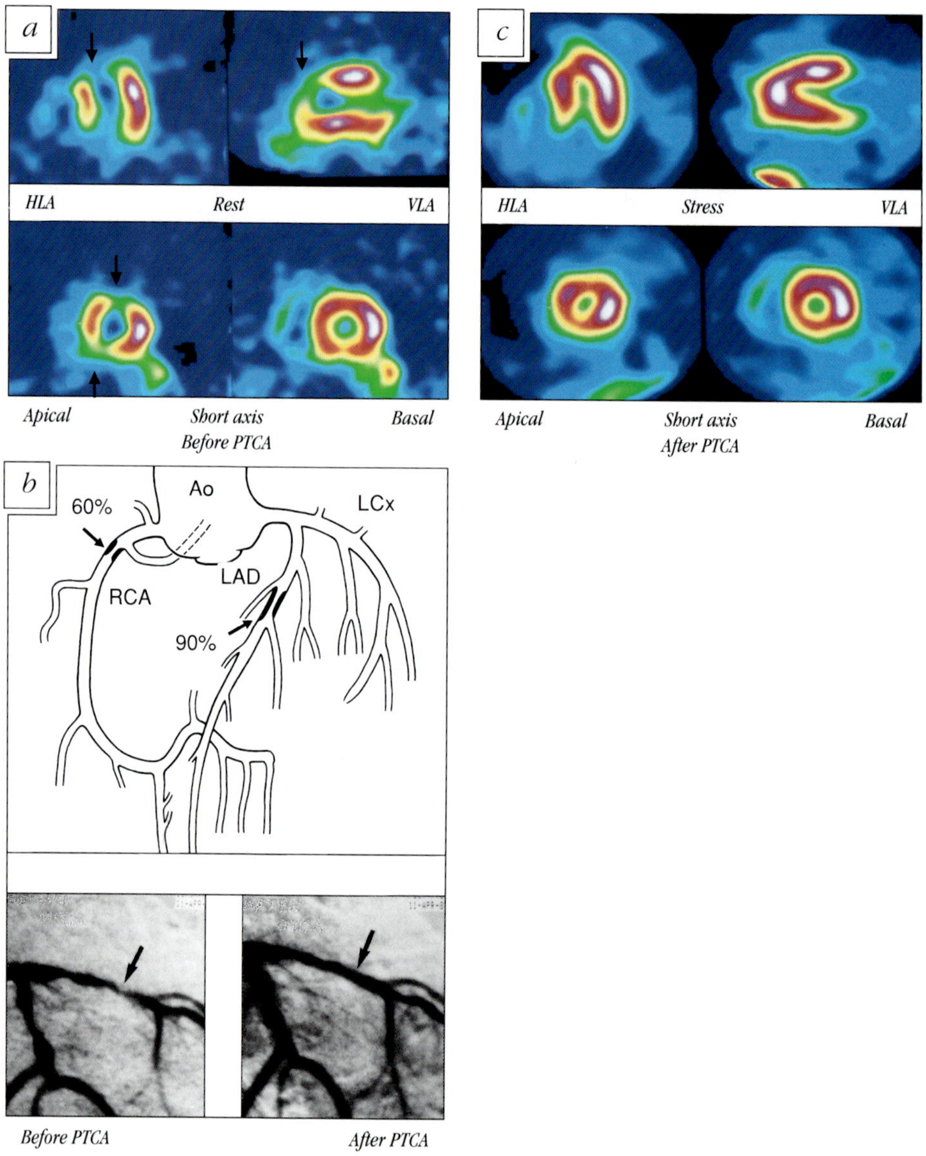

Four months later the patient described recurrent chest pain associated with moderate physical activities and stress perfusion imaging recorded defects in the same vessel territory as before (Fig. VIII.10d, arrows). Restenosis of the LAD and progression of the RCA disease were confirmed (Fig. VIII.10e, arrow) and the patient was referred for double bypass surgery.

Postoperative tomographic control performed 2 months later showed the successful revascularization of the LAD and RCA vessel territories (Fig. VIII.10f).

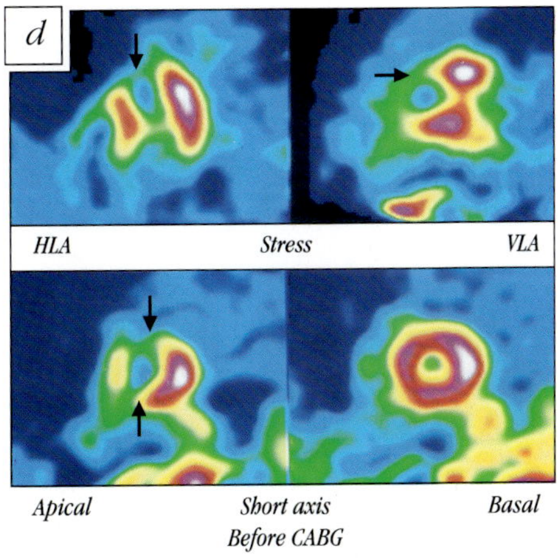

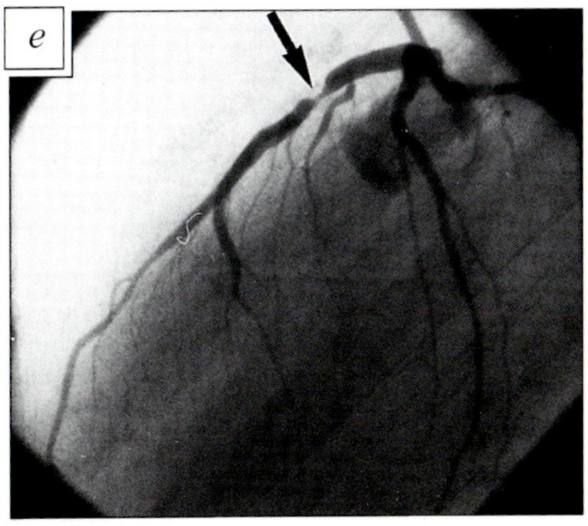

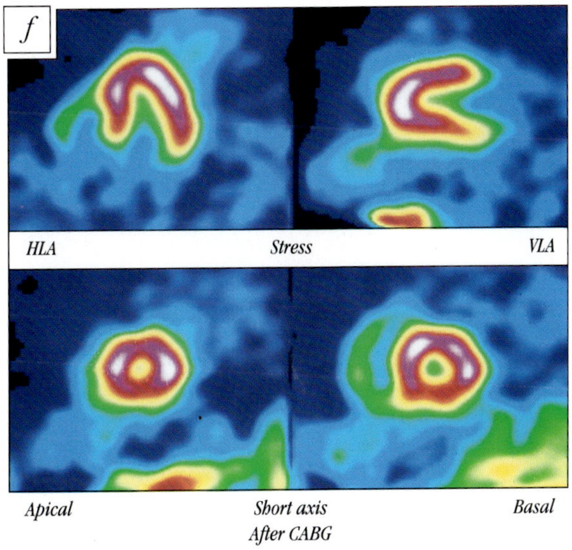

Case Study VIII.11

Recurrence of myocardial ischaemia after CABG

Mrs DV (58 years old) was submitted to double bypass surgery in April 1991. Her preoperative stress tomographic study showed large perfusion abnormalities in the anteroapical and inferior walls of the LV (Fig. VIII.11a, arrows). The coronary angiogram showed the presence of significant lesions on the LAD and RCA (Fig. VIII.11b, arrows).

Myocardial imaging performed 2 months after surgery to document the results of the procedure demonstrated a normal exercise perfusion pattern and a decreased ventricular size suggesting functional improvement (Fig. VIII.11c).

In October 1991, the patient described recurrence of typical chest pain induced by exercise. Scintigraphic evaluation revealed sestamibi exercise defects in the anteroseptal wall of the LV and the angiogram revealed severe LAD graft stenosis (Figs. VIII.11d,e, arrows). An angioplasty of the bypass was successfully performed.

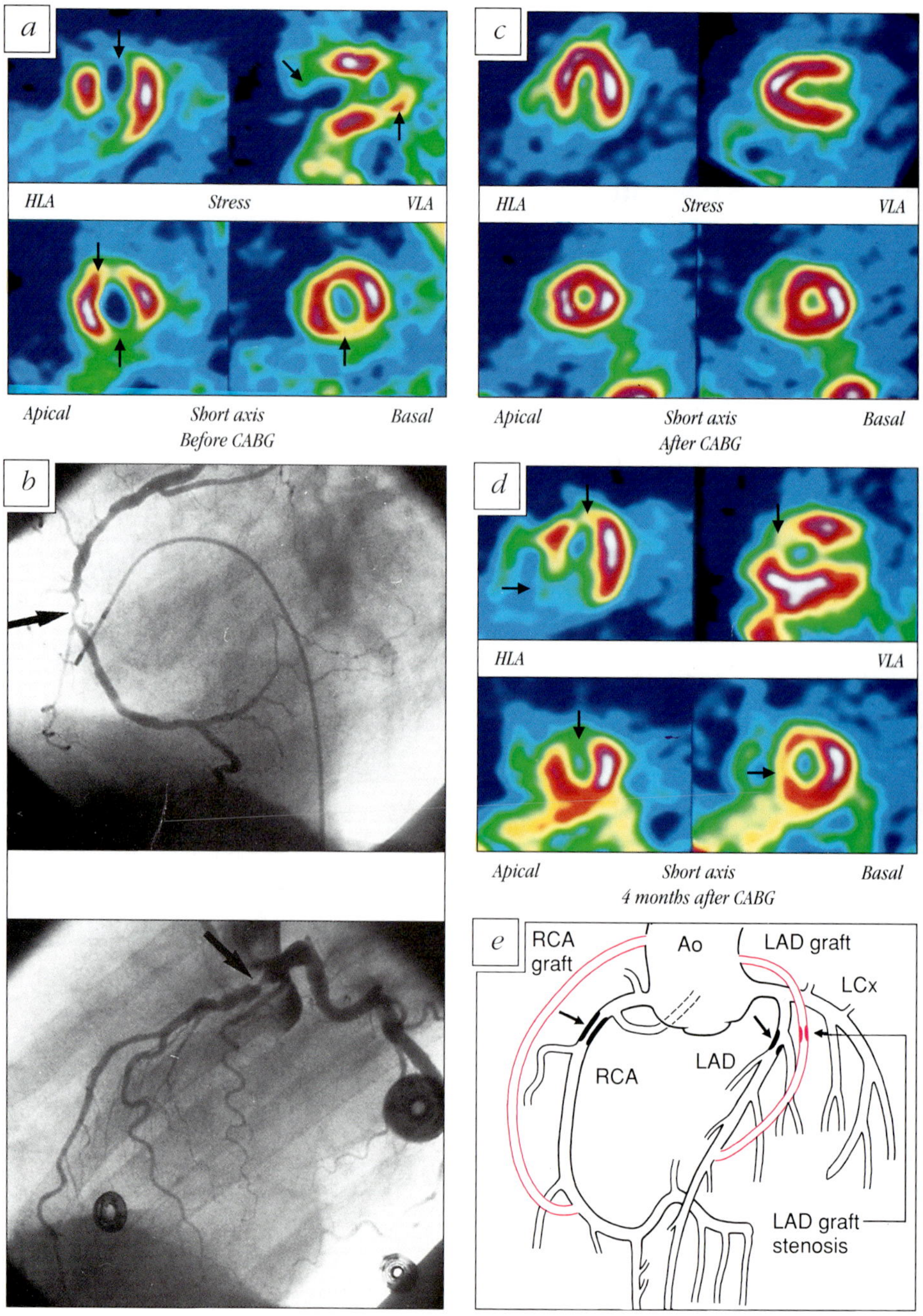

9 ASSESSMENT OF MYOCARDIAL INFARCT PATIENTS

Clinical Background

Clinical evidence of previous myocardial infarction may disappear with time. Retrospective diagnosis may be difficult in some patients when the ECG normalizes or becomes non-specific due to changes related to conduction disturbances or pacemakers. It is important to demonstrate the presence of coronary artery disease (CAD) as this diagnosis carries important therapeutic and prognostic information and is essential for the patient's management.

Information about infarct size and location, also of primary interest in assessing prognosis, can only be grossly obtained from conventional data, while direct evaluation is available using scintigraphic techniques and has been shown to be of prognostic significance.

In patients with a suspected acute infarction the ECG and pattern of cardiac enzymes, as well as the history, help us to differentiate between an acute infarction and chest pain of non-cardiac origin. Circumstances occur, however, when the enzyme pattern is equivocal (due to trauma or to a long delay after the onset of symptoms) and/or the ECG data are not pathogmonic.

Myocardial imaging has been used as a diagnostic and prognostic test in these equivocal cases. It has also been advocated as a means to rule out myocardial ischaemia and/or infarction and help in the early triage of acute patients.

Assessment of Size and Location of Myocardial Infarction

The location of a myocardial infarction correlates well with the ECG abnormalities in most of the patients admitted with an acute myocardial infarction. However, in some types of infarction, especially those caused by lesions of the circumflex coronary artery, the ECG changes can be minimal or even absent, while in other cases the ECG abnormalities are only present initially. In non-Q-wave infarction the ECG changes can be misleading and are only seen in the acute phase, while in subacute or old infarctions no abnormalities are seen. The ECG also lacks sufficient sensitivity to diagnose a second infarction.

In patients with abnormal initial activation as left bundle branch block (LBBB), pacemaker rhythm or Wolff–Parkinson–White syndrome, the ECG is mostly unable to provide any clue as to the location or even the presence of an acute myocardial infarction. Only a poor correlation has been found between the ECG abnormalities and size and extent of myocardial infarction in patients with abnormal or normal initial activations.

Before the era of thrombolytic therapy a correlation was found between infarct size and the maximal blood levels of the enzymes creatine phosphate kinase (CPK) or lactate dehydrogenase (LDH) in the acute phase of a myocardial infarction, at least if the patient was admitted soon after the onset of chest pain. This relationship has become less clear, however, since the introduction of fibrinolysis. In patients admitted in the subacute phase of an acute myocardial infarction the enzyme levels no longer have any value because the maximum value may have been missed or the values may have already normalized. In these patients admitted with a history of chest pain and an ECG compatible with a recent infarction, it is important to know if the infarction is 3 days or 3 weeks old because the treatment will differ. This can be done with acute infarct imaging using ^{99m}Tc pyrophosphate or ^{111}In antimyosin.

The infarct size and location have prognostic implications. Numerous studies[1–7] have demonstrated, both experimentally and clinically, the value of myocardial imaging in the assessment of infarct size and the importance of these parameters in describing these patients' prognoses. In fact, as demonstrated by Becker et al,[7] the knowledge of infarct size and left ventricular ejection fraction provides the best tool to distinguish between high-, intermediate- and low-risk groups.

Identification of patients without transmural infarction can be misleading as patients with posterior or posterolateral infarction frequently have transmural lesions without Q-waves, and are misdiagnosed on the ECG. Myocardial perfusion scans show large defects in these cases typical of transmural infarctions.

Selection of Patients for Admission to the Coronary Care Unit

Optimal medical management requires all patients with chest pain of potential cardiac origin to be admitted to the emergency room, or even better to the coronary care unit, unless myocardial ischaemia and infarction have been ruled out as a cause of symptoms. However, only around 30–50% of these patients are ultimately proved to have acute cardiac disease, but the time needed to exclude it may be long in some patients, during which the use of unnecessary but very expensive facilities is required. As early cardiac imaging can differentiate patients with ischaemic heart disease (that is ,patients with a perfusion defect either reversible or irreversible, acute or chronic) from patients without ischaemic heart disease (patients with no defect), this approach has been advocated as a cost-effective means to select patients for admission in the coronary care unit. The wide availability and ease of preparation of technetium-labelled compounds could be factors contributing to the extension of the use of this approach.

Aims of Sestamibi Studies

In patients with a definite or suspected old myocardial infarction information is needed to confirm the presence, size and location of the infarction.[8] Of particular importance is whether it extends in *one or more flow areas* of the different coronary arteries.[9] This information can be provided by myocardial perfusion imaging as demonstrated by the case studies given below. Also of importance are the functional repercussions of the infarction on ventricular size and regional and global left ventricular function. To obtain this information an independent echocardiographic or radionuclide angiogram study can be performed; however, the same information can be obtained by first-pass or gated acquisition concomitantly with the sestamibi perfusion study. In patients admitted with a suspected myocardial infarction the sestamibi study cannot differentiate either between an old or acute infarction, or between ischaemia and scar tissue. However, a normal distribution of the radioactive tracer excludes a myocardial infarction.

Clinical Points

- Infarct size and location have important prognostic significance.
- Right and left ventricular function after myocardial infarction determine prognosis.
- All these parameters can be determined with sestamibi.

References

1 HOLMAN BL, CHISHOLM RJ, BRAUNWALD E, The prognostic implications of acute myocardial infarction scintigraphy with ^{99m}Tc-pyrophosphate, *Circulation* (1978) **57**:320.
2 SILVERMAN KJ, BECKER LC, BULKLEY BH et al, Value of early thallium-201 scintigraphy for predicting mortality in patients with acute myocardial infarction, *Circulation* (1980) **61**:996.
3 ONG L, GREEN S, REISER P et al, Early prediction of mortality in patients with acute myocardial infarction: A prospective study of clinical and radionuclide risk factors, *Am J Cardiol* (1986) **57**:33.
4 SHAH PK, PICHLER M, BERMAN DS et al, Left ventricular ejection fraction determined by radionuclide ventriculography in early stages of first transmural myocardial infarction. Relation to short-term prognosis, *Am J Cardiol* (1980) **45**:542.
5 DEWHURST NG, HANNAN WJ, MUIR AL, Prognostic value of radionuclide ventriculography after myocardial infarction, *Q J Med* (1981) **49**:479.
6 ABRAMS DS, STARLING MR, CRAWFORD MH et al, Value of non-invasive techniques for predicting early complications in patients with clinical class II acute myocardial infarction, *J Am Coll Cardiol* (1983) **2**:818.
7 BECKER LC, SILVERMAN KJ, BULKLEY BH et al, Comparison of early thallium-201 scintigraphy and gated blood pool imaging for predicting mortality in patients with acute myocardial infarction, *Circulation* (1983) **67**:1272.
8 AHMAD M, LOGAN KW, MARTIN RH, Doughnut pattern of technetium-99m pyrophosphate myocardial uptake in patients with acute myocardial infarction. A sign of poor long-term prognosis, *Am J Cardiol* (1979) **44**:13.
9 BOTVINICK EH, PEREZ-GONZALEZ JF, DUNN R et al, Late prognostic value of scintigraphic parameters of acute mayocardial infarction size in complicated myocardial infarction without heart failure, *Am J Cardiol* (1983) **51**:1045.

Case Study IX.1

Transmural myocardial infarction

Mr DN, known to have an inferior wall myocardial infarction in the past, was admitted to hospital because of chest pain.

The ECG showed sinus bradycardia (heart rate 55 beats/min) and signs of an old inferior wall myocardial infarction (Fig. IX.1a). The enzymes remained normal and the ECG remained unchanged. An exercise test was performed which showed significant ST–T segment changes in the precordial leads without chest pain (Fig. IX.1a) and the sestamibi planar scintigraphy performed at stress and at rest showed a fixed inferoposterolateral defect corresponding to the infarct (Figs. IX.1b,c, arrows).

The infarction was responsible for abnormal wall motion well visualized on the planar gated acquisition in the left anterior oblique (LAO) 40° projection (Fig. IX.1d, arrows).

Because of the unknown origin of the chest pain and conflicting data of scan and ECG, a coronary angiogram was performed which showed single vessel disease of the right coronary artery (RCA) (Fig. IX.1e, arrow).

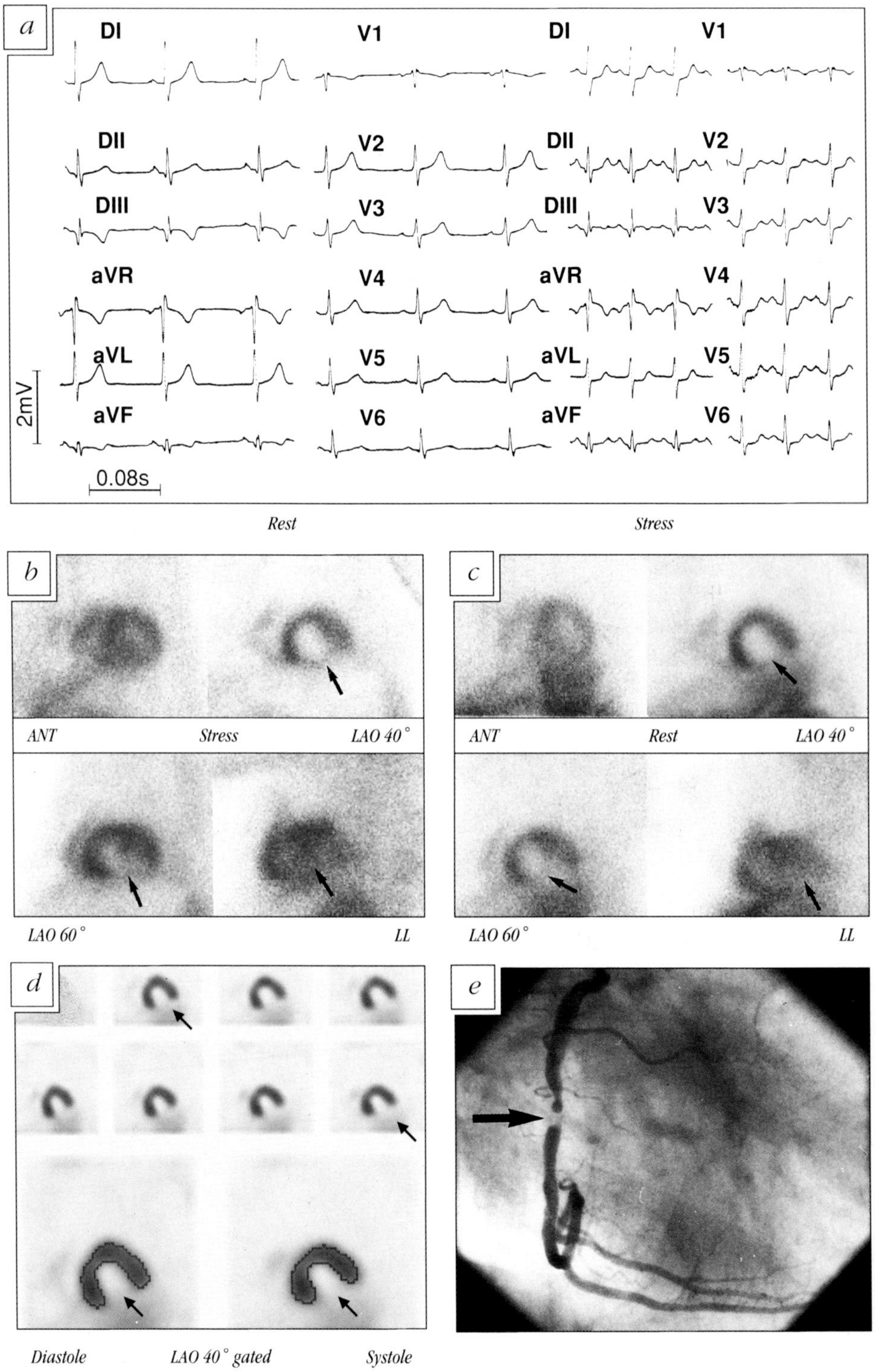

Case Study IX.2

Inferior myocardial infarction with small perfusion defect

The patient is a male smoker (49 years old) who was treated for 2 years for hypertension and lipid disorders. In November 1991 he developed transmural myocardial infarction.

Because of the minor ECG abnormalities, it was decided to remain conservative. The CK enzyme level rose to 500 units/litre. The course was uneventful and a stress ECG combined with a sestamibi study and an angiography was realized before hospital discharge. The ECG at rest showed signs of an inferior myocardial infarction (Fig. IX.2a). No changes occurred with exercise.

Stress and rest scintigraphy demonstrated the presence of small perfusion defects identical in extent and in severity in the inferoposterior wall of the LV (LAO 60° view, Figs. IX.2b,c, arrows).

An angiogram revealed the occlusion of the proximal RCA partially reperfused by collateral vessels coming from the left anterior descending (LAD) vessel territory (Fig. IX.2d, arrow).

These results indicated that the patient should continue on medical therapy.

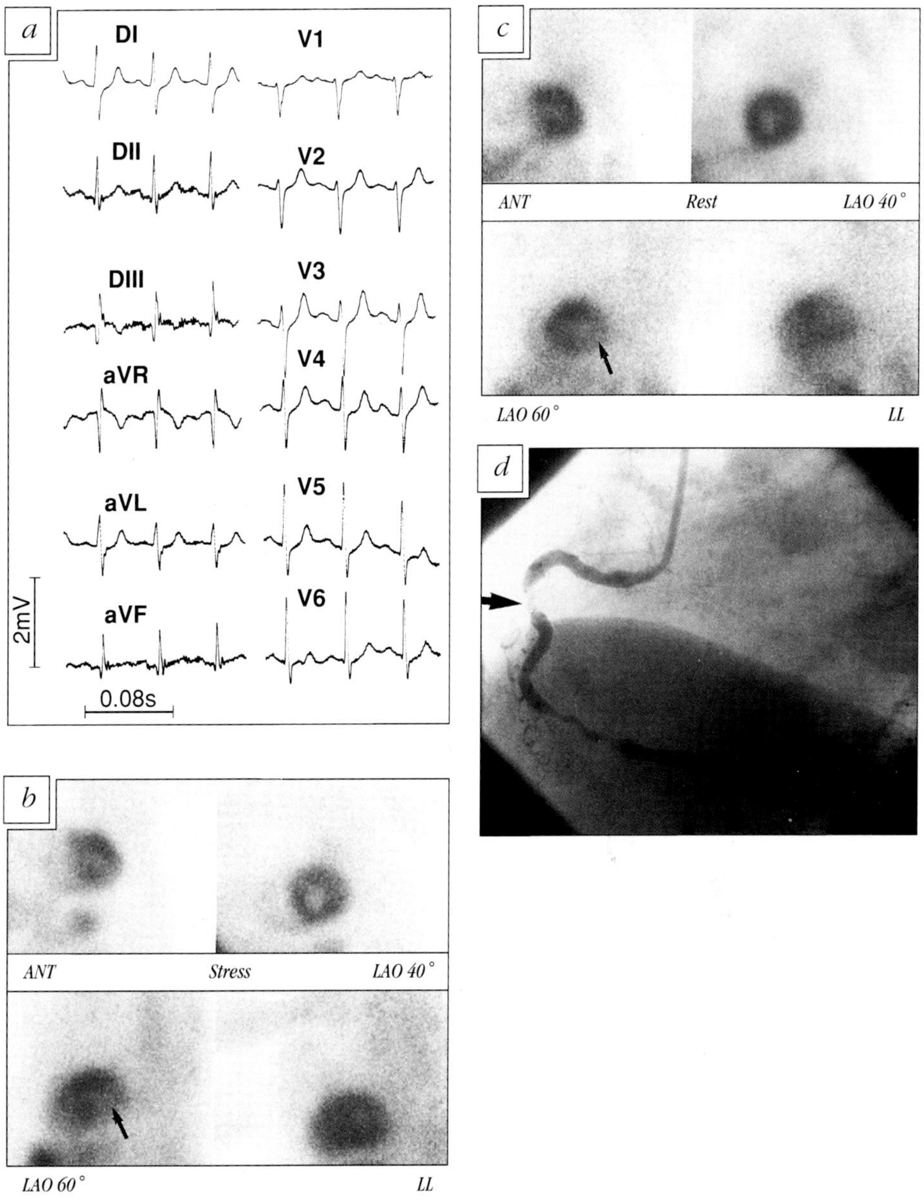

Case Study IX.3

Transmural inferior myocardial infarction with large perfusion defects

Mr KJ (61 years old) presented an inaugural precordial chest pain at home while he was painting. Pain persisted for 1 h radiated to his shoulders and to his back but finally subsided. The patient remained asymptomatic for a few hours. Chest pain recurred during the night and he was admitted to the hospital for further investigations.

The ECG showed ST elevations in the inferior leads and in the right precordial leads compatible with an inferoposterior myocardial infarct with RV involvement (Fig. IX.3a) and biological data indicated a significant rise in the CK–MB isoenzyme serum level. The patient was treated by heparin, nitrates and calcium antagonists.

The coronary angiogram performed on day 8 demonstrated occlusion of the RCA. The area distal to the occlusion was not perfused by collateral vessels (Fig. IX.3b).

To evaluate the extent of perfusion abnormalities and to assess prognosis, a rest and stress sestamibi tomography was performed 2 weeks after the acute event. It showed perfusion defects in the inferior and in the inferoposterior walls of the LV. No significant changes were observed at stress consistent with a myocardial infarction without residual ischaemia (Figs. IX.3c,d, arrows).

The patient was referred for medical therapy and follow-up.

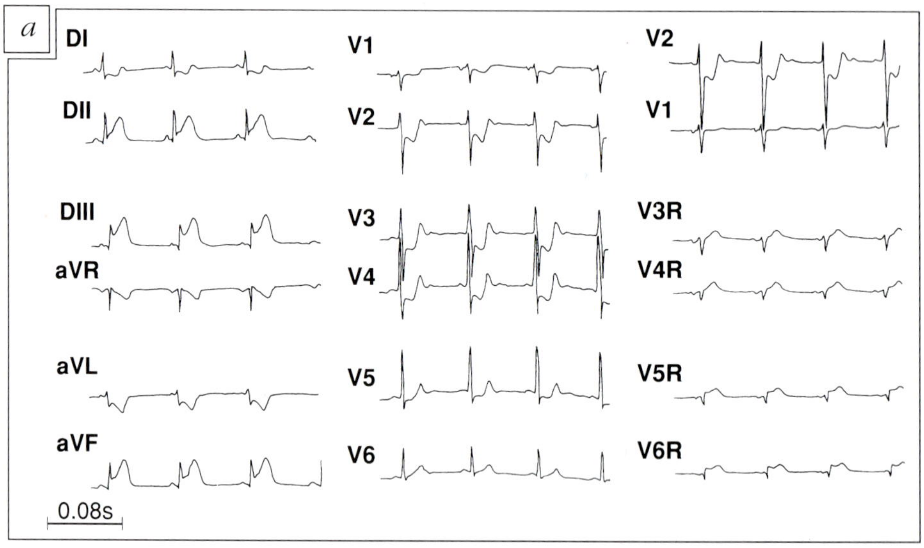

Admission ECG

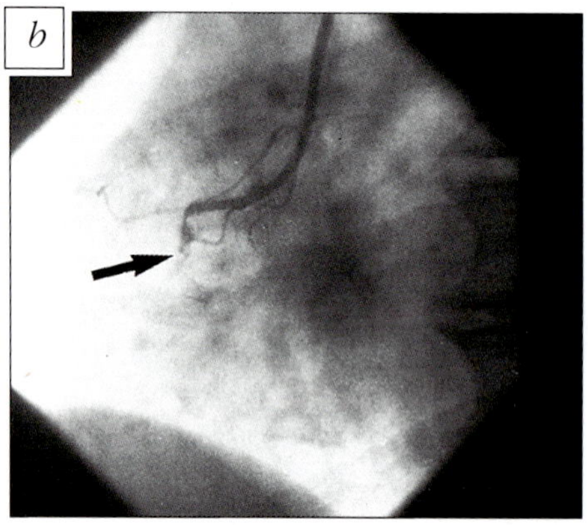

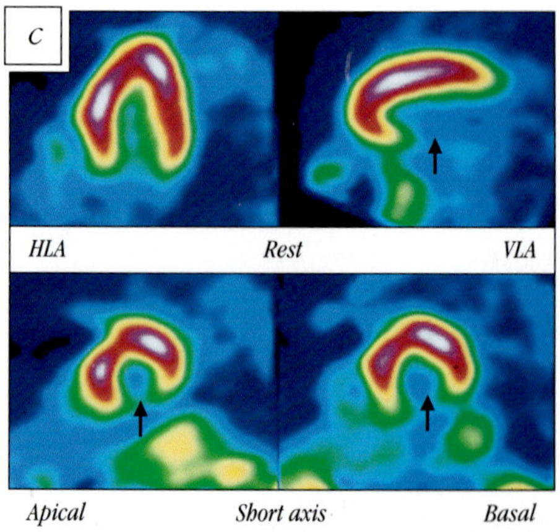

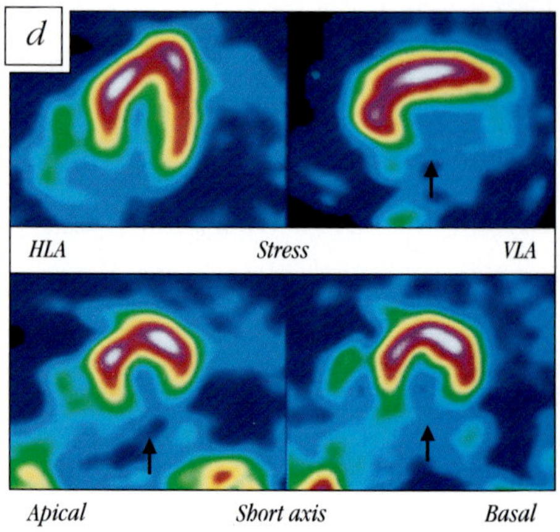

Case Study IX.4

Subacute myocardial infarction

The patient, a 57-year-old male known to have diabetes mellitus, developed at home left precordial chest pain radiated to his arms, his throat and his back which persisted for more than 1 h. Pain occurred while he was watching a cricket match on television. Two weeks later he came to the hospital for treatment of his diabetes mellitus.

The ECG at that time showed small Q-wave and T-wave changes in the inferior leads compatible with a recent inferior wall infarction (Fig. IX.4a). To analyse myocardial perfusion, a rest and stress sestamibi scintigraphy study was done. Similar sestamibi defects were observed at rest and at stress in the inferoapical and in the posterolateral walls of the LV (Figs. IX.4b,c, arrows).

This myocardial scar was responsible for inferoapical abnormal wall motion visualized on the gated LAO 40° projection (Fig. IX.4d, arrows).

The coronary angiogram demonstrated the presence of single RCA occlusion (Fig. IX.4e, arrow).

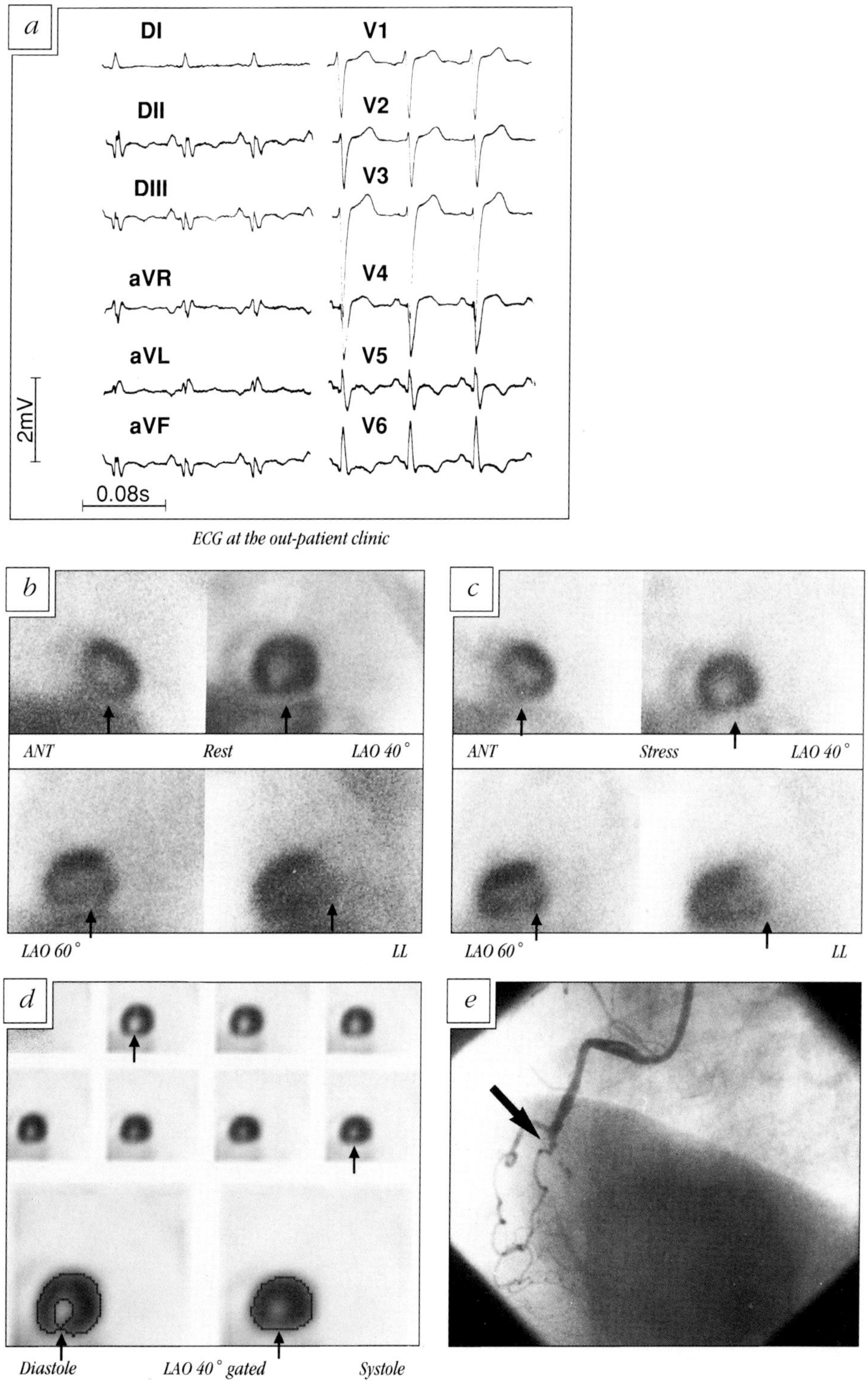

ECG at the out-patient clinic

Case Study IX.5

Interest of sestamibi imaging for detecting necrosis in a second vessel territory in a patient with previous myocardial infarction

Mr AJ, a 56-year-old male, developed in 1988 an inferior myocardial infarction. He remained asymptomatic for 3 years. In October 1991 he presented again with chest pain of more than 1 h duration, not relieved by short-acting nitrates.

The ECG at admission showed an old inferior myocardial infarction and a slow R progression in the precordial leads (Fig. IX.5a).

A sestamibi study performed at rest and at stress to assess regional myocardial perfusion demonstrated perfusion defects in the inferior, in the inferoposterior and in the anteroseptal walls of the LV (Figs. IX.5b,c, arrows), suggesting also an anteroseptal myocardial infarction.

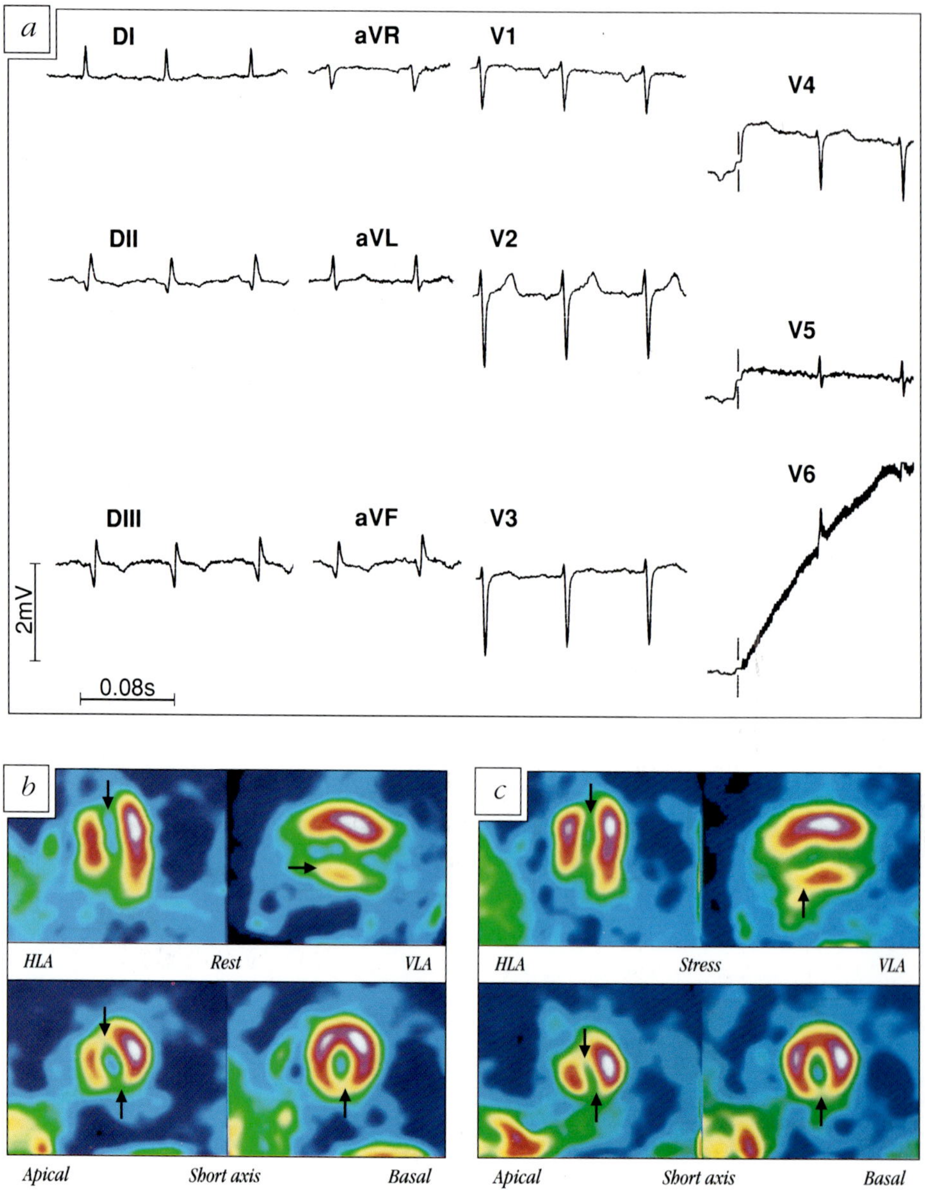

A radionuclide angiography was realized, to evaluate ventricular function, and showed anterior akinesis of the LV, on the amplitude image, in the right anterior oblique (RAO) view (Fig. IX.5d, arrow).

Results of coronary angiography performed a few days later indicated severe stenosis of the LAD coronary artery and occlusion of the RCA (Figs. IX.5e,f, arrows).

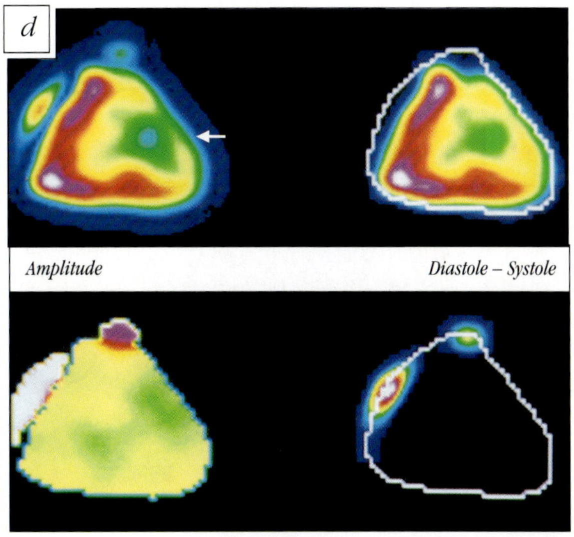

Phase *Equilibrium* *Systole – Diastole*

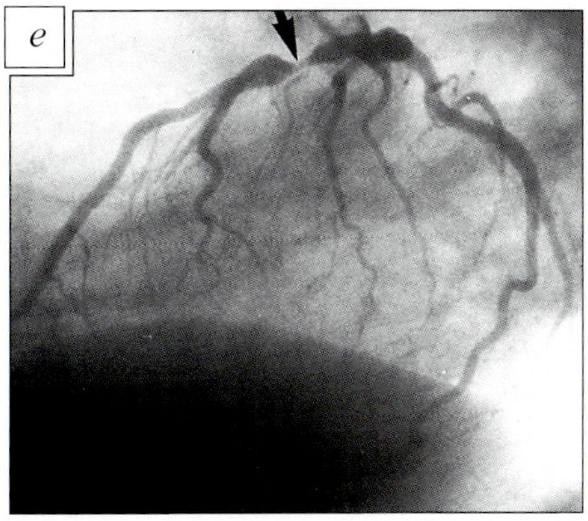

Left coronary arteries

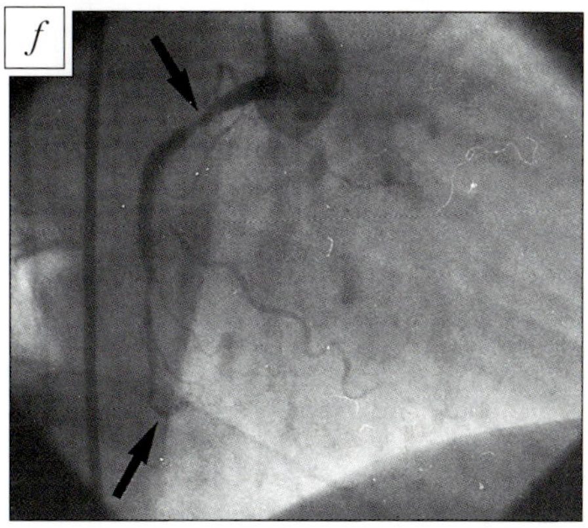

RCA

Case Study IX.6

Non-diagnostic ECG in the presence of LBBB

Mr JPL, a 68-year-old male smoker known to have hypertension, developed chest pain radiating to his right shoulder. Pain disappeared in 30 min. During the pain, the patient complained of dyspnoea, nausea and palpitations. The next morning, chest pain recurred while he was eating breakfast. He was admitted to hospital.

The patient's blood sample indicated a significant rise in the CK–MB isoenzyme level but the ECG was not conclusive because of LBBB.

To locate the infarction, a ^{99m}Tc pyrophosphate scan was performed which showed pathological uptake in the anteroseptal region (Fig. IX.6a, arrows). Before discharge, an exercise test combined with tomographic imaging showed ECG changes; however, they were insignificant because of the LBBB (Fig. IX.6b).

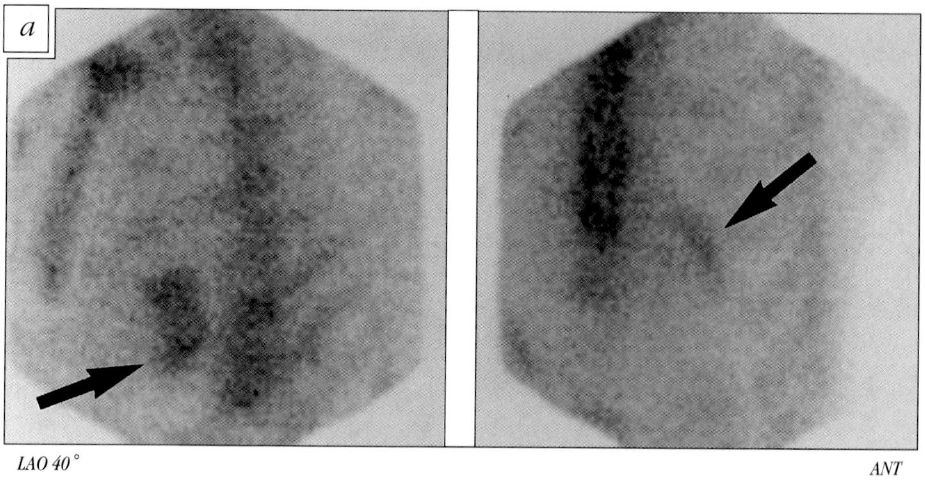

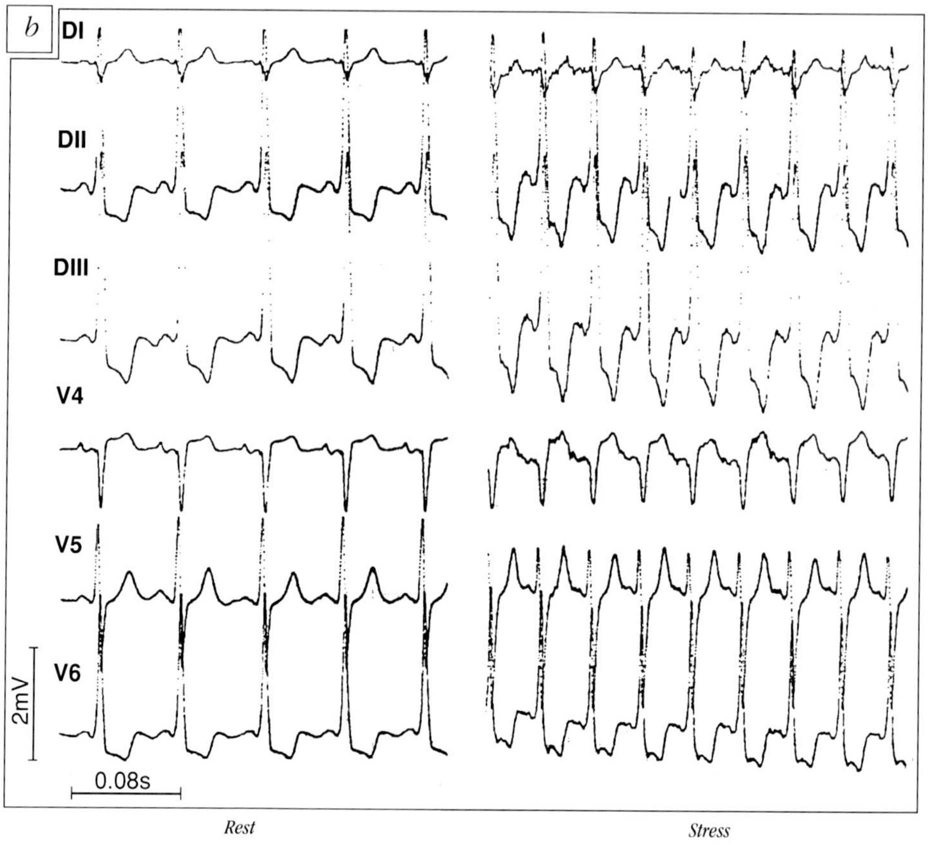

Tomography at stress showed sestamibi defects in the anteroseptal wall of the LV (Fig. IX.6c, arrows). At rest, the perfusion pattern was similar to that at stress and did not suggest myocardial ischaemia surrounding the infarcted area (Fig. IX.6d, arrows).

Coronary angiography showed an occlusion in the mid-LAD (Fig. IX.6e, arrow).

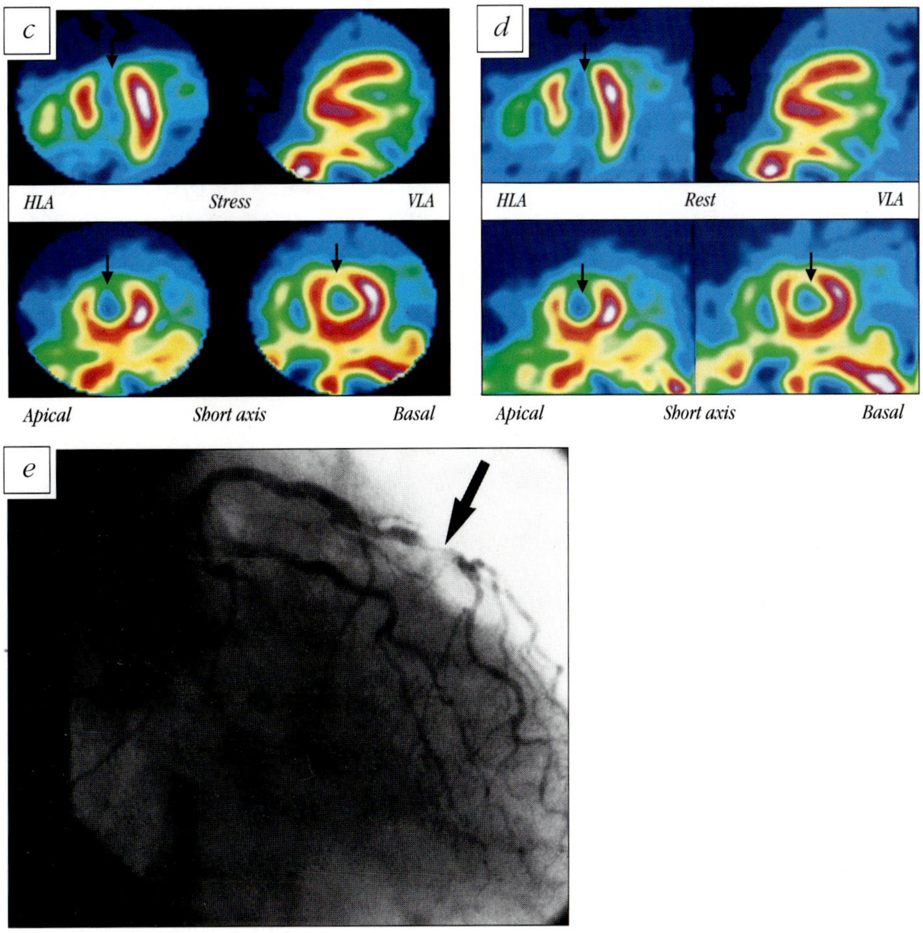

Case Study IX.7

Old transmural myocardial infarction with small perfusion defects

Mr WM (47 years old) came to the out-patient clinic because he developed left precordial chest pain radiating to his left upper limb during exercise.

Pain did not react when short-acting nitrate was administered sublingually.

The ECG performed at rest was normal (Fig. IX.7a), as were laboratory data.

The scintigraphic evaluation showed identical small defects on rest and stress sestamibi tomograms in the three orthogonal projections, corresponding to myocardial infarction in the LAD vessel territory (Figs. IX.7b,c, arrows).

Angiographic data confirmed the presence of single vessel disease with a diagonal stenosis of 95% (Fig. IX.7d). Because the patient was now free of complaint and in a low-risk group he was only given medical treatment.

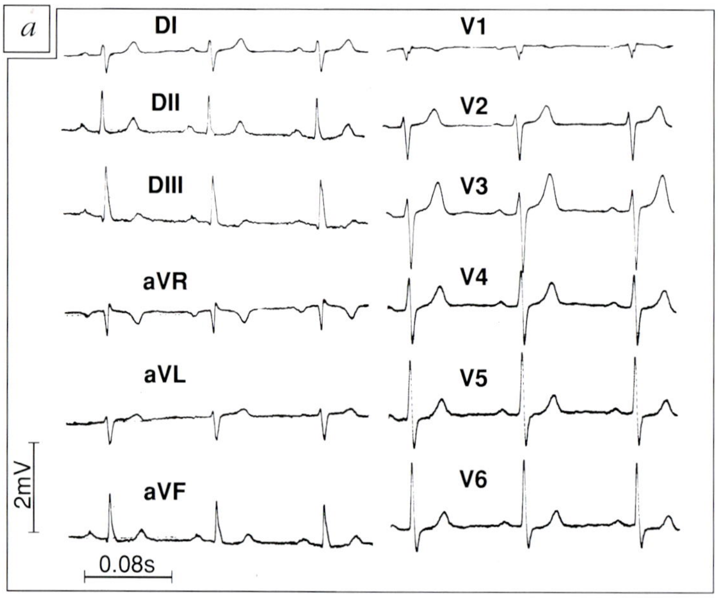

Admission ECG

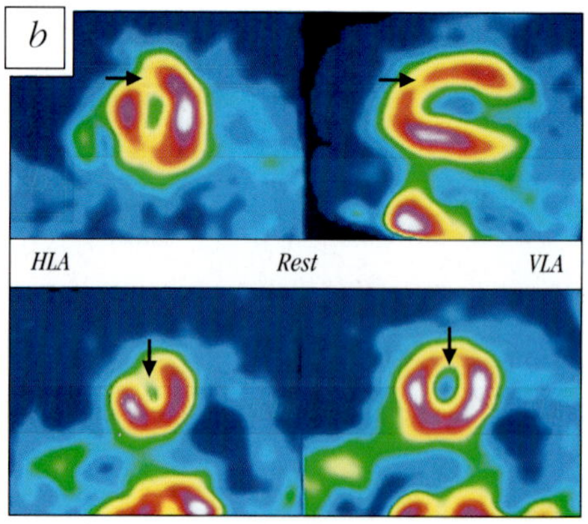

Apical *Short axis* *Basal*

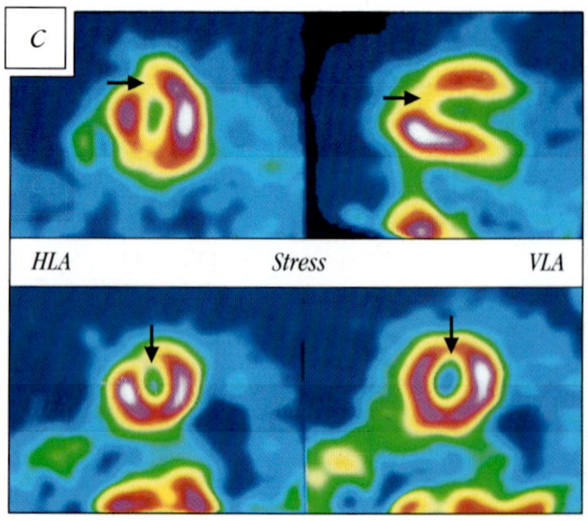

Apical *Short axis* *Basal*

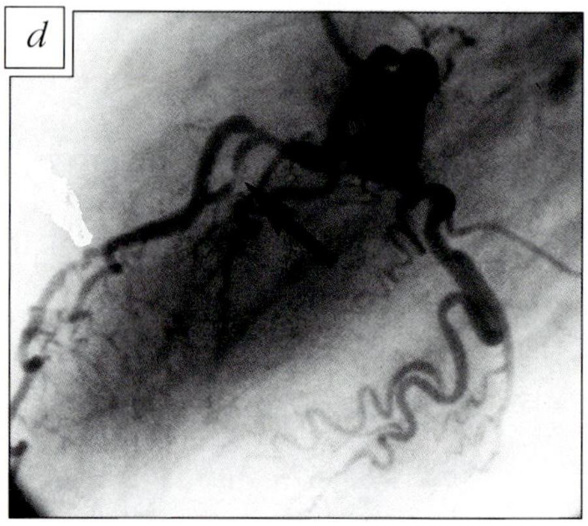

Case Study IX.8

Inconclusive ECG in the presence of Wolff–Parkinson–White syndrome

This case concerns a 67-year-old patient with Wolff–Parkinson–White syndrome who presented with typical precordial chest pain. His cardiovascular risk factors included a positive familial history, hypertension and dyslipaemia.

As his ECG was uninterpretable (Fig. IX.8a), myocardial perfusion imaging was performed immediately after admission and showed small perfusion defects in the inferoposterior wall of the LV localizing the area at risk (Fig. IX.8b, arrows). Because of the small size of the defects, no thrombolytic therapy was given.

Before discharge, a sestamibi exercise test was done. The perfusion pattern was similar to the pattern found just after admission (Fig. IX.8c, arrows) and the rest study also showed the same abnormalities. It was therefore decided to treat conservatively.

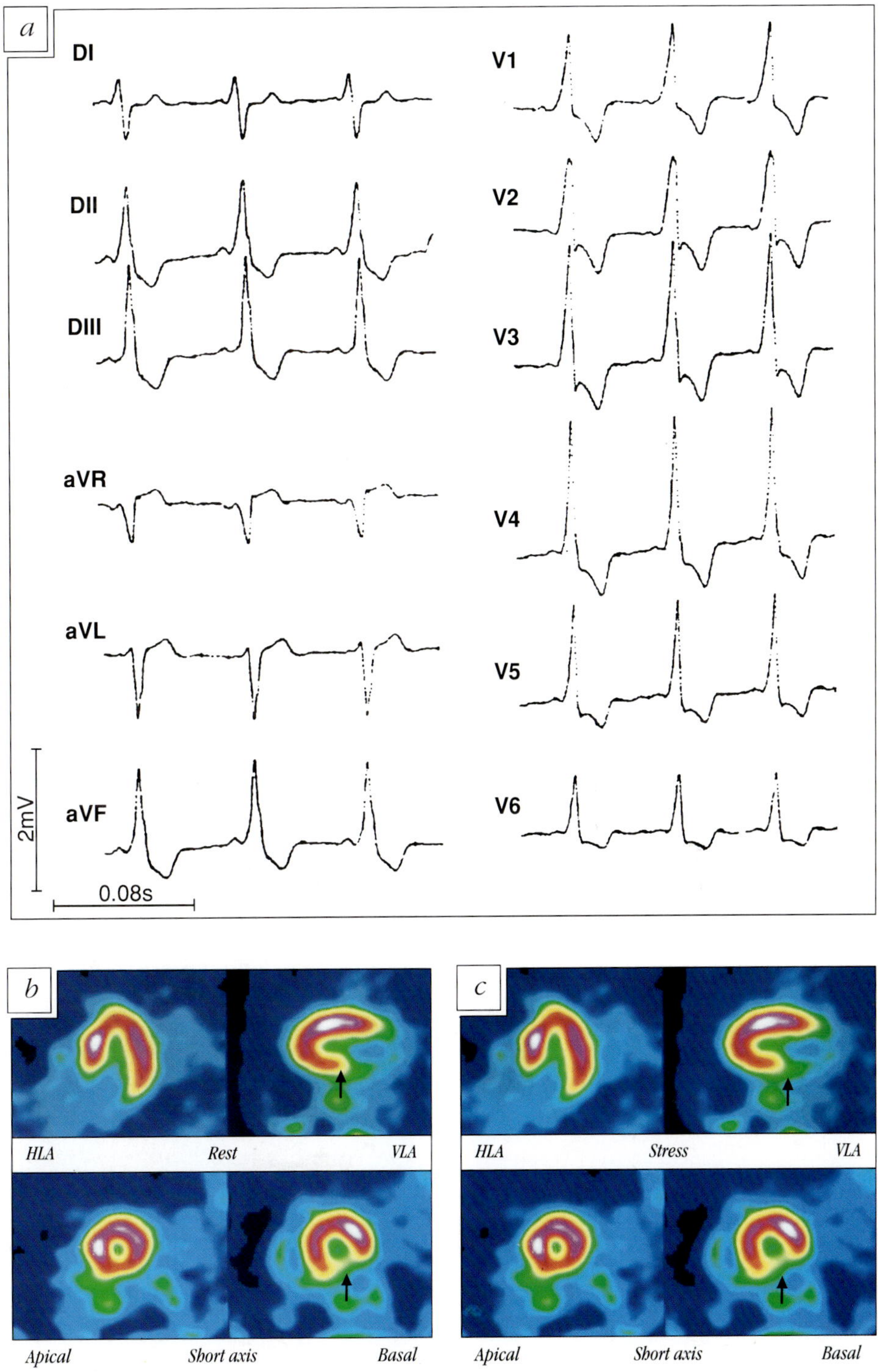

Case Study IX.9

Interest of pyrophosphate and sestamibi imaging in the acute phase of myocardial infarction

Mr PG visited the out-patient clinic because he had experienced precordial chest pain 2 days earlier. Pain started when he was taking a nap and was still present.

The ECG showed a subacute anteroseptal infarction (Fig. IX.9a). To gain information as to the size of the myocardial infarction, a pyrophosphate study was performed. Pathological uptake was observed in a large area (Fig. IX.9b, arrows).

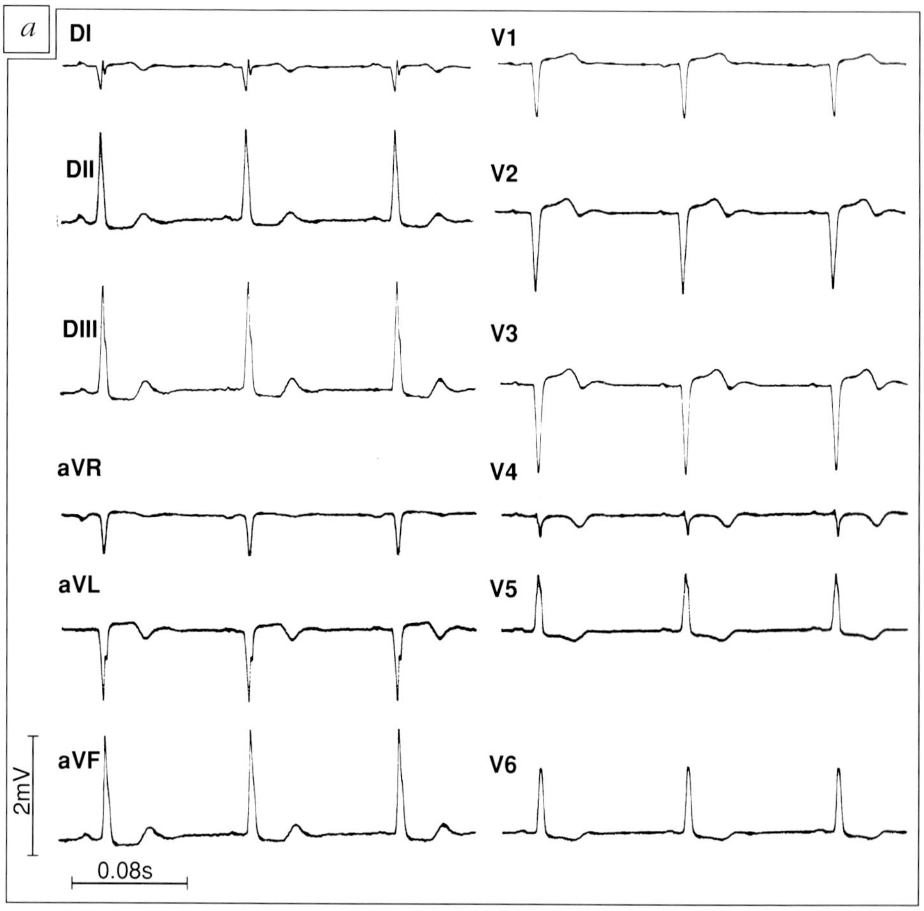

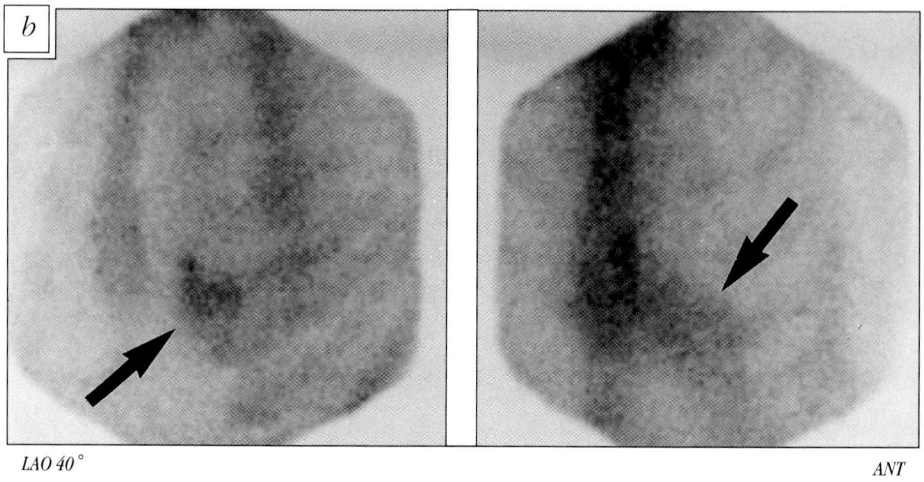

A sestamibi study performed before discharge at stress and at rest demonstrated abnormal perfusion pattern in the anteroseptal wall of the LV, corresponding to myocardial infarction without ischaemia (Fig. IX.9c, arrows).

Because he developed secondary ventricular tachycardia, a coronary angiography was made which demonstrated a subocclusion of the proximal LAD coronary artery (Fig. IX.9d, arrow).

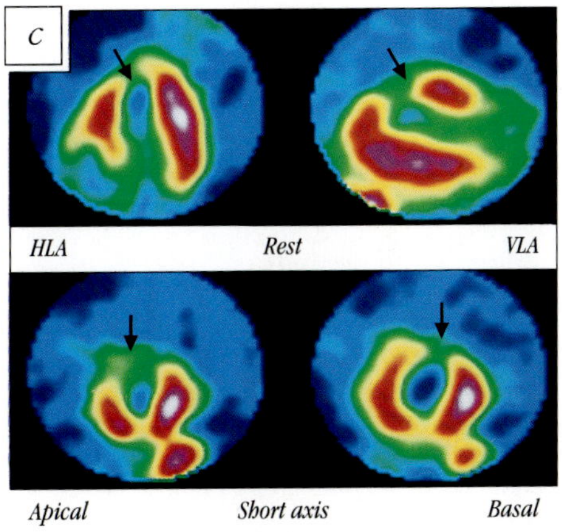

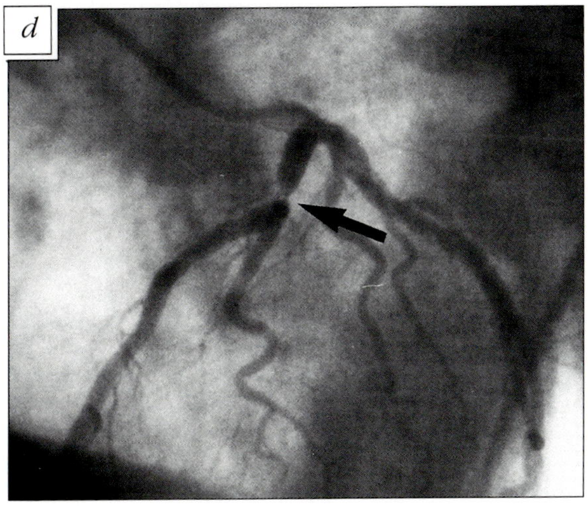

Case Study IX.10

Interest of myocardial perfusion imaging in posterolateral myocardial infarction in presence of non-diagnostic ECG

Mr JF is 74 years old and suffers from paroxysmal atrial fibrillation. He complained of precordial chest pain and nausea when he was driving his car. Two months earlier he had visited the out-patient clinic.

His pulse rate was irregular (±80 beats/min) and his blood pressure 166/95 mmHg. Routine blood investigation was normal.

Sestamibi tomography performed at rest and at stress clearly demonstrated perfusion defects in the lateral, in the inferoposterior and in the inferior walls of the LV corresponding to myocardial infarction (Figs. IX.10a,b, arrows), while the ECG showed no significant ST–T segment changes (Fig. IX.10c).

Coronary angiography showed an occlusion of the left circumflex (LCx) coronary artery (Fig. IX.10d, arrow).

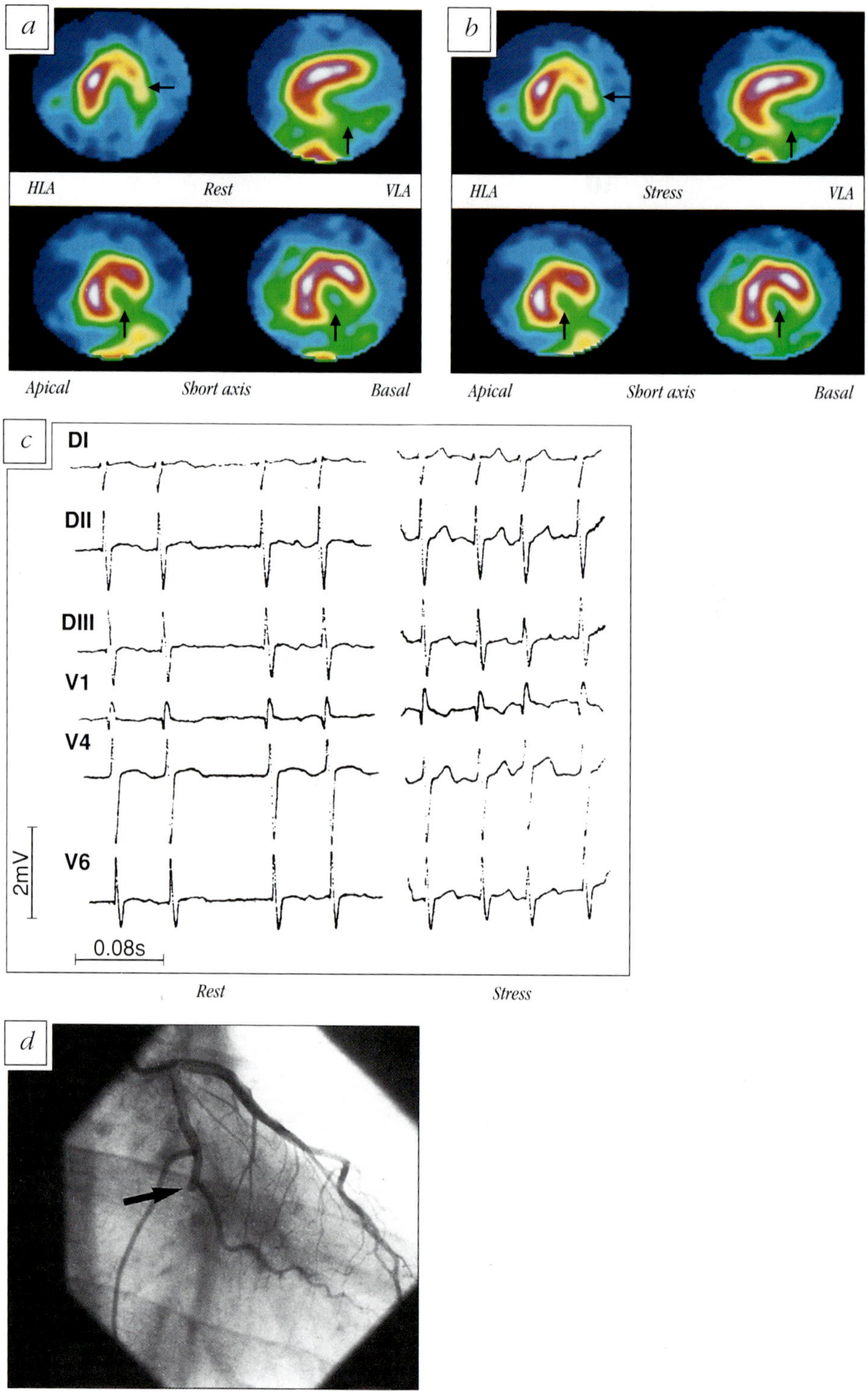

10 ASSESSMENT OF POST-MYOCARDIAL INFARCTION PATIENTS

Clinical Background

Patients surviving an acute myocardial infarction remain at increased risk of cardiovascular complication, and their prognosis should be more precisely defined. From past studies,[1–3] it is known that approximately 10% of patients with an acute myocardial infarction die during the year following their hospital discharge. Most deaths, of which about 50% are sudden, occur within 3–6 months after the acute event. The extent of myocardial damage (that is the infarct size) and the left ventricular ejection fraction are the major determinants of prognosis (see Chapter 9).

Not only do the infarct size and left ventricular function have prognostic implications, but the presence or absence of residual ischaemia is also important. If ischaemia is present, then further information is necessary about its extent and location – whether it is around or at a distance from the acute myocardial infarction. Ischaemia at a distance, in another coronary artery perfusion bed, has more severe prognostic implications than the presence of ischaemia in the region of the infarcted area.[4]

Complications of infarction in the acute phase include rhythm disturbances caused by electrical instability, aneurysmal formation of the left ventricle (LV), valvular leakage resulting from ischaemic papillary muscle dysfunction or rupture, as well as rupture of the free wall or of the interventricular septum. Radionuclide angiography, an accurate technique used to evaluate overall cardiac function and to detect areas of dysfunction, can also recognize the formation of an aneurysm, measure the regurgitation fraction and estimate the size of a left-to-right shunt in the case of an intraventricular septal rupture. Information on regional myocardial function can also be derived using wall motion data. However, following successful reopening of an occluded vessel, salvaged myocardium can remain akinetic and therefore may be difficult to differentiate from necrotic muscle. Special studies are necessary in these cases to assess myocardial viability. Stunned myocardium will eventually show wall motion improvement after revascularization, but complete recovery may be delayed for months.

Clinical Problem

Since the recognition of the importance of assessing infarct size and dysfunction and of detecting residual ischaemia, the number of patients routinely undergoing exercise testing combined with radionuclide study, 24-h registration, signal-averaging ECG and coronary angiography has increased substantially. In the past exercise tests were done only until 70% of the maximum predicted heart rate was achieved; in most clinics a symptom-limited exercise test is now performed before discharge.[5]

The exact amount at which to perform exercise tests is still controversial, and investigations have been done to determine the prognostic value of such tests performed as early as 3 days after the acute onset of chest pain.[6] The main value of the exercise test is to provide information about the exercise tolerance of a patient. This has of course prognostic significance, but does not detect the presence, site and extent of residual ischaemia. Combining these exercise tests with radionuclide imaging provides a tool to measure not only the exercise tolerance, but also the presence, the size, and location of the area of residual ischaemia. This allows differentiation between absence of ischaemia, ischaemia in the region of the myocardial infarction and ischaemia at a distance from the myocardial infarction. In spite of the progress made with these non-invasive techniques, the number of patients who undergo a coronary angiogram before discharge has also increased. Coronary angiography, however, displays only the anatomy of the coronary arteries, giving no further information about the functional relevance of these stenoses.[7]

The functional significance of a stenosis in the infarct-related vessel is especially difficult to appreciate. Thrombolytic therapy has a high success rate in opening the occluded vessel but spontaneous fibrinolysis and reopening can also occur, although usually later. The degree of residual stenosis after fibrinolysis is unpredictable, and the viability status of the infarcted territory is quite variable. Radionuclide studies are capable of detecting the presence of residual myocardial ischaemia in or around the area of infarction as well as at a distance, and therefore of evaluating the significance of a lesion. Radionuclide studies can also differentiate between necrotic and viable tissue.

Investigations in patients with acute myocardial infarction are mainly designed to define management and to assess the possibility of improving the outcome by intervention. These investigations, percutaneous transluminal coronary angioplasty (PTCA) and coronary artery bypass graft (CABG), are now widely available and may be preferred to medical therapy depending on several parameters. Invasive interventions are preferred when large ischaemic areas around or at a distance from the acute myocardial infarction are detected.

Aim of sestamibi studies

After myocardial infarction, we need to evaluate the repercussion of necrosis, infarct size and left ventricular function (wall motion), to assess the extent of the coronary disease and the presence or absence of residual ischaemia. Studies with sestamibi allow us to answer these questions. Comparison of images obtained after injection of sestamibi at peak exercise and at rest give information about the presence, extent and location of ischaemia. By acquiring these images in gated mode, we can also gain information about regional left ventricular wall motion. Use of the first-pass technique in combination with the injection at rest also provides information about the right ventricle and about central circulatory dynamics. Persistence of ventricular dysfunction in areas of restored perfusion is suggestive of myocardial stunning. Persistence of a mild to moderate perfusion defect at rest can represent partial myocardial necrosis or can be evidence of a residual severe stenosis. Therefore evaluation of myocardial viability should be pursued to define the need for further revascularization.

Clinical Points

- **Major determinants of prognosis after myocardial infarction are infarct size, left ventricular ejection fraction and the presence or absence of residual ischaemia at a distance.**
- **All these variables can be determined with sestamibi scintigraphy.**

References

1 THE MULTI-CENTER POST-INFARCTION RESEARCH GROUP, Risk stratification and survival after myocardial infarction, *N Engl J Med* (1983) **309**:331.

2 NORRIS RM, BAINABY PF, BRAND PWT et al, Prognosis after recovery from first acute myocardial infarction determinants of reinfarction and sudden death, *Am J Cardiol* (1984) **53**:406.

3 FIORETTI P, BROWER RW, SIMOONS ML et al, Prediction of mortality during the first years after acute myocardial infarction from clinical variables and stress test at hospital discharge, *Am J Cardiol* (1985) **55**:1313.

4 PYROR DB, BRUCE RA, CHAITMAN BR et al, Task Force I: Determination of prognosis in patients with ischemic heart disease, *J Am Coll Cardiol* (1989) **14**: 1016.

5 JUNEAU M, THÉROUX P, GOLLES S et al, Maximal versus low level exercise testing after Q and non Q wave myocardial infarction, *J Am Coll Cardiol* (1991) **17**:21.

6 TOPOL EJ, JUNI JE, O'NEIL WW et al, Exercise testing three days after onset of acute myocardial infarction, *Am J Cardiol* (1987) **60**:958.

7 GIBSON RS, WATSON C, Events after uncomplicated myocardial infarction: A prospective study comparing predischarge exercise, thallium 201 scintigraphy and coronary angiography, *Circulation* (1983) **68**:321.

Case Study X.1

Small transmural inferior wall myocardial infarction without residual ischaemia

Mr A, a 53-year-old male, who smoked more than 25 cigarettes a day for more than 35 years, was admitted with an acute inferior wall infarction probably due to a distal occlusion in the right coronary artery (RCA) (no ST–T segment elevation in lead V4R, Fig. X.1a). His subsequent course was uneventful and the maximal AST level was 135 units/litre.

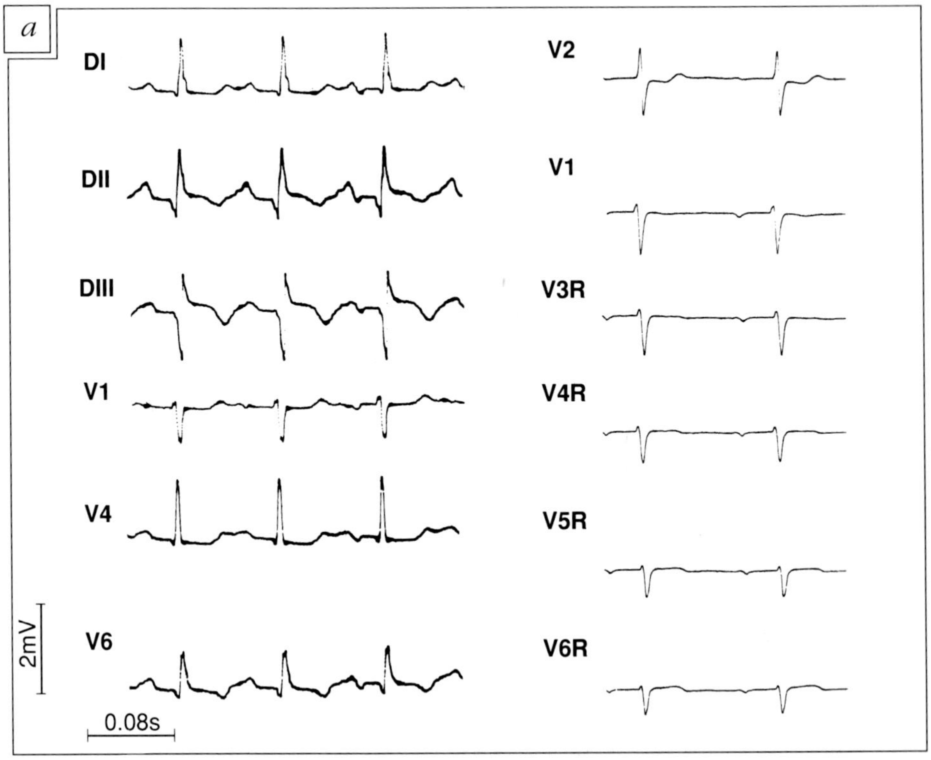

Before discharge, a treadmill exercise test combined with sestamibi scintigraphy was performed. The patient stopped after the second minute of stage IV of the Bruce protocol because of fatigue. The maximal heart rate was 150 beats/min and significant ST–T changes were seen in leads V4 and V6 (Fig. X.1b).

The sestamibi scans performed at rest and after exercise showed the same perfusion defect in the inferoposterior wall (Figs. X.1c,d, arrows) with no sign of residual ischaemia either in the region of or at a distance from the infarction.

Considering the small size of the infarction and the absence of residual symptoms or ischaemia as demonstrated by the sestamibi scan, it was decided to treat conservatively and discharge the patient without further exploration.

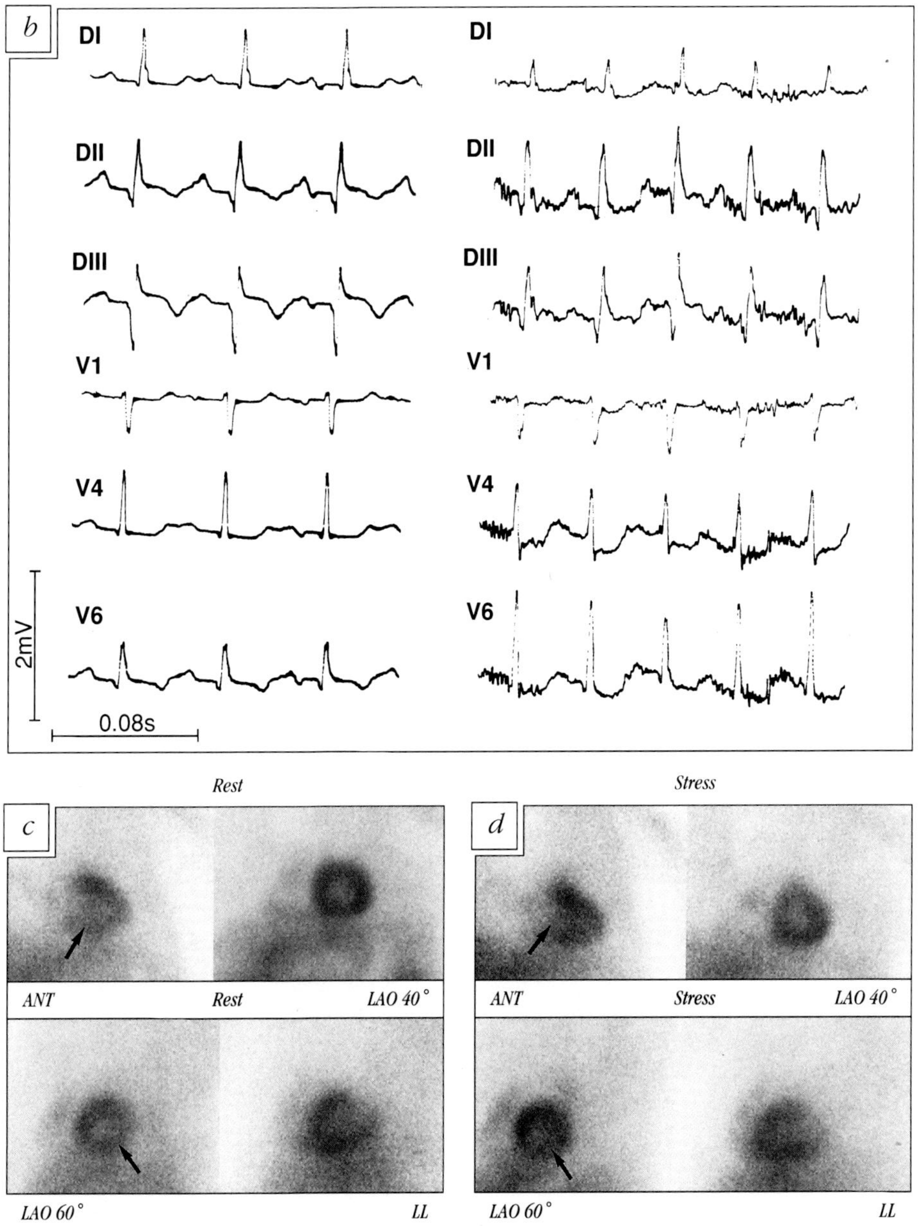

Case Study X.2

Transmural infarction without residual ischaemia

Mrs B, 63 years old and known to have stable anginal complaints, was admitted to hospital with chest pain unresponsive to nitrate administered sublingually. When she arrived in the hospital the pain had already been present for 12 h.

The ECG showed a picture of an acute inferoposterior infarction (Fig. X.2a). In spite of the delay, but because of the persistence of chest pain, thrombolytic therapy was administered but was not successful. Pain persisted and the ECG remained the same.

An angiogram performed on an emergency basis revealed a 99% stenosis in the RCA (Fig. X.2b, arrow) and a stenosis of approximately 60% in the left anterior descending (LAD) artery. The RCA was dilated successfully (Figs. X.2c,d, arrows) but ECG and enzymatic signs of an inferoposterior infarction persisted (Fig. X.2e).

Before discharge, an exercise test combined with tomographic sestamibi imaging was performed. A fixed defect in the inferolateroposterior wall compatible with the infarction without signs of ischaemia in the flow area of the LAD was found (Figs. X.2f,g, arrows).

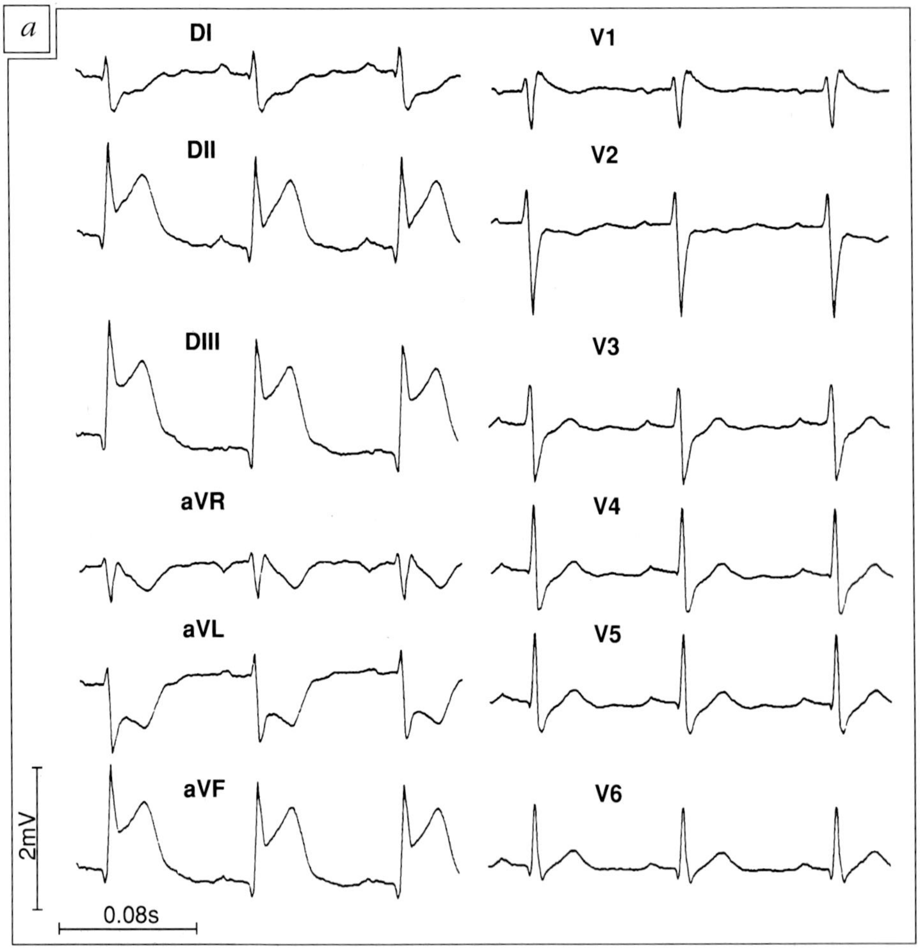

At admission

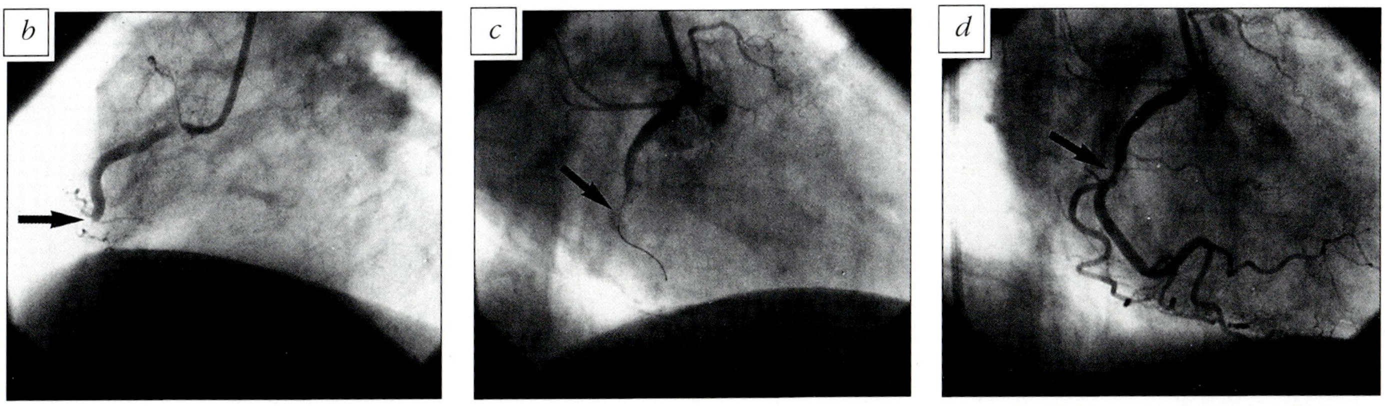

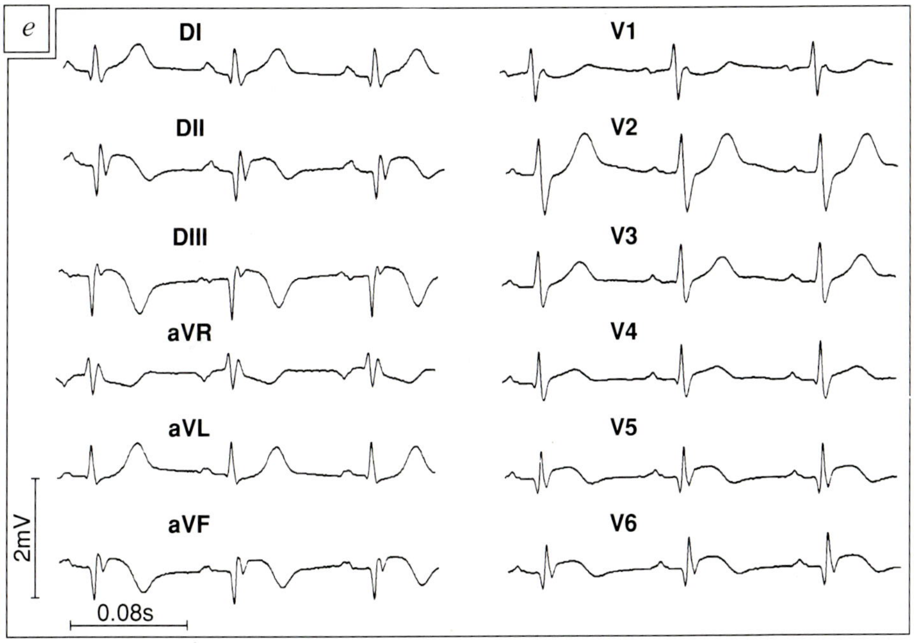

After angioplasty

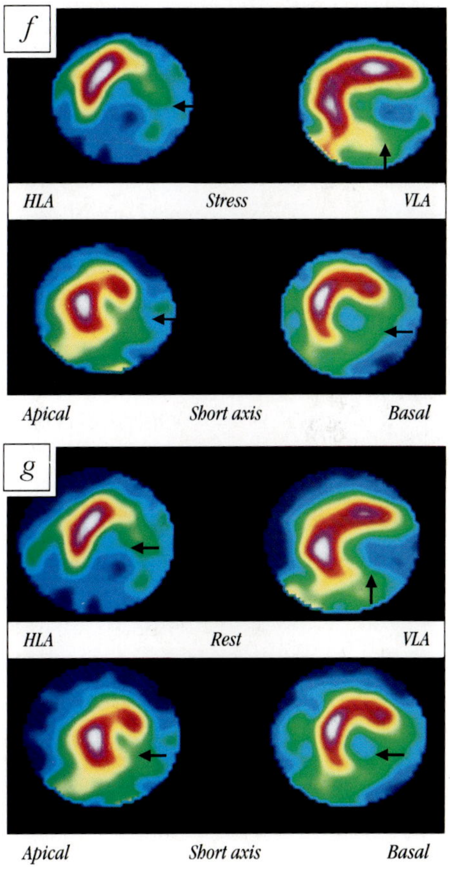

Case Study X.3

Transmural myocardial infarction with a left ventricular aneurysm and secondary ventricular fibrillation

Mrs L, a 62-year-old female, was admitted to hospital with an acute anteroseptal infarction (ECG, Fig. X.3a).

Treatment with intravenous streptokinase was unsuccessful, so the patient was brought to the catherization laboratory for investigation. An occluded proximal LAD was found (Fig. X.3b, arrow) which could not be passed by a guide wire catheter. She developed an anteroseptal infarction with signs of left ventricular dysfunction. The ECG showed intermittent right bundle branch block (Fig. X.3c), with a horizontal axis. Radionuclide ventriculography performed 4 days after admission showed increased systolic and diastolic volumes, dyskinesia of the anteroseptal wall and an abnormal left ventricular ejection fraction (27%, Fig. X.3d, arrows).

A rest and stress sestamibi tomographic scan demonstrated a large anteroseptal myocardial infarction with no additional ischaemia (Figs. X.3e,f, arrows).

Ten days after admission ventricular tachycardia started which deteriorated to ventricular fibrillation requiring defibrillation. These complications were heralded by the development of right bundle branch block, by the low left ventricular ejection fraction (<40%) and by the left ventricular aneurysm.

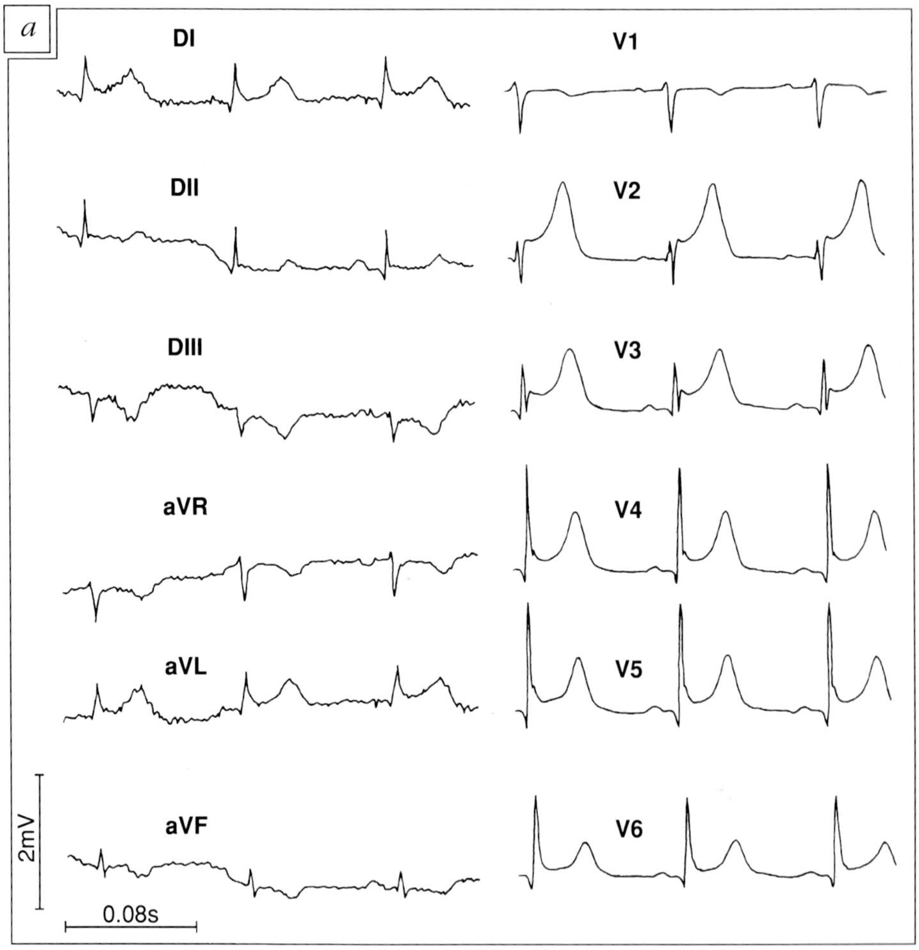

At admission

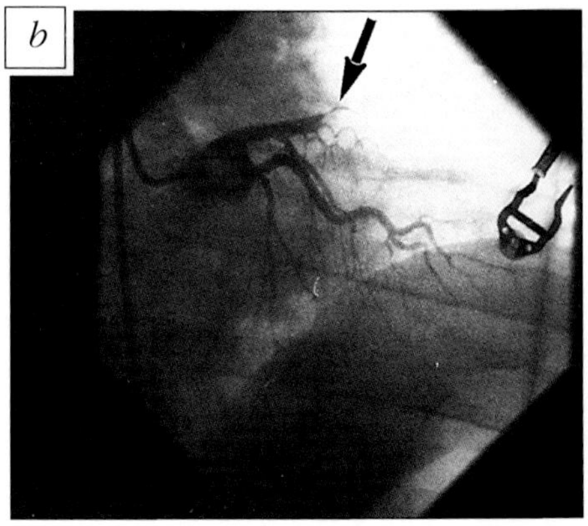

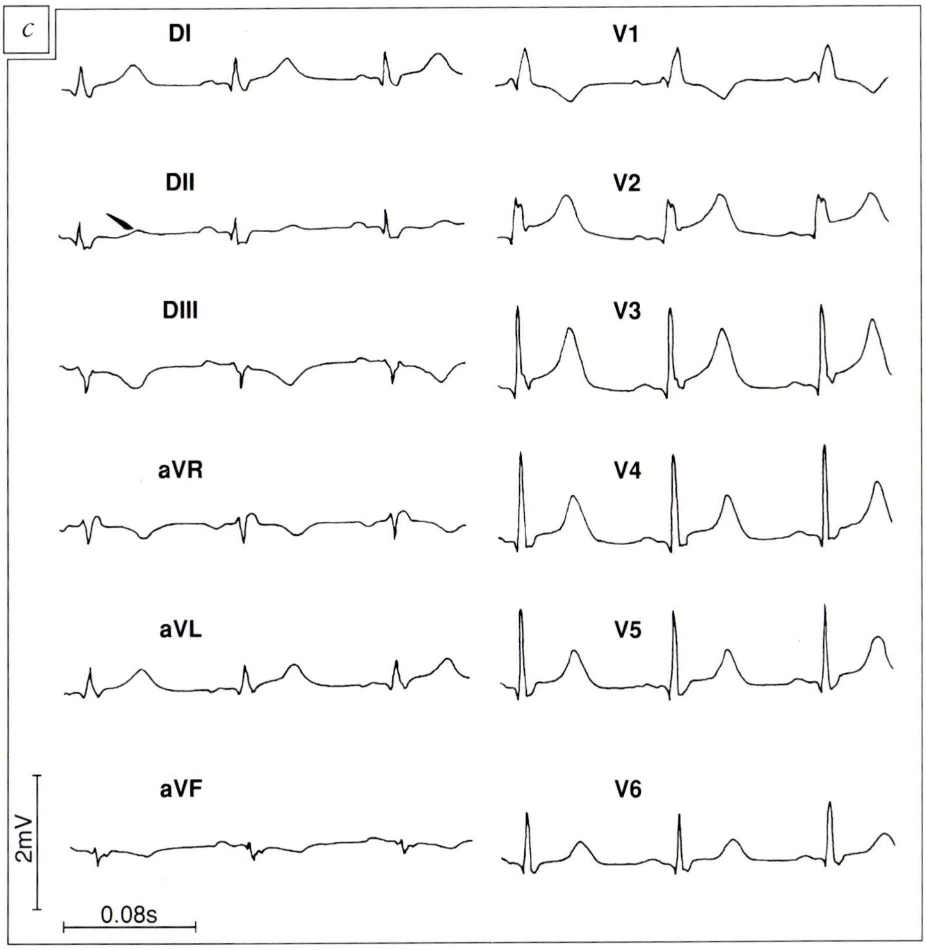
c
DI
DII
DIII
aVR
aVL
aVF
V1
V2
V3
V4
V5
V6
2mV
0.08s

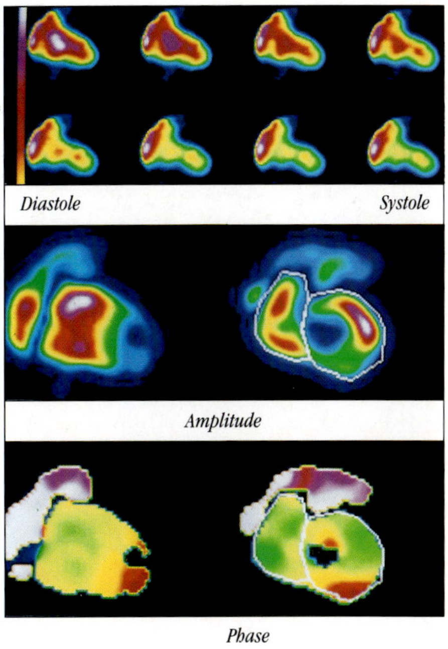
Diastole
Systole
Amplitude
Phase

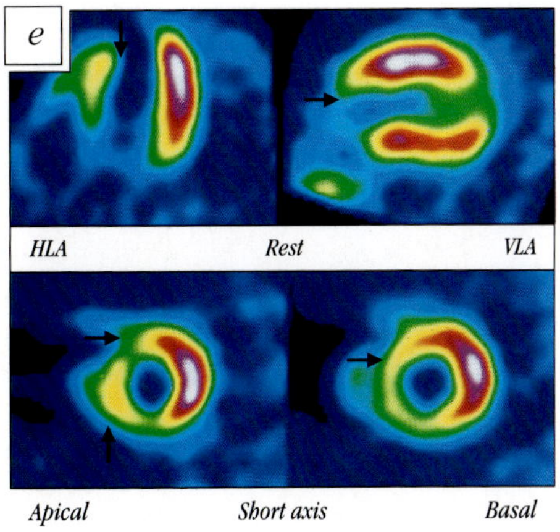
e
HLA
Rest
VLA
Apical
Short axis
Basal

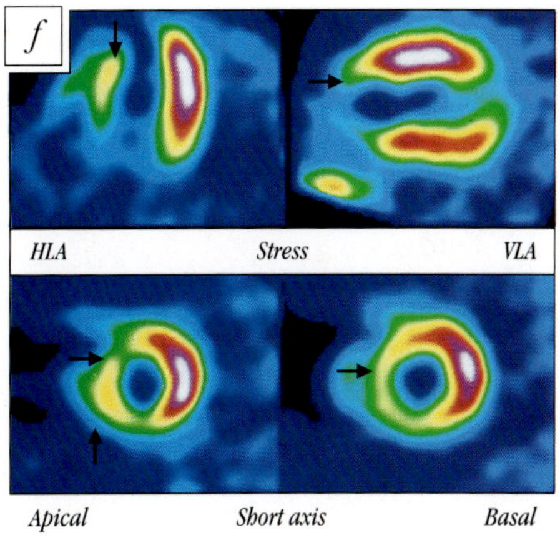
f
HLA
Stress
VLA
Apical
Short axis
Basal

Case Study X.4

Anterior wall myocardial infarction with residual ischaemia

Mrs C suffered an acute anterior wall myocardial infarction for which she received successful thrombolytic therapy. Coronary angiography showed luminal irregularities in the RCA and a 70% lesion in the left circumflex (LCx) artery, while the LAD showed a stenosis of approximately 50% (Fig. X.4a, arrows).

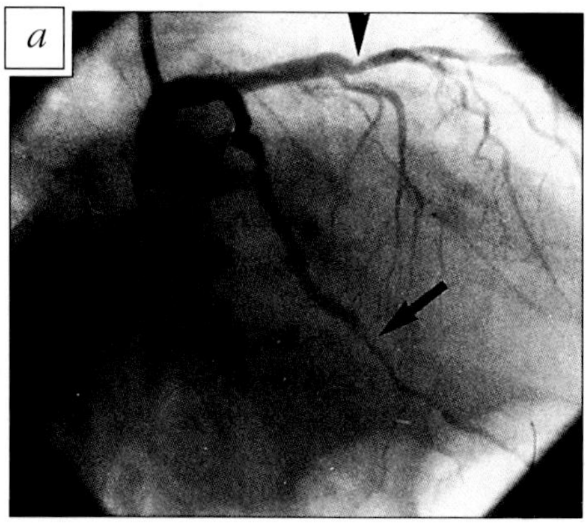

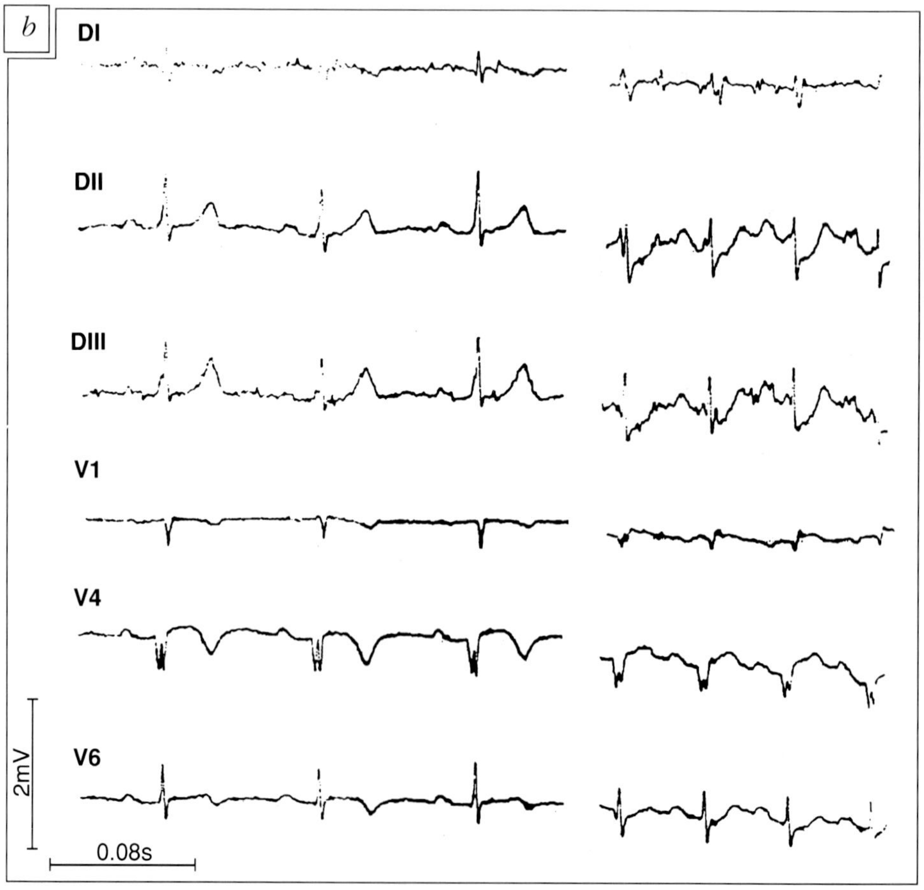

Rest *Stress*

The exercise test was performed on a treadmill 2 weeks after the myocardial infarction. She walked up to 1 min of Stage III of the Bruce protocol. The heart rate went up to a maximal value of 140 beats/min and there was a normal blood pressure response. The ECG showed pseudonormalization of a negative T-wave in leads V4 and V6 (Fig. X.4b). Sestamibi tomography demonstrated larger perfusion defects at stress than at rest (in the anteroseptal wall of the LV) corresponding to myocardial ischaemia around the infarct area (Figs. X.4c,d, arrows). The LCx stenosis was not considered as functionally significant and this opinion was confirmed by the normal perfusion pattern in that area.

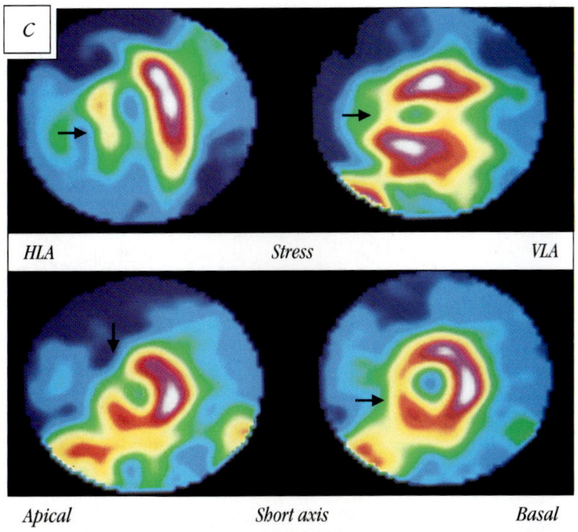

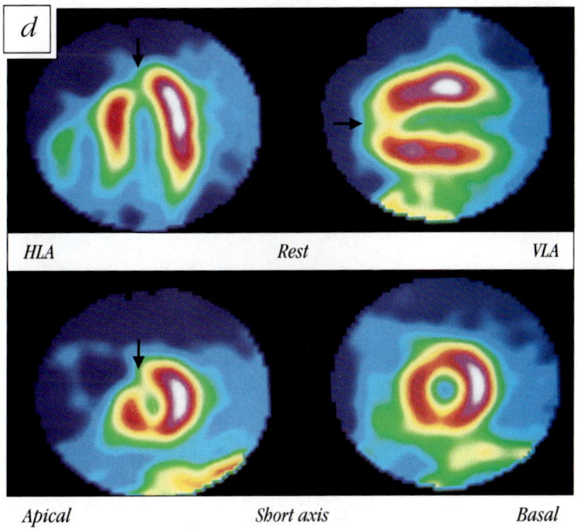

Case Study X.5

Transmural myocardial infarction with residual ischaemia

Mr G, 67 years old, was admitted 2 weeks earlier with an acute inferior wall myocardial infarction treated successfully by thrombolysis.

A treadmill exercise test was performed. He walked until the end of stage IV of the Bruce protocol. The heart rate went up to 150 beats/min. The patient stopped because of fatigue. The ECG showed ST elevation in leads DII and DIII, suggestive of abnormal inferior wall motion (Fig. X.5a). Sestamibi demonstrated stress defects in the inferoposterior and lateral walls of the LV while at rest perfusion defects were smaller and involved only the inferoposterior wall (Figs. X.5b,c, arrows).

In this patient the inferior myocardial infarction was treated successfully by fibrinolysis, but signs of residual ischaemia in the periphery of the infarct were present. However, because of the absence of anginal complaints, and because the patient showed good exercise tolerance, it was decided to keep him on medical therapy with regular follow-up.

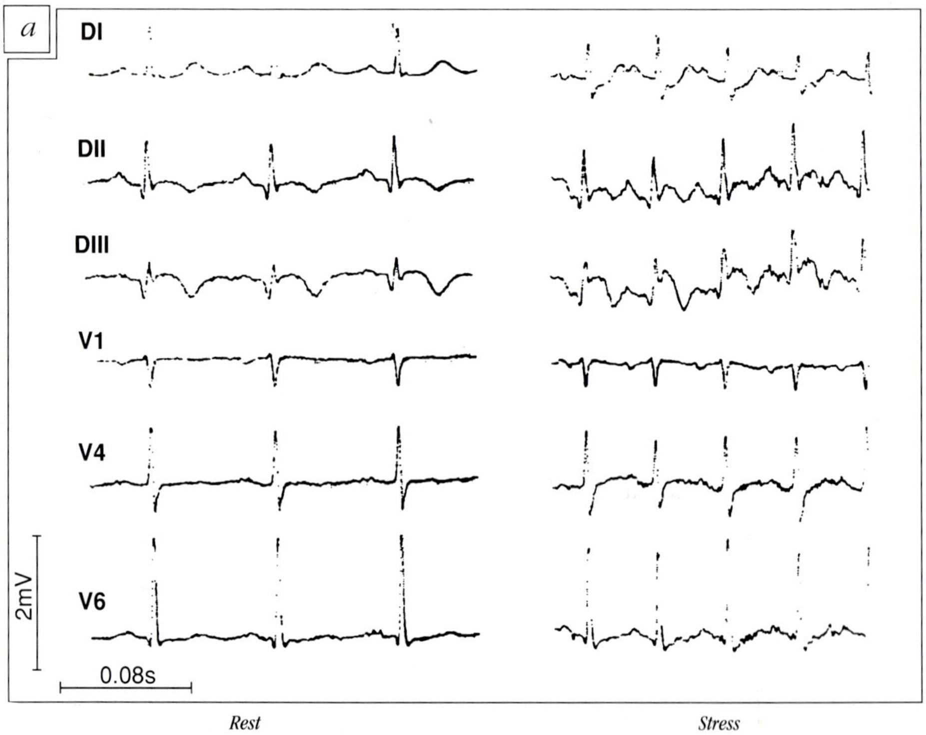

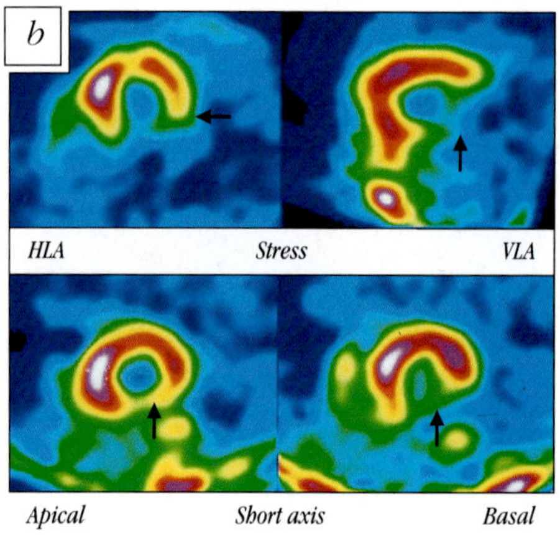

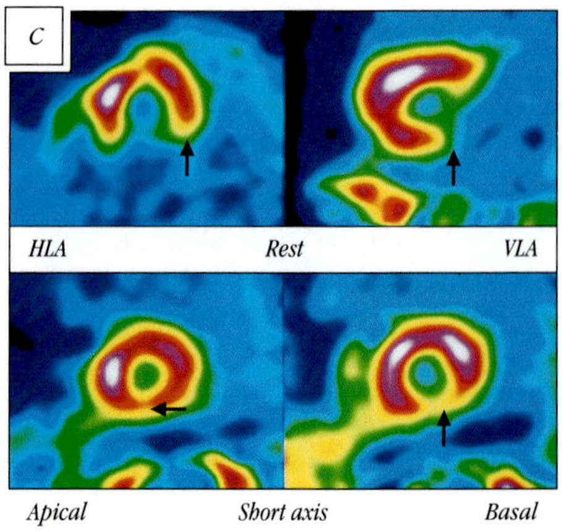

Case Study X.6

Myocardial infarction with residual ischaemia in another vessel territory

Mr LM suffered in the past from a small inferior wall myocardial infarction. He then complained of recurrent chest pain radiating to his left shoulder and a stress sestamibi study was performed.

The ECG at rest showed aspecific ST–T wave changes (Fig. X.6a). The patient exercised to a workload of 90 W. His pulse rate went to 100 beats/min with a normal blood pressure response. He stopped for dyspnoea and angina pectoris. The ECG recorded during stress and recovery showed significant changes in several leads (Fig. X.6a).

The sestamibi tomogram showed stress perfusion defects involving the lateral, the inferoposterior and the inferior walls of the LV (Fig. X.6b, arrows). At rest smaller defects involving the inferior and the inferoposterior walls only were present, suggestive of an inferior myocardial infarction with lateral ischaemia (Fig. X.6c, arrows).

The coronary angiogram showed triple vessel disease and the patient was referred for CABG (Figs. X.6d,e, arrows).

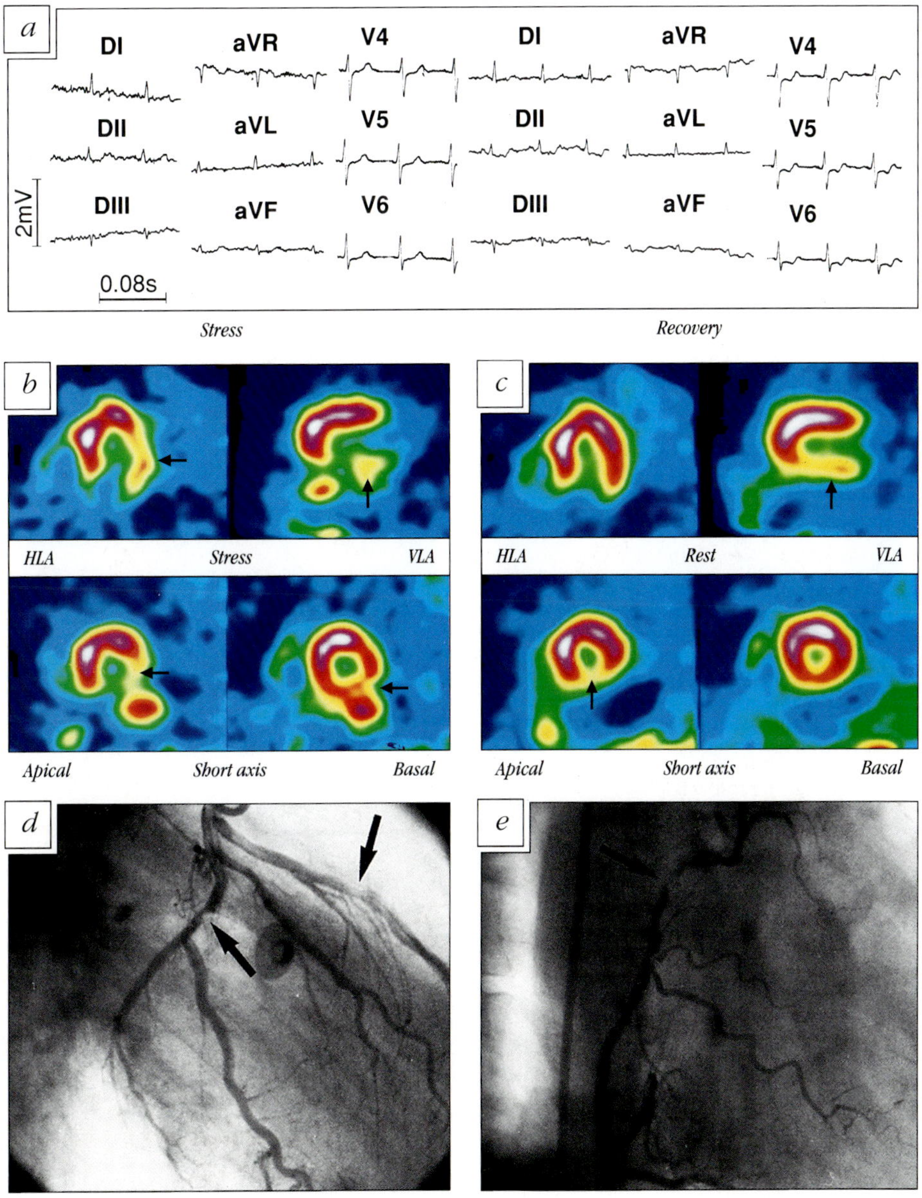

Case Study X.7

Myocardial infarction probably resulting from coronary artery spasm

A 29-year-old female visited the casualty department of our hospital because of episodes of chest pain.

The ECG showed an AV nodal escape as well as a sinus rhythm with signs suggestive of a recent inferoposterior wall myocardial infarction (Fig. X.7a).

The patient was referred to the coronary unit where the pain became exaggerated and the ECG showed new signs of an acute AS infarction (Fig. X.7b). Thrombolytic therapy was given as the pain did not react on administration of nitroglycerin intravenously.

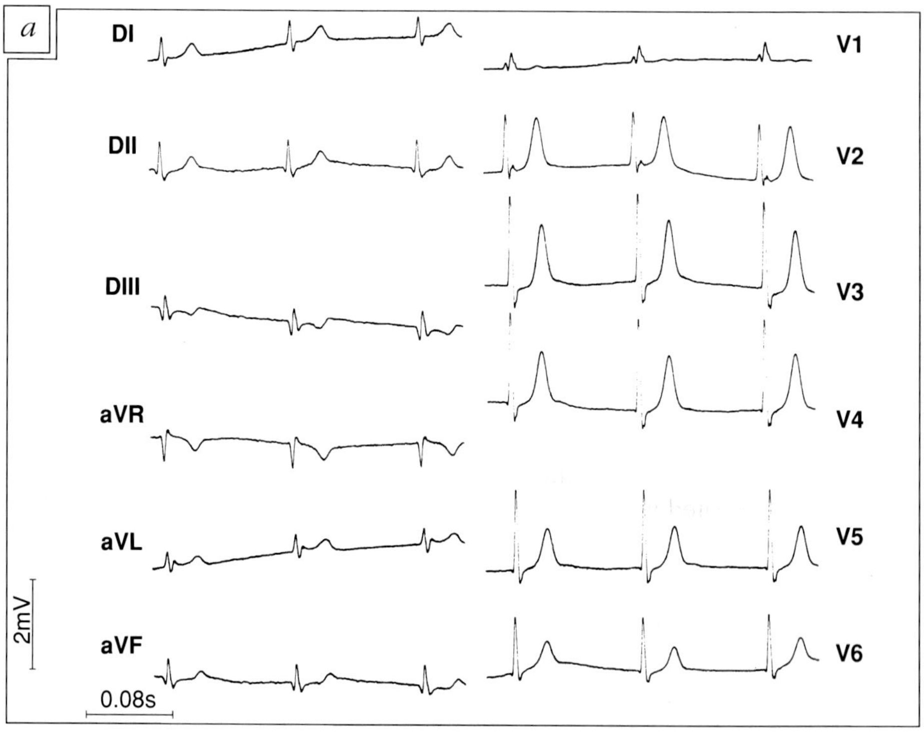

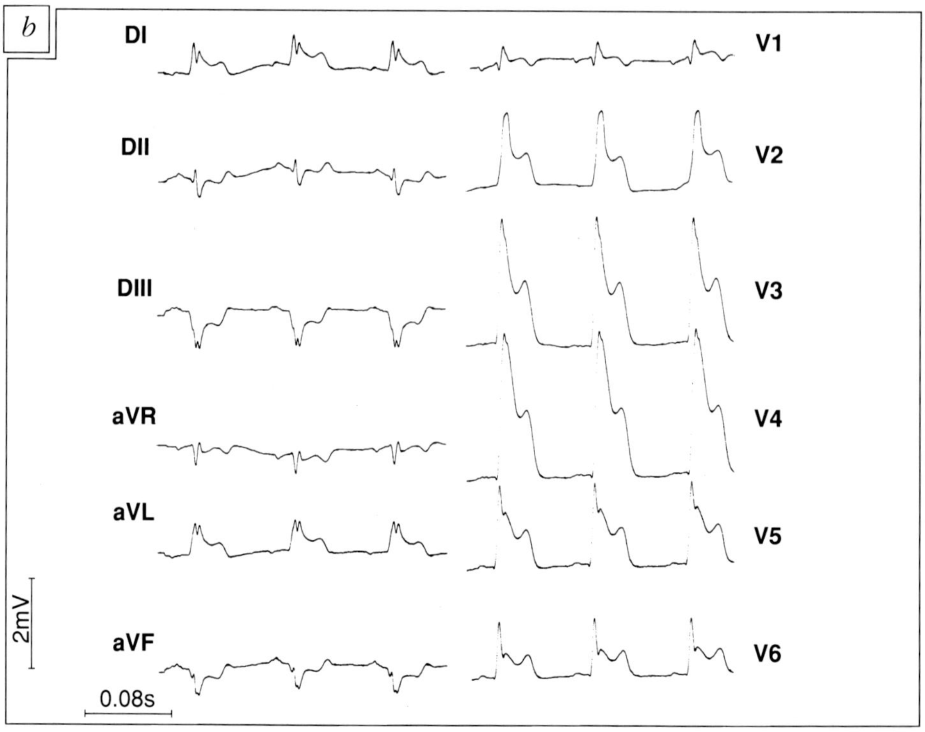

The pain disappeared after 15 min and the ECG returned to baseline (Fig. X.7c). There was no enzyme rise and a sestamibi tomographic scan showed a fixed defect in the inferoposterior wall of the LV corresponding to myocardial infarction without residual ischaemia (Figs. X.7d,e, arrows). The perfusion pattern was normal in the LAD territory, implying successful thrombolysis.

Catheterization demonstrated hypokinesia of the inferior wall with normal coronary arteries and the patient is now treated with high doses of calcium antagonists.

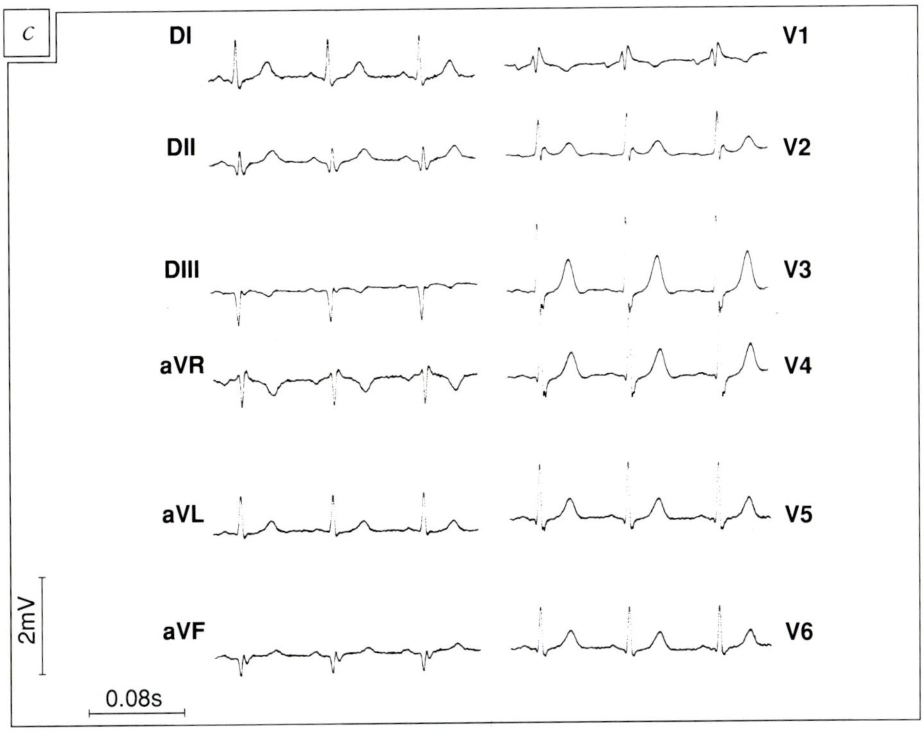

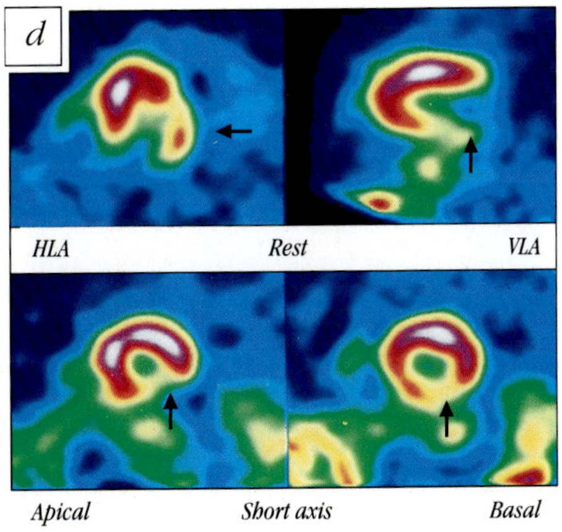

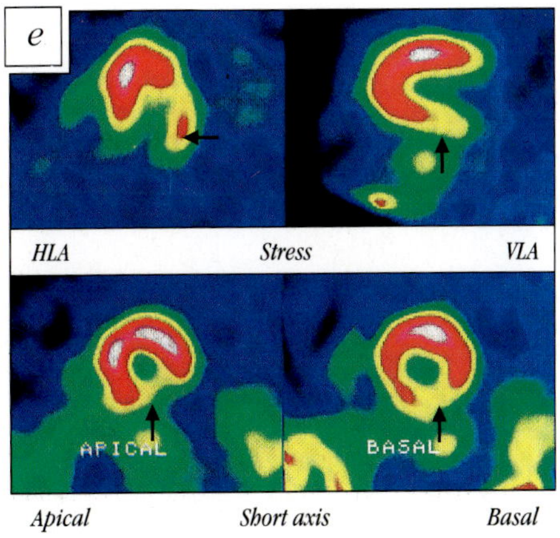

Case Study X.8

Transmural myocardial infarction with myocardial ischaemia inducing ventricular arrhythmia

A 59-year-old male known to have had an inferior wall myocardial infarction for 3 years experienced recurrent anginal complaints with exercise and in the cold for 6 weeks.

Exercise test combined with sestamibi imaging was done. Several ventricular premature beats (VPB) were present at rest (Fig. X.8a). He reached the second minute of stage III of the Bruce protocol and stopped because of chest pain. The ECG showed significant ST–T segment changes. Sestamibi was injected but thereafter the patient developed ventricular tachycardia (Fig. X.8b) which deteriorated to ventricular fibrillation. After defibrillation and resuscitation, sinus rhythm was restored and ECG changes were even more marked (Fig. X.8c). Sestamibi scan showed an irreversible inferior wall defect and a reversible posterolateral defect compatible with ischaemia in the LCx vessel territory (Figs. X.8d,e, arrows). The coronary angiogram confirmed these data as it showed an occluded RCA and significant stenosis of the LCx (Fig. X.8f, arrows).

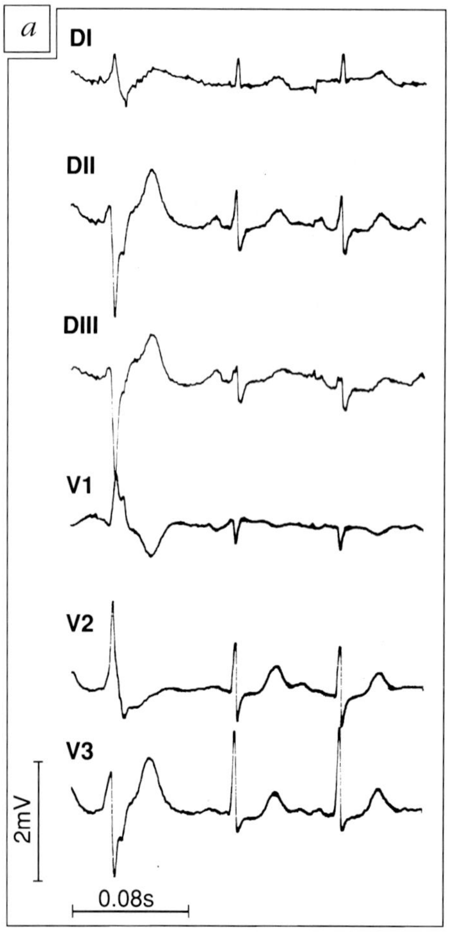

Rest

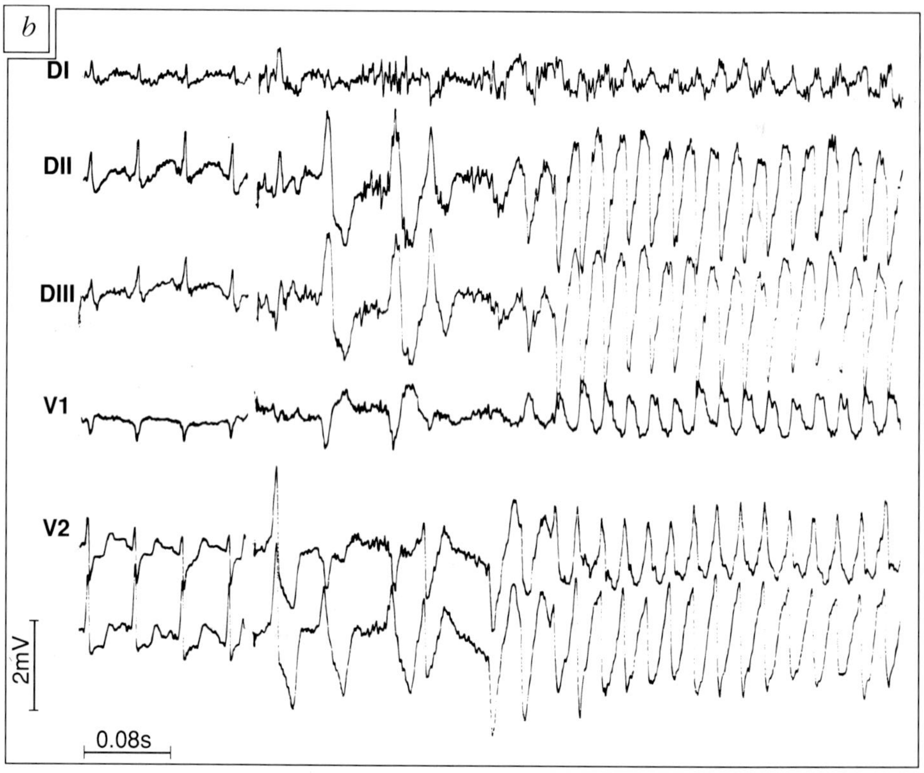

Peak exercise

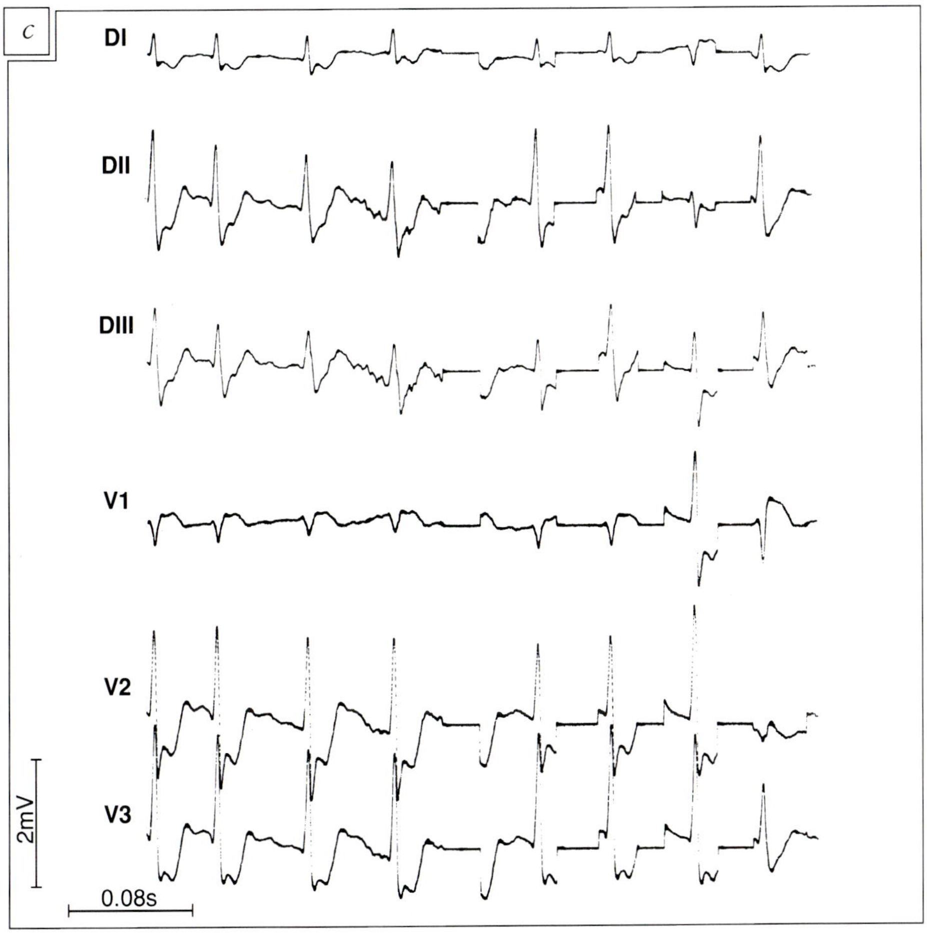
c
DI
DII
DIII
V1
V2
V3
2mV
0.08s

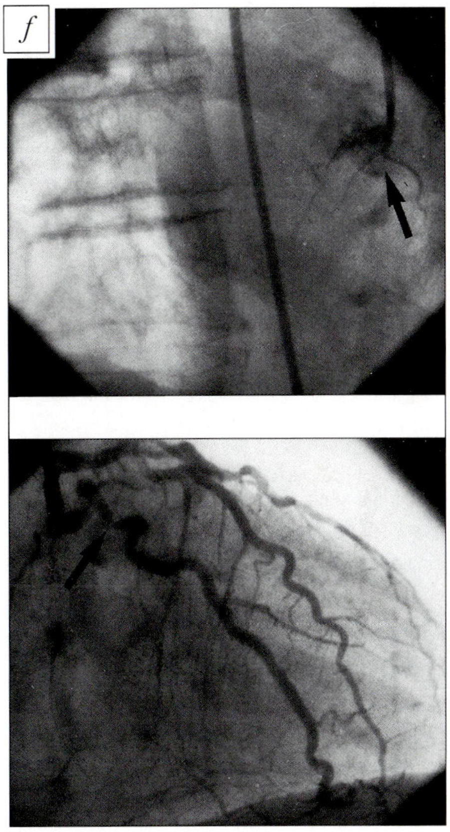
f

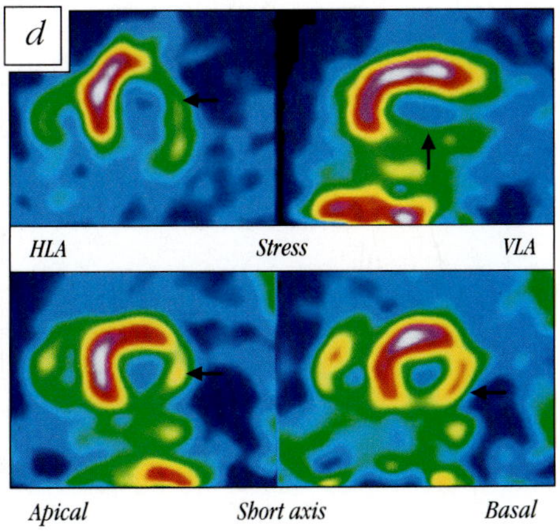
d
HLA
Stress
VLA
Apical
Short axis
Basal

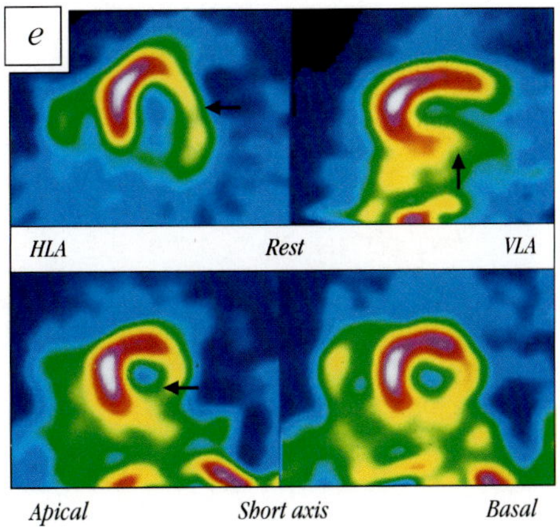
e
HLA
Rest
VLA
Apical
Short axis
Basal

Case Study X.9

Large inferoposterior myocardial infarction

A 35-year-old male had a long episode of anginal complaints 2 weeks before he visited the outpatient cardiology clinic for the first time.

After this episode the patient remained free of complaints. However, his ECG showed signs of an old inferoposterior infarction (Fig. X.9a). To detect the presence or absence of residual ischaemia, an exercise test combined with planar sestamibi scintigraphy was done.

Rest and stress images showed the same inferoposterior perfusion defect, compatible with the ECG and corresponding to myocardial infarction (Figs. X.9b,c, arrows). In spite of these results, but with regard to his young age, a coronary angiogram was made which showed a subtotal stenosis in the proximal part of the right dominant coronary artery (Fig. X.9d, arrow), but no other lesion in the left system.

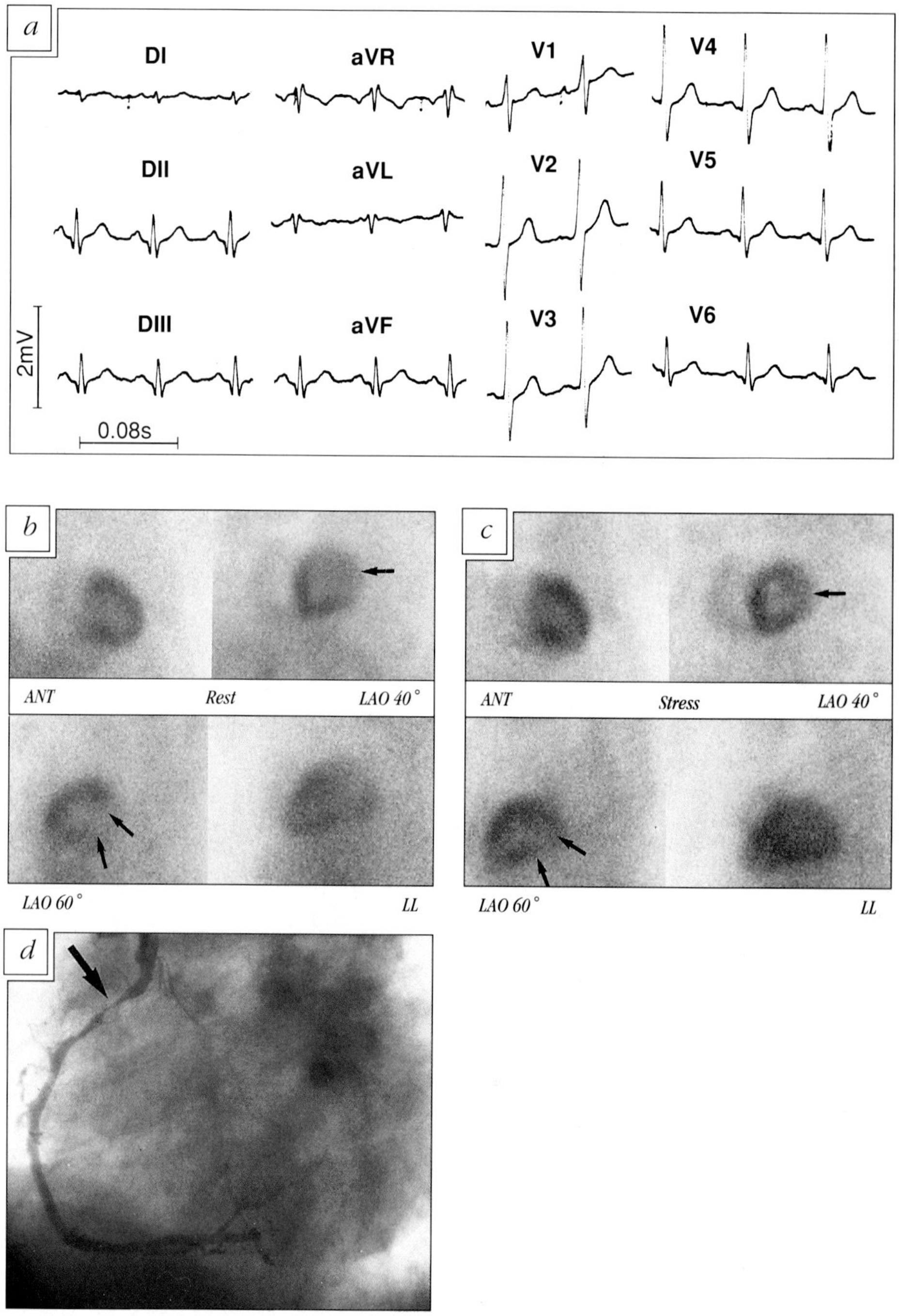

11 ASSESSMENT OF THE EFFICACY OF THROMBOLYSIS

Clinical Background

Concepts of ischaemia and infarction: historical development

Myocardial necrosis as a consequence of acute myocardial infarction remains a major cause of death and morbidity in patients with coronary disease. During the evolutionary process to myocardial necrosis, initial reversible phases lead to 'completed infarction' at the end of a continuum of myocardial injury.

In patients with acute myocardial infarction (AMI) the long-term outcome has been evaluated in many studies. Clearly defined goals of current approaches base their principles on a proven clear relationship between infarct extent and future complications and outcome.[1–3]

Cardiology in the 1990s will therefore include an active therapeutic component to modify the chain of events at an early stage of evolving infarction. One of the major determinants is final ventricular function as a result of the relationship between 'areas at risk', i.e. the territories of irreversibly damaged myocardium versus the additional tissue which may have been spared or salvaged by an intervention but may still be in jeopardy from future ischaemic events.[4]

Thus, early interventions, such as thrombolysis or percutaneous transluminal coronary angioplasty (PTCA), to salvage myocardium otherwise threatened by necrosis, play an important role in the treatment of AMI. In addition, individual risk stratification plays a major role in many interventional strategies.[5–7]

Although the experimental and conceptual determinants of the area at risk are well defined, the clinical situation is far more complex and more difficult to assess (see Table 11.1).

- The acute event is often the result or the end point of a long history of coronary disease with perhaps multiple lesions.
- Collateral supply, vascular tone and sensitivity to humoral or neural stimuli may be different.

Table 11.1
Variables of ischaemia and necrosis. It is almost impossible to predict the severity and extent of ischaemic injury.

Time and site of flow reduction
Collateral flow
Vascular tone
Heart rate and metabolic demand
Hypertrophy
Sensitivity to humoral and neural stimuli
Wall stress at time of ischaemia

Hypertrophy, heart rate and wall stress are additional variables affecting the extent of necrosis. Severity and extent of an ischaemic injury are therefore difficult to predict and highly variable, even when time and site of occlusion are known. Also, autopsy data of non-survivors of AMI reveal a significant variability in the extent of the area of necrosis within the area at risk.

Assessment of the area at risk

Although history, ECG and enzyme studies are still cornerstones for the diagnosis of MI, these conventional indicators may exhibit inherent conceptual limitations. Late ventricular function has been shown to be one important prognostic parameter. The described development of new therapeutic regimens following the concepts of at least partial salvage of myocardium to reduce infarct size has led to widespread acceptance and clinical use of strategies such as thrombolysis and PTCA. The aims of these regimens are to reduce damage, modify prognosis and avoid further ischaemia. To achieve these aims it is important to have suitable methods and criteria with which to identify early those patients who have benefited from an intervention, and to stratify those who are likely to need aggressive treatment for the prevention of future damage.

Radionuclide methods have been shown to be helpful in this respect, as they can be performed non-invasively at the bedside. Perfusion imaging with ^{201}Tl before and following reperfusion has shown reduction of the perfusion abnormalities by thrombolytic treatment but has been hampered by the physiological properties of the tracer, in particular the 'redistribution' phenomenon. Ventricular function has been shown to be quite variable shortly after the event and serial assessments of ventricular function have shown a significant variability of the late functional outcome due to ongoing repair processes and partial or complete spontaneous restoration of blood flow.[8,9]

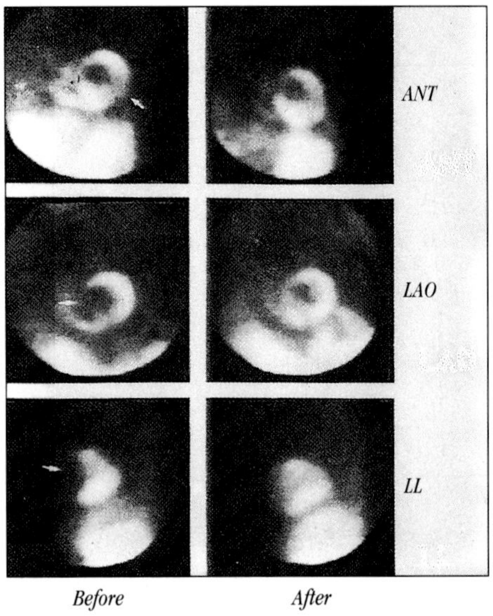

Figure 11.1
Assessment of the area at risk before and after thrombolytic therapy: pre-treatment images show large perfusion abnormality in the anteroseptal walls; post-treatment injection delineates major salvage by improvement of perfusion. (From Wackers et al[8], with permission.)

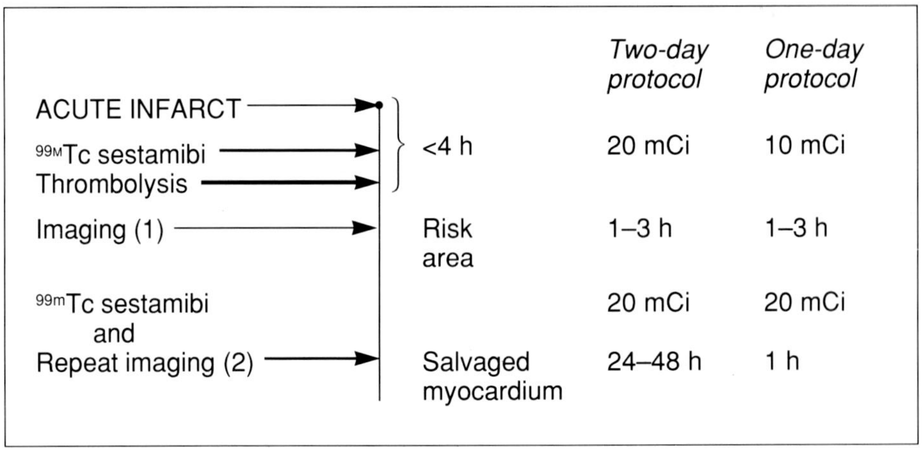

Figure 11.2
Serial ^{99m}Tc sestamibi imaging for assessment of thrombolysis showing two- and one-day protocols.

Aims of Sestamibi Studies

With the advent of the radiotracer sestamibi, for the first time an approach is available that can document the status of perfusion (at the time before an intervention), allow later imaging of this initial area at risk without delaying essential treatment, and facilitate the assessment of individual treatment effects by comparative images obtained after a second injection (Fig. 11.1).[9]

Figure 11.2 illustrates such an approach that has already been tested by several institutions, in particular in a multicentre trial involving investigators at Yale University School of Medicine, the Mayo Clinic and Baylor College of Medicine. These studies clearly demonstrate that sestamibi can provide information on the myocardial area at risk and the extent of myocardial salvage after thrombolysis.[10,11]

Additionally, a preceding first-pass study (by acquisition of the same injected dose of the late study when the patient has stabilized) can be used to evaluate function shortly after thrombolysis.

Case XI.2 highlights an alternative approach where no acute, i.e. pre-treatment, sestamibi study is done, but where an intermediate (24–48 h) study is used to document the status of perfusion following the intervention. An additional pre-discharge exercise study will then be used to assess recurrent ischaemia as an aid to risk stratification.

Findings of these important studies indicate that:

- Patients with AMI, whether or not treated with thrombolysis, show a marked variation of area at risk. It is noteworthy that the extent of that initial perfusion defect could not be predicted by clinical variables in the emergency room, the location of infarction, or the site of occlusion of the infarct-related artery.
- Patients with open infarct-related arteries showed a significantly larger decrease in defect size than patients with an occluded artery. Equally important, patients with sestamibi perfusion defect sizes <30% on planar imaging had open infarct-related vessels, providing potential important information for later management.
- Sestamibi imaging at various time points (18–48 h, 6–14 days) (Fig. 11.3) following the acute event also demonstrated further late decrease in defect size (before discharge), suggesting either continued improvement of blood flow or resolution of metabolic derangements in ^{99m}Tc sestamibi transport or intracellular binding.
- Other studies using SPECT techniques found a significant correlation ($r = -0.82$, $P = 0.0002$) between the final amount of hypoperfused myocardium (that evident at 6–14 days) and the late resting ejection fraction and confirm the ability of such an approach to document the amount of salvage as well as the amount of hypoperfused myocardium (Fig. 11.4).[11]

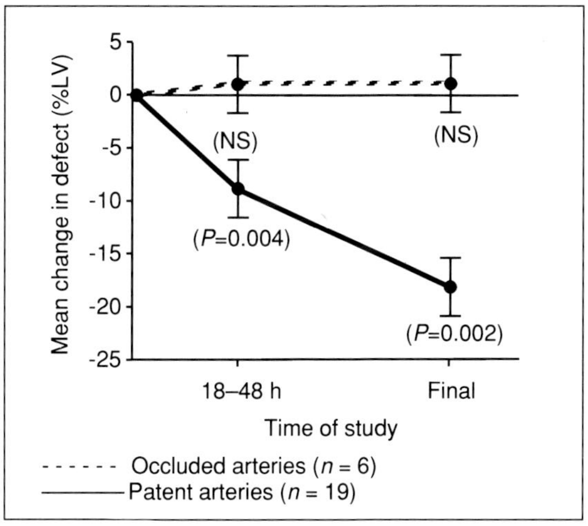

Figure 11.3
Sequential change in SPECT ^{99m}Tc sestamibi defect size. (From Pellikka et al,[12] with permission.)

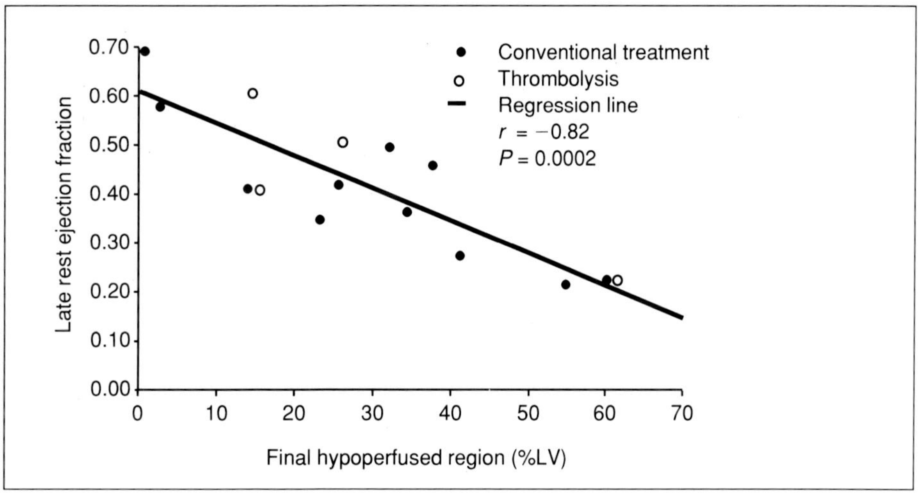

Figure 11.4
Final ^{99m}Tc sestamibi defect size vs late rest ejection fraction. (From Gibbons et al,[11] with permission)

Summary

In summary, the amount of myocardium 'at risk' is an important parameter in the assessment of myocardial ischaemia and injury. This myocardium 'at risk' shows a wide variation from patient to patient and cannot be predicted by other frequently used approaches, such as clinical presentation in the emergency room, the location of infarction or the site of angiographic occlusion.

Sestamibi permits non-invasive assessment of the amount of hypoperfused myocardium, when injected during acute occlusion early in evolving MI, prior to administration of the therapeutic thrombolytic agent. This approach is feasible without further delaying therapy due to the characteristics of the tracer. When a decrease in the extent of the sestamibi perfusion defect is observed, successful reperfusion and salvage of jeopardized myocardium are suggested.

Clinical Points

- ^{99m}Tc sestamibi defect size during coronary occlusion delineates the 'area at risk'.
- Myocardium 'at risk' after MI varies greatly.
- A decrease in ^{99m}Tc sestamibi defect indicates reperfusion and myocardial salvage.

References

1 CIGARROA RG, LANGE RA, HILLIS LD, Prognosis after acute myocardial infarction in patients with and without residual antegrade coronary blood flow, *Am J Cardiol* (1989) **64**:155.

2 GELTMAN EM, EHSANI A, CAMPBELL MK, SCHECHTMANN K et al, The influence of location and extent of myocardial infarction on long term ventricular dysrhythmia and mortality, *Circulation* (1979) **60**:805.

3 KANNEL WB, SORLIE P, MCNAMARA PM, Prognosis after initial myocardial infarction: the Framingham study, *Am J Cardiol* (1979) **44**:53.

4 MULTICENTER POSTINFARCTION RESEARCH GROUP, Risk stratification and survival after myocardial infarction, *N Engl J Med* (1983) **309**:331.

5 TIMI RESEARCH GROUP, Immediate vs delayed catheterization and angioplasty following thrombolytic therapy for acute myocardial infarction, *JAMA* (1988) **260**:2849.

6 ISAM STUDY GROUP, A prospective trial of intravenous streptokinase in acute myocardial infarction (ISAM): mortality, morbidity, and infarct size at 21 days, *N Engl J Med* (1986) **314**:1465.

7 WILLIAMS DO, BORER J, BRAUNWALD E, Intravenous recombinant tissue-plasminogen activator in patients with acute myocardial infarction: a report from the NHLBI thrombolysis in acute myocardial infarction trial, *Circulation* (1986) **73**:338.

8 WACKERS FJ, GIBBONS RJ, VERANI MS et al, Serial quantitative planar technetium-99m isonitrile imaging in acute myocardial infarction, *J Am Coll Cardiol* (1989) **14**:861.

9 Kayden DS, MALTERA JA, ZARET B, WACKERS FJT, Demonstration of reperfusion after thrombolysis with technetium-99m isonitrile myocardial imaging, *J Nucl Med* (1988) **29**:1865.

10 WACKERS FJT, Thrombolytic therapy for myocardial infarction: assessment of efficacy by myocardial perfusion imaging with technetium-99m sestamibi, *Am J Cardiol* (1990) **66**:36E.

11 GIBBONS RJ, VERANI MS, BEHRENBECK T et al, Feasibility of tomographic Tc-99m-hexakis-2-methoxy-2-methylpropyl-isonitrile imaging for the assessment of myocardial area at risk and the effect of treatment in acute myocardial infarction, *Circulation* (1989) **80**:1277.

12 PELLIKKA PA, BEHRENBECK T, SVERANI M et al, Serial changes in myocardial perfusion using tomographic technetium-99m-hexakis-2-methoxy-2-methylprop-yl-isonitrile imaging following reperfusion therapy of myocardial infarction, *J Nucl Med* (1990) **31**:1269.

Case Study XI.1

Interest of sestamibi imaging to document the value of thrombolysis

A 50-year-old male arrived in the emergency department suffering from chest pain that had been present for the last 2 h. He was overweight and smoked 30 cigarettes a day. There was no known history of myocardial infarction and the ECG showed ST abnormalities in the anterior leads and supraventricular and ventricular arrhythmias (Fig. XI.1a).

The patient was admitted to the CCU and experienced further chest pain. The ECG changed and showed ST-segment elevation from lead V1 to lead V6 (Fig. XI.1b). This was an impending anterior myocardial infarction requiring rapid thrombolytic treatment. To evaluate the area at risk and the results of the thrombolytic therapy, sestamibi was injected prior to thrombolysis. This did not delay the treatment as imaging could start after treatment was underway. The first sestamibi study performed in these conditions demonstrated an extensive anteroseptal area at risk in the anterior and LAO 40° projections (Fig. XI.1c, left panel). The follow-up study performed 1 day later indicated a practically complete salvage of the myocardium (Fig. XI.1c, right panel). The first angiogram performed 60 min after the beginning of tissue plasminogen activator (TPA) infusion still showed a complete proximal LAD occlusion correlating with the initial set of images obtained 1 h later (Figs. XI.1d and XI.1c, left panel). Angiographic control performed 24 h after infusion revealed an open infarct-related vessel with a high-grade proximal LAD stenosis (Fig. XI.1e). These findings also correlated with the significant improvement of myocardial perfusion observed on the second set of perfusion images (Fig. XI.1c, right panel). As the patient exhibited exercise-induced ischaemia on pre-discharge exercise-ECG test, the high-grade LAD lesion was subsequently dilated successfully with PTCA (Figs. XI.1f,g).

This case study highlights the value of sestamibi in measuring the area at risk and in documenting the results of thrombolytic therapy.

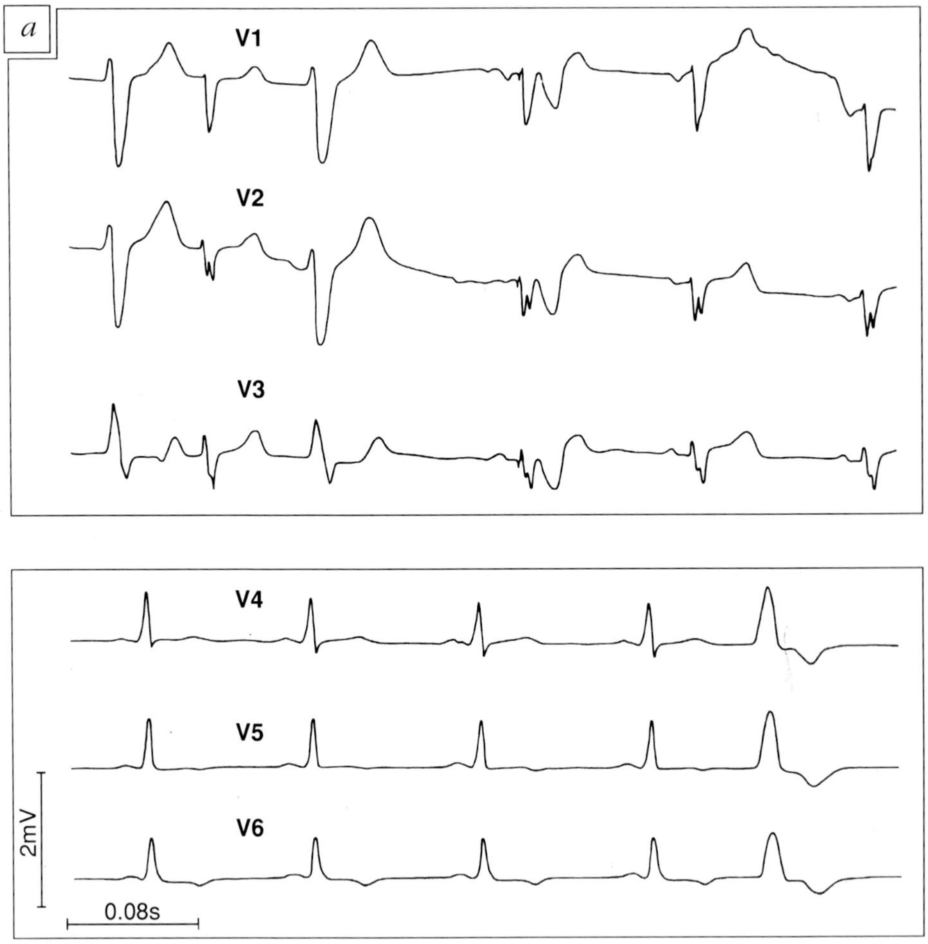

ECG at admission

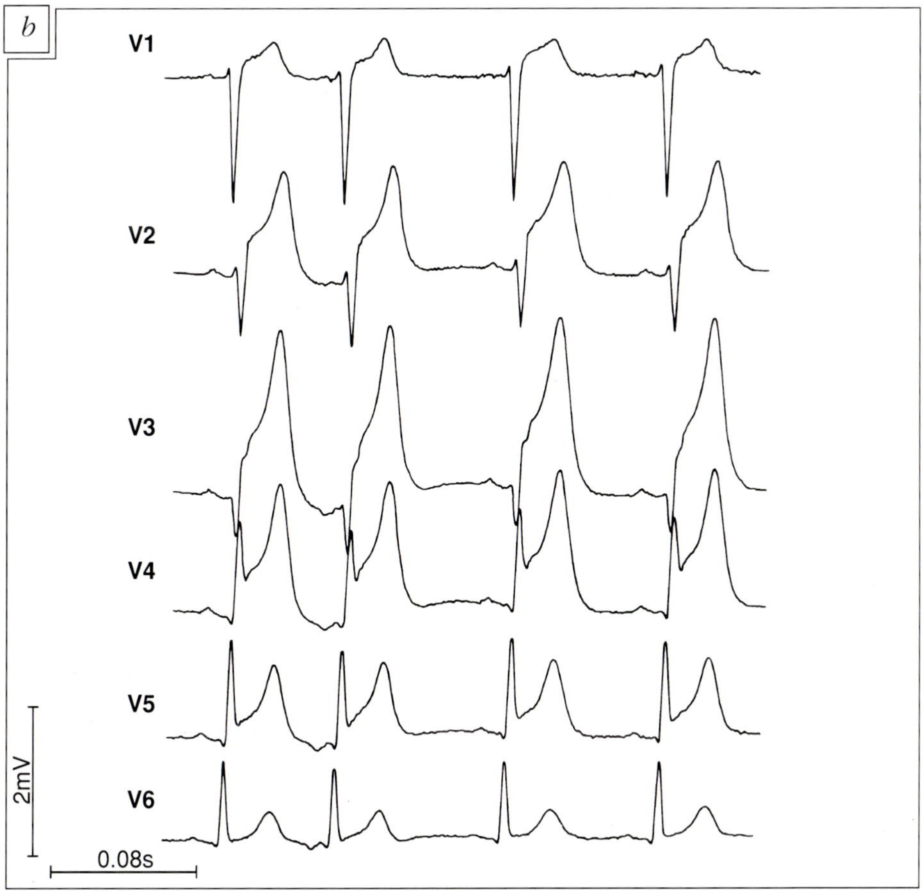

ECG during pain

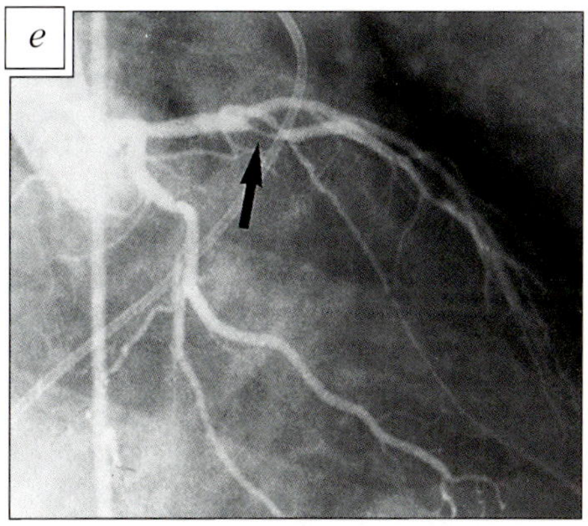

24 h after TPA

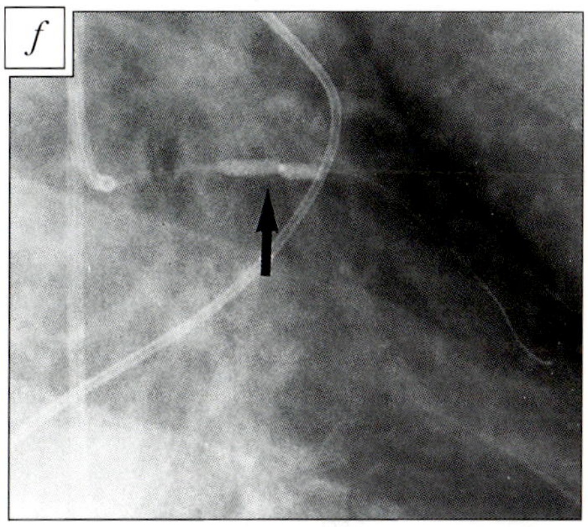

During PTCA

Anterior

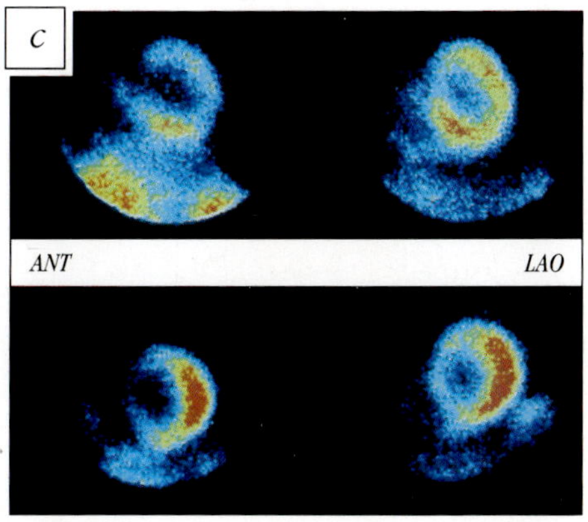

Before TPA *After TPA*

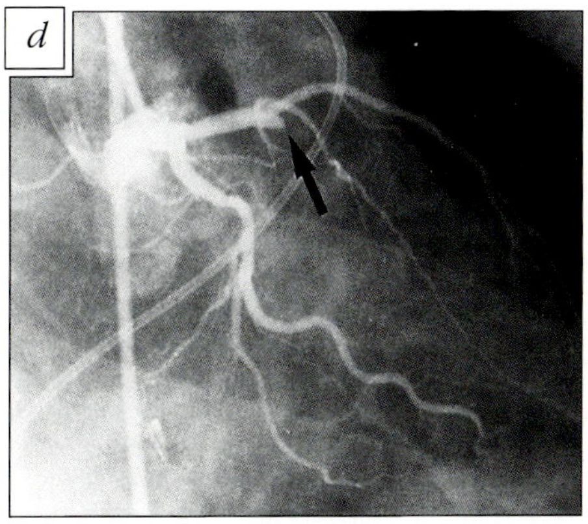

1 h after TPA

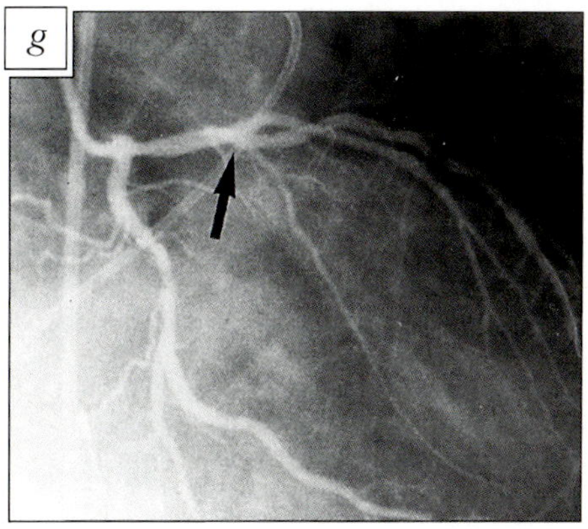

After PTCA

Case Study XI.2

Example of reocclusion after thrombolysis

This 62-year-old woman, obese and with hyperlipidaemia, was admitted with clinical signs of inferior myocardial infarction and was treated with thrombolysis. Maximal CK was 468 units/litre and she recovered quickly. Myocardial imaging was carried out about 24 h after the acute event to assess the amount of perfusion abnormality. The ECG at that time exhibited small Q-waves in leads DII, DIII and aVF and negative T-waves (Fig. XI.2a). Planar scintigraphy demonstrated a small perfusion defect in the inferoapical wall of the LV (Fig. XI.2b, upper panel). When the patient developed atypical chest pain and non-definitive ECG changes characterized by rotation counterclockwise and some T-wave changes (Fig. XI.2c), sestamibi was again injected to monitor potential perfusion changes. A significantly larger perfusion defect with loss of apparent initial gain was noted in the same area and also in the inferoposterior wall of the LV on the LL projection, suggesting reocclusion despite atypical symptoms (Fig. XI.2b, lower panel). Subsequent angiography showed complete RCA occlusion (Fig. XI.2d, arrow).

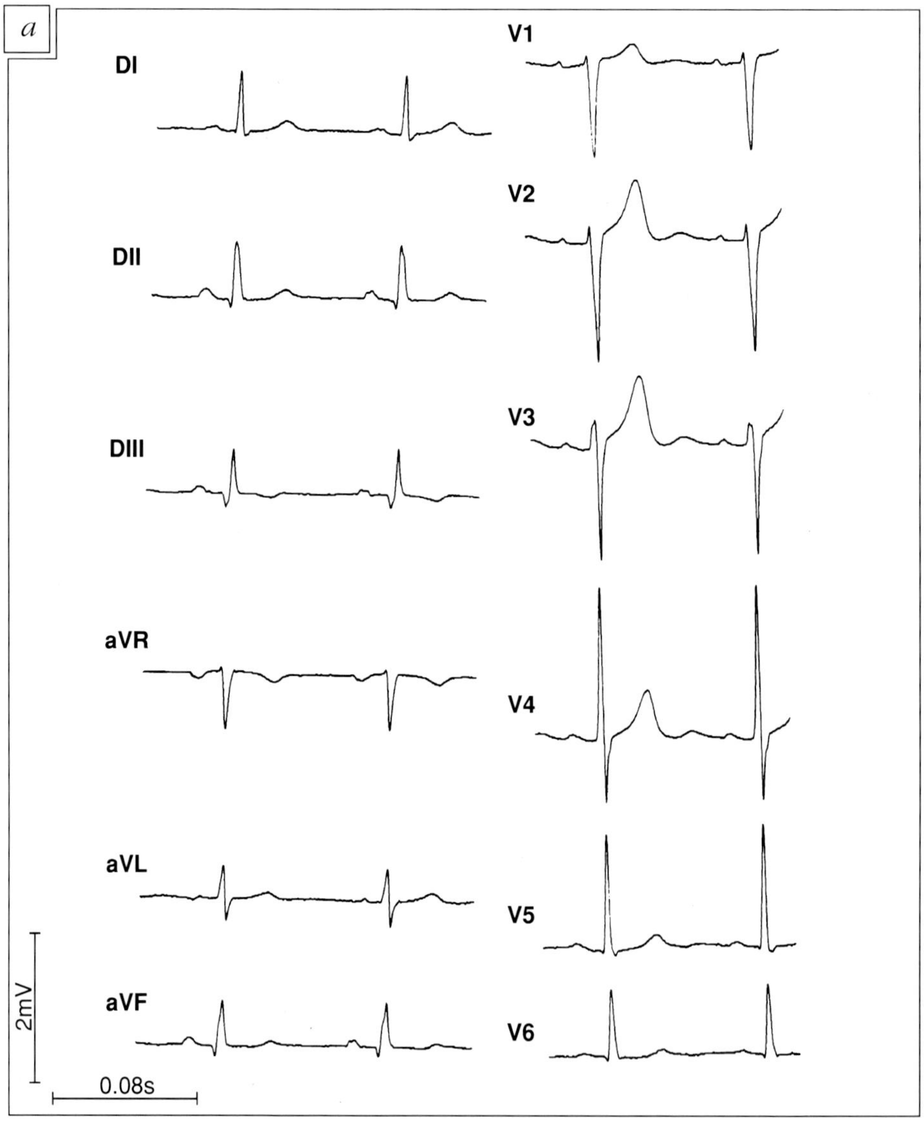

24 hours

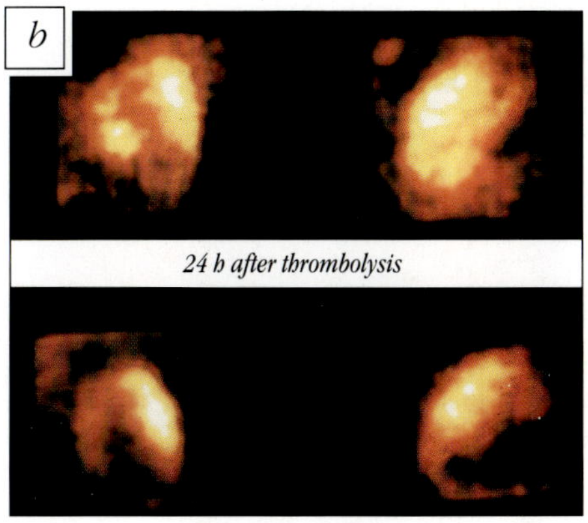

ANT 48 h after thrombolysis LL

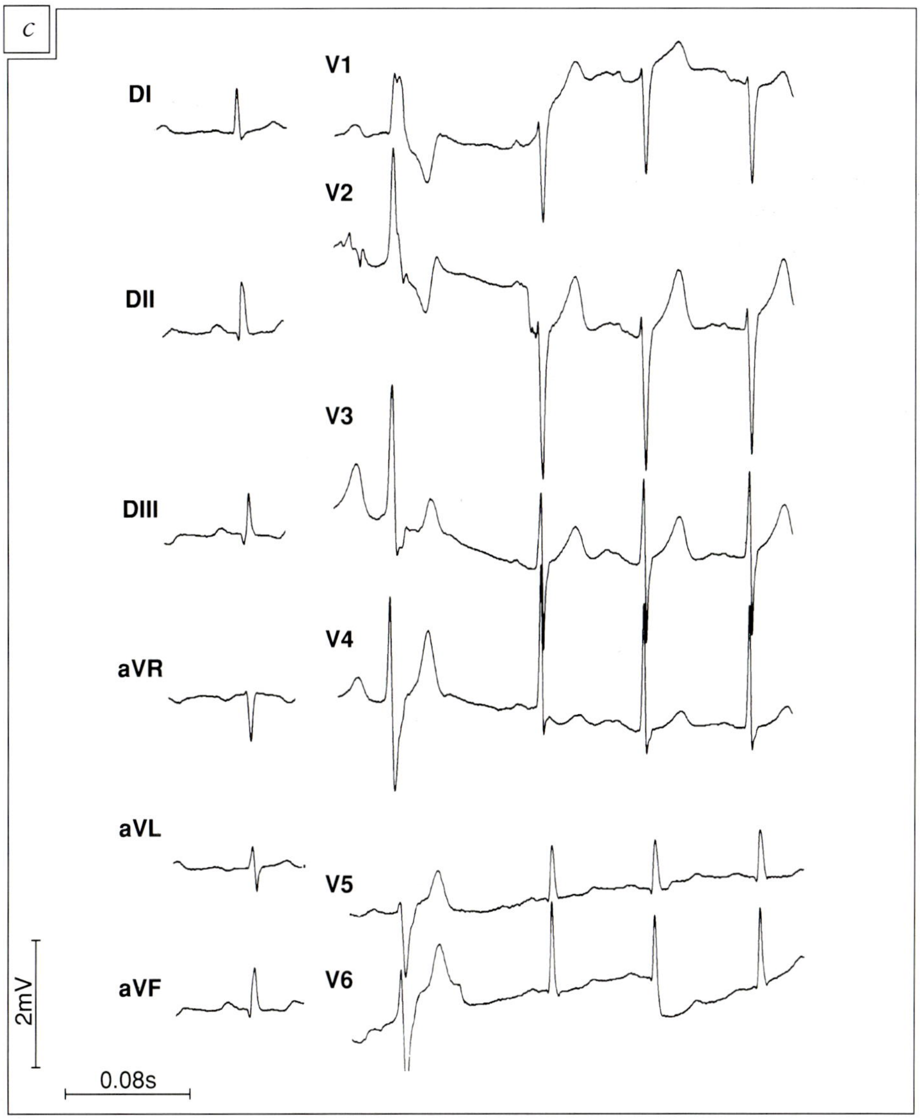

48 hours

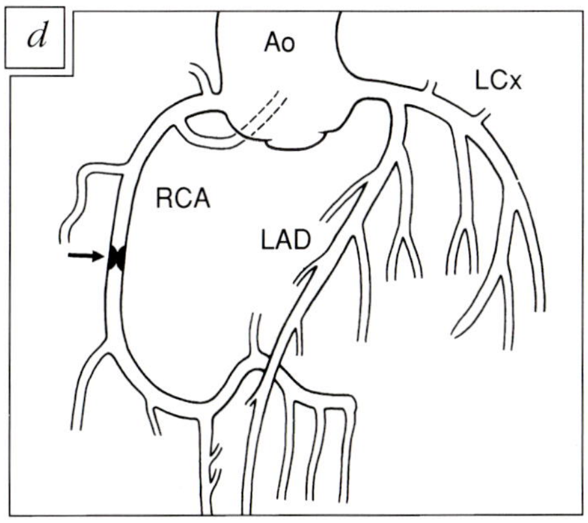

Case Study XI.3

Partial myocardial salvage after thrombolysis

On a rainy Tuesday a truck driver, a heavy smoker for years, experienced some pain at the precordium after changing a tyre on the highway, but continued his journey as he attributed the symptoms to his work on the truck. When home, retrosternal pain became more severe and while he waited for the ambulance, he collapsed. Brought to the hospital, the ECG showed massive ST elevation in all anterior leads. Some Q-waves were already apparent, but the pain persisted (Fig. XI.3a). CPK at that time was 95 units/litre, which is slightly above the normal limit (80 units/litre). Despite a period of around 6½ h having elapsed after onset of symptoms, because of ongoing ischaemia, thrombolysis was carried out. CPK values rose to 1335 units/litre but dropped fairly rapidly.

Planar scintigraphy was performed with sestamibi after injection before onset of thrombolytic treatment. Images obtained in the anterior and in the LAO 60° views 2 h later showed a large perfusion defect in the anteroseptal regions with virtually no uptake in the anteroapical segment (Fig. XI.3b, upper panel).

Images 24 h later after re-injection of the radiotracer still showed a significant defect, especially in the anteroapical segment, but clear improvement in the anteroseptal and partial improvement in the anterolateral regions (Fig. XI.3b, lower panel).

a

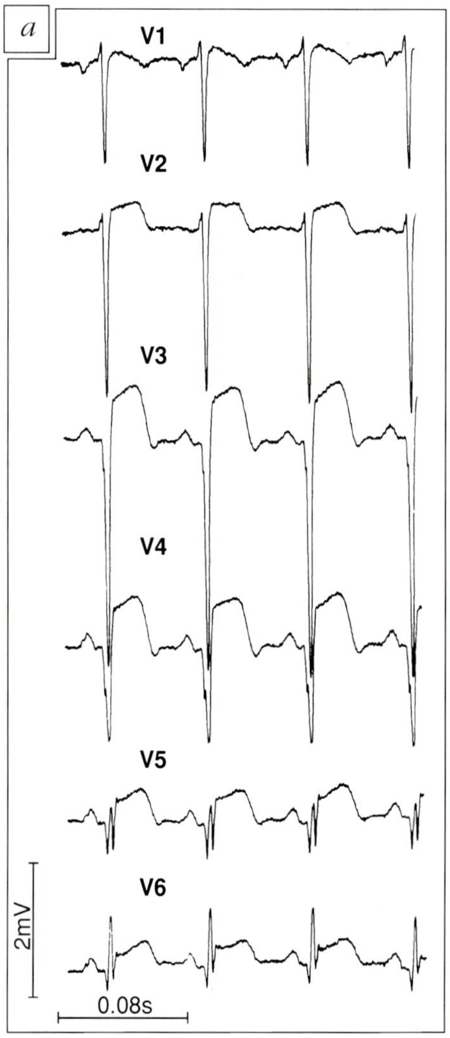

ECG at admission

b

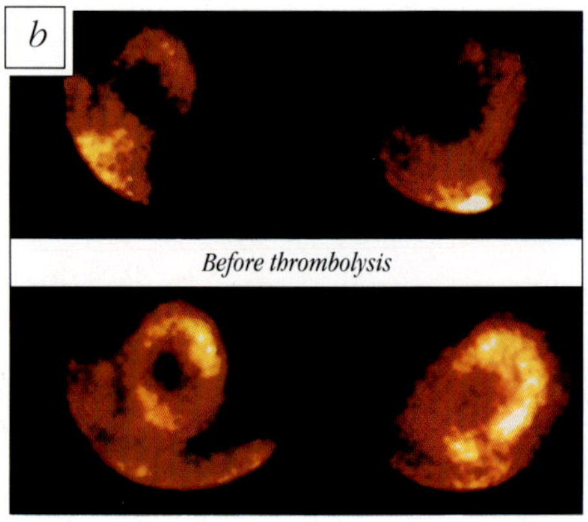

Before thrombolysis

ANT *After thrombolysis* *LAO 60°*

This information suggested at least partial salvage within the area at risk and demonstrated possible intervention benefit despite a longer time between onset of ischaemia and treatment.

Based on the evidence of partial salvage, coronary angiography was performed showing a very proximal, high-grade LAD stenosis, close to the left main segment of the vessel, and a diagonal branch narrowing. Both were dilated by PTCA (LAD – PTCA shown on angiographic image sequence) (Figs. XI.3c,d,e, arrows).

In summary, this case study illustrates the potential of this approach to judge interventional success on a patient-by-patient basis.

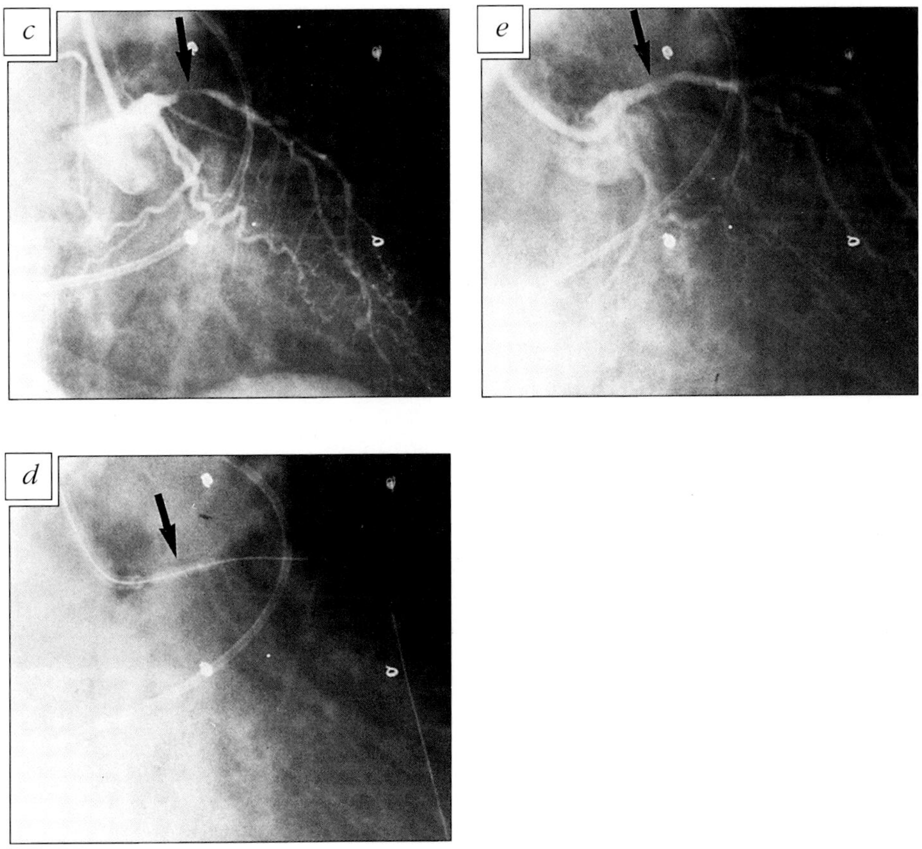

12 PROGNOSIS OF PATIENTS WITH CORONARY ARTERY DISEASE

Clinical Background

Although it has markedly improved over the last decade, the diagnosis of coronary artery disease (CAD) still implies an ominous prognosis. We have learned, however, that this prognosis varies widely among different subsets of patients and we have identified the principal risk factors.[1]

The principal risk factors for the presence of CAD also influence the outcome. They can readily be determined by the cardiologist, whether in the out-patient's clinic or in the hospital. They include:

1 Family history for CAD, positive or negative.
2 Age and sex of the patient.
3 Cholesterol level.
4 Presence of high blood pressure.
5 Presence of diabetes mellitus.
6 And last but not least, whether or not the patient smokes.

Correcting some of those risk factors can alter the prognosis in patients with known disease. For instance, cessation of smoking has a more significant effect, even in patients post-myocardial infarction, than most other interventions including coronary artery bypass grafting! Also crucial to determining prognosis among patients with known CAD are factors requiring specific cardiological investigations. Indeed, prognosis is related not only to the extent of CAD, but even more to the functional consequences of disease on myocardial function. The extent of left ventricular dysfunction, global and regional, is probably the principal prognostic factor in symptomatic patients. Presence or absence of ventricular arrhythmias, although linked to the presence of left ventricular dysfunction, has been shown to be an independent risk factor.

Clinical Problem and Aims of Sestamibi Studies

The task of every cardiologist is therefore to assess each patient's prognosis. More specifically, there is a need to recognize patients at high risk, in whom consideration should be given to more invasive procedures, and patients with low or very low risk, in whom no further testing but only regular follow-up is indicated.

As seen earlier, clinical history can give clues as far as risk factors are concerned, but other techniques, including nuclear cardiology techniques, are indicated to determine the extent of CAD, the level of left ventricular function, and to exclude cardiac arrhythmias.

Using nuclear cardiology techniques, we are able to gather information about the number of coronary arteries that are involved (see Chapter 4), the extent of myocardium that is at risk, and the presence or absence of scar tissue (see Chapter 9). Patients at high risk have large defects or defects pointing to multiple vessel disease or to proximal lesions. In particular, patients with defects in the proximal LAD territory (septum + anterolateral wall) and patients with left main equivalent defects (anterior + posterolateral defects) have a poorer prognosis. Also the presence of reversible abnormalities, isolated or in combination with fixed perfusion defects, implies more severe risk than fixed defects alone[2–7] (see Case Studies IV.3, IV.4, IV.6, VIII.8, X.1 and X.9).

Signs of altered left ventricular function during exercise such as transient cardiac dilatation or tracer lung uptake (mainly seen with thallium, but also recognizable with sestamibi if imaging is done early) also correspond to an increased risk.[8]

Analysis of left and right ventricular function is usually performed using radionuclide ventriculography and is most useful in patients after a myocardial infarction. In these patients the level of left ventricular function is the best predictor of prognosis.[9] Patients with CAD and diffuse severe hypokinesia have a poorer prognosis than patients with focal wall motion abnormalities, even if these abnormalities include aneurysmal formation. Patients with diffuse left and right ventricular dilatation and dysfunction are at especially high risk. The incidence of complications such as mitral inçompetence, ventricular septal rupture, aneurysm or presence of apical thrombi further add to the risk.[10,11]

Patients at low risk are equally easy to categorize using nuclear cardiology techniques.[8] Generally, the perfusion defect is small or not appreciable. At the least, a non-reversible perfusion defect is manifest. Overall, left ventricular function remains good and wall motion abnormalities are not extensive. The left ventricular ejection fraction does not drop with exercise. In patients after successful revascularization, no residual ischaemia can be documented.

Conclusion

Radionuclide investigations of perfusion and function can provide major clues regarding patients at high and low risk in the course of CAD. Although not yet always documented using sestamibi, these non-invasive criteria have proven at least as accurate or more accurate than standard angiographic or other criteria of prognosis.

References

1 Rahimtoola SH, Clinical overview of management of chronic ischemic heart disease, *Circulation* (1991) **84**:I81.

2 Brown KA, Prognostic value of thallium-201 myocardial perfusion imaging, *Circulation* (1991) **83**:363.

3 Iskandrian AS, Hakki AH, Kane-Marsch S, Prognostic implications of exercise thallium-201 scintigraphy in patients with suspected or known coronary artery disease, *Am Heart J* (1985) **110**:135.

4 Kaul S, Lilly DR, Gascho JA et al, Prognostic utility of the exercise thallium-201 test in ambulatory patients with chest pain: comparison with cardiac catheterization, *Circulation* (1988) **77**:745.

5 Fleg JL, Terstenblith G, Zonderman AB et al, Prevalence and prognosis significance of exercise-induced silent myocardial ischemia detected by thallium scintigraphy and electrocardiography in asymptomatic volunteers, *Circulation* (1990) **81**:428.

6 Okada RD, Boucher CA, Kirshenbaum HK et al, Improved diagnostic accuracy of thallium-201 stress test using multiple observers and criteria derived from interobserver analysis of variance, *Am J Cardiol* (1980) **46**:619.

7 Weiner DA, Ryan TJ, McCabe CH et al, Value of exercise testing in determining the risk classification and the response to coronary artery bypass grafting in three-vessel coronary artery disease: a report from the Coronary Artery Surgery Study (CASS) registry, *Am J Cardiol* (1987) **60**:262.

8 Gibson RS, Watson DD, Craddock GB et al, Prediction of cardiac events after uncomplicated myocardial infarction: a prospective study comparing predischarge exercise thallium-201 scintigraphy and angiography, *Circulation* (1983) **68**:321.

9 Multicenter Postinfarction Research Group, Risk stratification and survival after myocardial infarction, *N Engl J Med* (1983) **309**:331.

10 Gibbons RJ, Rest and exercise radionuclide angiography for diagnosis in chronic ischemic heart disease, *Circulation* (1991) **84**:I93.

11 Jones RH, Johnson SH, Bigelow C et al, Exercise radionuclide angiography predicts death in patients with coronary artery disease, *Circulation* (1991) **84**:I52.

13 SESTAMIBI AS A CLINICAL RESEARCH TOOL

The excellent physical characteristics of sestamibi and its pharmacokinetic properties, in particular its low degree of redistribution, have led to new possibilities that are currently being explored by several investigators. These cover both cardiac and non-cardiac applications, like the imaging of parathyroid adenomas and hyperplasia (Case Study XIII.1), the differential diagnosis of thyroid cold nodule, the diagnosis of recurrent brain tumour, etc.[1,2]

Among the new cardiac applications, the use of sestamibi injected during acute coronary symptoms to assess the area at risk of myocardial infarction and serve as baseline to document the success of reperfusion therapy, has already been described in Chapter 11.

Acute injection with delayed imaging also forms the basis for 'differential diagnosis of chest pain' described in Chapter 6. The same principle applies to several clinical and research situations. Intravenous injection in the catheterization laboratory at the time of balloon angioplasty has been used to document the acute functional perfusion bed corresponding to a complete occlusion at the site of a given lesion and validate the concept of acute injection and delayed imaging to estimate the area at risk in man (Case Study XIII.2).[3] These studies have also demonstrated that the size of exercise-induced myocardial ischaemia is not predictive of the size of the total area at risk.[4]

Combined injection of a perfusion tracer, for example, thallium, selectively in the coronary artery, distal to the site of occlusion, and of another tracer, sestamibi, intravenously at the time of balloon occlusion, allows double labelling, positive and negative, of this perfusion bed. In the absence of collaterals, the distribution of these tracers demonstrates no overlap. In the presence of collaterals, however, significant overlap is observed as the intravenously injected sestamibi perfuses whole or part of the coronary bed distal to the point of occlusion. This approach appears attractive for the study of the importance of the collateral circulation (Case Study XIII.3).[4]

Selective intracoronary injection has also been used to determine the size of the myocardial area perfused by a coronary artery. This approach has important educational value by demonstrating the wide variability of myocardial blood supply and coronary anatomy (Case Study XIII.4). It could also potentially be used to differentiate between viable and necrotic myocardium. Although selective intracoronary injection is not usually used for this indication, the absence of overlap between the different coronary artery beds might be useful in some cases.[5]

Finally, selective coronary injection has been used in patients with refractory ventricular rhythm disturbances in whom selective alcohol injection was planned to destroy the site of origin of the tachycardia. Verification by selective coronary branch injection of sestamibi, of the area perfused by the artery supplying the arrhythmogenic area is helpful to assess the safety of the alcoholization procedure.[5]

As previously described by Gewirtz et al in the experimental animal, changes in heart size and geometry can be responsible for changes in myocardial images unrelated to changes in perfusion.[6] Indeed, geometric changes and partial volume effect can result in artefactual zones of hypofixation mainly in the apex. Use of sestamibi has allowed a similar demonstration in man in a patient with aortic valve regurgitation and exercise-induced left ventricular dilatation in the absence of coronary lesions. Immediate post-exercise imaging following previous rest injection of sestamibi demonstrates similar cardiac dilatation and apical hypoperfusion as exercise injection, although the resting sestamibi images were normal (Case Study XIII.5).

Gated perfusion imaging, although logistically more demanding, can be performed as a result of the increased photon flux of technetium-labelled perfusion agents. The potential applications should be divided among those making use of the increased resolution to improve the diagnostic accuracy of perfusion imaging and those utilizing the dynamic sequence to derive information about function as well as perfusion.

Several authors have pointed out the theoretical and practical advantages of frozen diastolic frames to assess myocardial perfusion, free of motion artefacts and less influenced by changes in partial volume effect. Indeed, the coexistence of a wall motion abnormality increases the 'visibility' of a perfusion defect, while on the contrary, functional recovery decreases the ability to visualize a similar perfusion defect on ungated imaging. Diastolic gating maximizes the ability to diagnose perfusion abnormalities in most instances and has been reported to be preferable to ungated images despite the loss in count density (Case Study XIII.6).[7]

Gating of planar images can be used to assess global left ventricular function as demonstrated by Najm and colleagues[8] (see also Case Study VI.3). The radionuclide fractional shortening described by these authors correlates with the left ventricular ejection fraction measured by contrast or radionuclide angiography. Regional wall motion can also be assessed on these images, but the influence of overall cardiac motion must be taken into account in the interpretation of wall motion data, especially if functional images such as difference or amplitude images are used. Evaluation of regional thickening using gated tomographic imaging probably provides a more accurate evaluation of regional wall motion, even though it is certainly influenced by changes in partial volume effect.

Simultaneous assessment of perfusion and function should be helpful in the differential diagnosis of myocardial infarction (MI), complete or incomplete, hibernating myocardium (or chronic myocardial ischaemia), acute myocardial ischaemia and stunned myocardium (persistently dysfunctioning reperfused myocardium).[9] Myocardial infarction is characterized by a combination of marked hypoperfusion and regional dysfunction having led to cell death and membrane disruption. Hibernating myocardium is closely related to MI but the degree of hypoperfusion should be less. Acute ischaemia is accompanied by transient hypoperfusion and dysfunction. Taking into account the absence of sestamibi redistribution, the combination of functional recovery with an abnormal perfusion should be the characteristic pattern of transient ischaemia. On the contrary, stunned myocardium is characterized by prolonged dysfunction despite re-established perfusion (Case Study XIII.7). The examples provided are illustrative of the suggested relationship between uptake and viability. Although more work is required on this question to evaluate the sensitivity, specificity and reproducibility of sestamibi to characterize viable and non-viable myocardium in different clinical conditions, the currently available data appear encouraging.[10] Caution remains appropriate, however, until the clinical relevance of these data is confirmed.

Another approach to combine viability and perfusion assessment has been proposed by the Group at Cedar Sinai. They propose the use of thallium at rest with early or delayed imaging followed by sestamibi at stress. It is also possible in this protocol to perform dual energy simultaneous acquisition of the stress and rest images with optimal comparative superimposition.[11]

Uptake of sestamibi in left ventricular myocardium is proportional to the mass of perfusable tissue. The same is also true for the right ventricle. Like thallium, sestamibi has been proposed to assess right ventricular hypertrophy and dilatation in patients with chronic pulmonary disease or congenital heart disease. Sestamibi, however, provides clearer images of the right ventricle than thallium and its value in diagnosing right ventricular perfusion abnormalities at rest and exercise has been reported. Although not all investigations have been successful, encouraging results have been presented in right myocardial ischaemia and infarction.

Conclusions

The physical and biological characteristics of sestamibi have encouraged investigators to explore new clinical applications using this tracer.

We have illustrated some of the cardiac applications in this chapter. Other applications, in particular non-cardiac applications, do exist, but are beyond the scope of this book.

References

1 O'Doherty JO, Kettle AG, Wells P et al, Parathyroid imaging with Technetium-99m-Sestamibi: preoperative localization and tissue uptake studies, *J Nucl Med* (1992) **33**:313.

2 Hassan IM, Sahweil A, Constantinides C et al, Uptake and kinetics of Tc-99m hexakis 2-methoxy isobutyl isonitrile in benign and malignant lesions in the lungs, *Clin Nucl Med* (1989) **14**:333.

3 Braat SH, De Swart H, Rigo P et al, Value of technetium MIBI to detect short lasting episodes of severe myocardial ischaemia and to estimate the area at risk during coronary angioplasty, *Eur Heart J* (1991) **12**:30.

4 Larock MP, Legrand V, Kulbertus H et al, Assessment of transient myocardial ischemia and of ventricular dysfunction, during PTCA, with MIBI tomography and angiography, *Eur J Nucl Med* (1990) **16**:400.

5 Braat SH, De Swart H, Janssen JH et al, Use of Technetium-99m Sestamibi to determine the size of the myocardial area perfused by a coronary artery, *Am J Cardiol* (1990) **66**:85E.

6 Gewirtz H, Grötte GJ, Strauss HW et al, The influence of left ventricular volume and wall motion on myocardial images, *Circulation* (1979) **59**:1172.

7 Corbett JR, Kahn JK, Akers MS et al, Improved detection of coronary stenosis with gated tomographic assessment of LV segmental perfusion and function with Tc-99m RP-30, *Circulation* (1988) **78**:II192.

8 Najm YC, Timmis AD, Maisey MN et al, The evaluation of ventricular function using gated myocardial imaging with Tc-99m sestamibi, *Eur Heart J* (1989) **10**:142.

9 Rahimtoola SH, The hibernating myocardium, *Am Heart J* (1989) **117**:211.

10 Sinusas AJ, Trautman KA, Bergin JD et al, Quantification of 'area at risk' during coronary occlusion and degree of myocardial salvage after reperfusion with technetium-99m methoxyisobutylisonitrile, *Circulation* (1990) **82**:1424.

11 Berman DS, Kiat H, Van Train K et al, Technetium-99m Sestamibi in the assessment of chronic coronary artery disease, *Sem Nucl Med* (1991) **21**:190.

Case Study XIII.1

Parathyroid imaging using ^{99m}Tc sestamibi

Parathyroid imaging is usually performed using thallium and technetium. It appears advantageous, however, to substitute sestamibi for thallium and ^{123}I for technetium. Using these isotopes, 3–4 h after iodine administration (for optimal image quality, although imaging could be performed earlier), sestamibi is injected and the patients studied 10–15 min later. Imaging of both isotopes is performed simultaneously in separate energy windows maximizing anatomical overlap and suppressing the need for realignment.

Normalization is performed by correlation analysis of the two images (in a large region of interest encompassing the thyroid by excluding the salivary glands) and followed by subtraction of the iodine image from the sestamibi image.

This technique results in clear images of parathyroid adenomas against a low background. In Fig. XIII.1a, the parathyroid adenoma is well visualized at the upper part of the right thyroid lobe (arrows). The salivary glands are also visualized on the difference image.

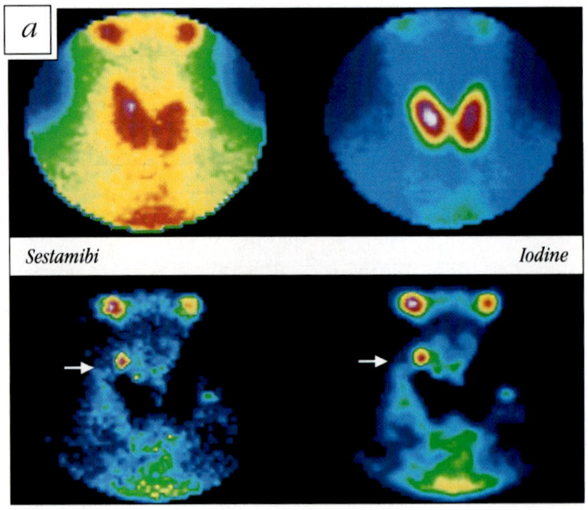

Subtraction (Sestamibi – Iodine)

Case Study XIII.2

Demonstration of the area at risk of complete coronary occlusion by imaging after sestamibi injection during PTCA

This patient with single vessel left anterior descending (LAD) stenosis had percutaneous transluminal coronary angioplasty (PTCA) for symptomatic angina pectoris interfering with his daily activities (Fig. XIII.2a, arrow). Sestamibi imaging performed before PTCA demonstrated a perfusion abnormality at stress in the LAD territory (Fig. XIII.2b, upper panel). Sestamibi was injected intravenously during the PTCA procedure and delayed imaging demonstrated a large perfusion defect reflecting the area at risk of an acute occlusion (Fig. XIII.2c, top panel). On the same figure, the resulting normal stress images after PTCA was illustrated (lower panel). Angiographic results after PTCA were also excellent (Fig. XIII.2d, arrow). Ventriculography performed during balloon occlusion demonstrated the functional consequences of acute myocardial ischaemia. A large antero-apical akinetic area was demonstrated in this right anterior oblique (RAO) projection ventriculogram (Fig. XIII.2e, lower panel, arrows) corresponding to the large perfusion defect.

This case illustrates the value of acute injection of sestamibi with delayed imaging to visualize the area at risk during an acute occlusion as also applied in the setting of acute MI.

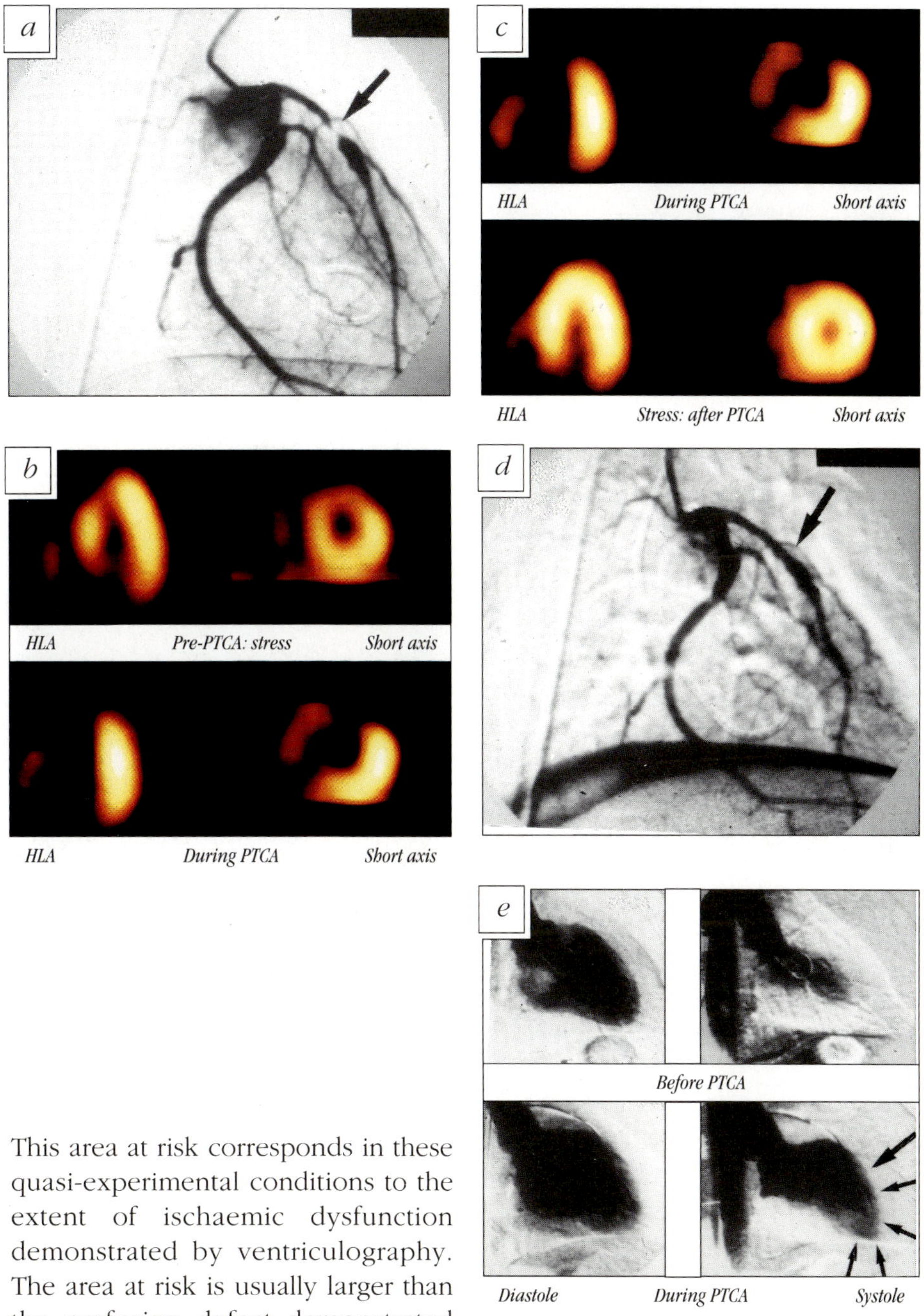

This area at risk corresponds in these quasi-experimental conditions to the extent of ischaemic dysfunction demonstrated by ventriculography. The area at risk is usually larger than the perfusion defect demonstrated during exercise-induced ischaemia, as the latter is influenced by the variable intensity of the exercise.

Case Study XIII.3

Demonstration of collateral blood flow by dual isotope imaging

This patient with anteroseptal ischaemia and stenosis was studied during the course of an LAD angioplasty. Contrast injection in the proximal left system at the time of balloon occlusion demonstrated collateral blood flow to the distal LAD beyond the balloon occlusion (Fig. XIII.3a, arrows). Intravenous sestamibi injection resulted in images demonstrating only mild anteroapical perfusion defects. The distribution of thallium injected directly in the LAD distal to the occlusion overlapped with sestamibi distribution (Fig. XIII.3b). The limited size of the perfusion defect during balloon occlusion and the presence of thallium/sestamibi overlap reflected the functional value of the collateral flow. In contrast, in a patient with LAD stenosis without angiographically demonstrated collaterals, the sestamibi perfusion defect was marked and no significant overlap with thallium was present (Fig. XIII.3c).

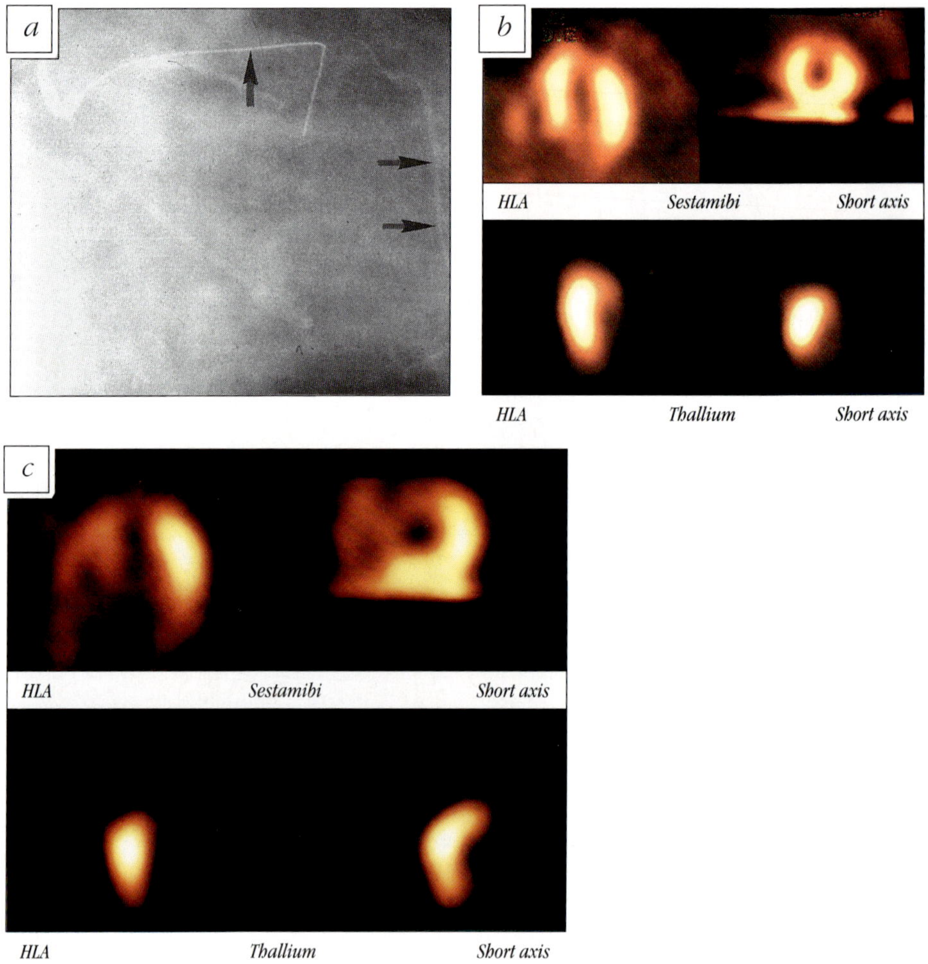

Case Study XIII.4

Large and small perfusion defects using intracoronary injection of sestamibi

Intracoronary injection of sestamibi can be performed at the time of coronary angiography to define, by delayed imaging, the perfusion territory of a given coronary artery or branch, as explained earlier in this chapter.

Figure XIII.4a displays the perfusion territory of a dominant right coronary artery (RCA) supplying, in addition to the right ventricle (RV), a large portion of the inferoposterior wall of the left ventricle (LV), as well as the inferior portion of the septum.

Figure XIII.4b displays another case in which the perfusion territory of the RV is smaller and mainly limited to the inferoposterior wall.

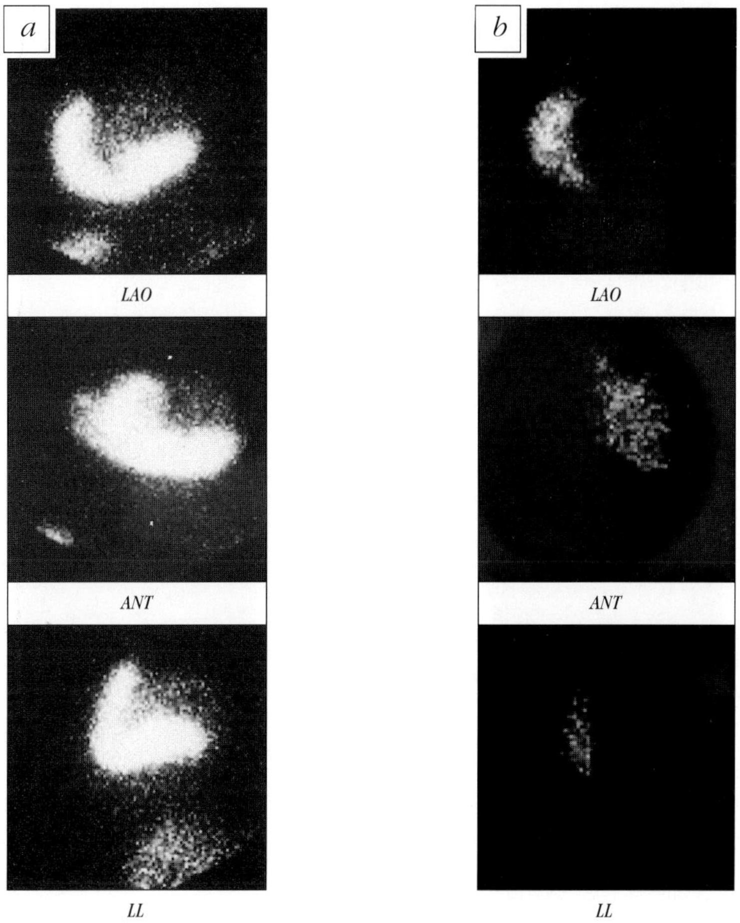

Case Study XIII.5

Changes in heart size and geometry responsible for an apical defect in a patient without CAD

A 64-year-old man with aortic valve disease and angina pectoris is studied by exercise myocardial scanning using ^{201}Tl. This study (Fig. XIII.5a, arrows) demonstrates an abnormal scan with left ventricular dilatation and an apical defect. These abnormalities disappear with redistribution while the LV diminishes in size (Fig. XIII.5b).

Cardiac catheterization demonstrated significant aortic regurgitation but the absence of coronary artery lesion. To confirm the hypothesis that the apical defect resulted from left ventricular dilatation and partial volume effect, the exercise test was repeated using ^{99m}Tc sestamibi pre-injected at rest and imaged at rest 1 h after injection, and subsequently after exercise without re-injection. The sestamibi rest study was normal (Fig. XIII.5c). With exercise, an apical defect developed again, together with left ventricular dilatation (Fig. XIII.5d, arrows).

In this case, the properties of sestamibi (absence of significant redistribution) allowed us to demonstrate the role of ventricular dilatation and partial volume effect on myocardial images and to distinguish these changes from perfusion abnormalities.

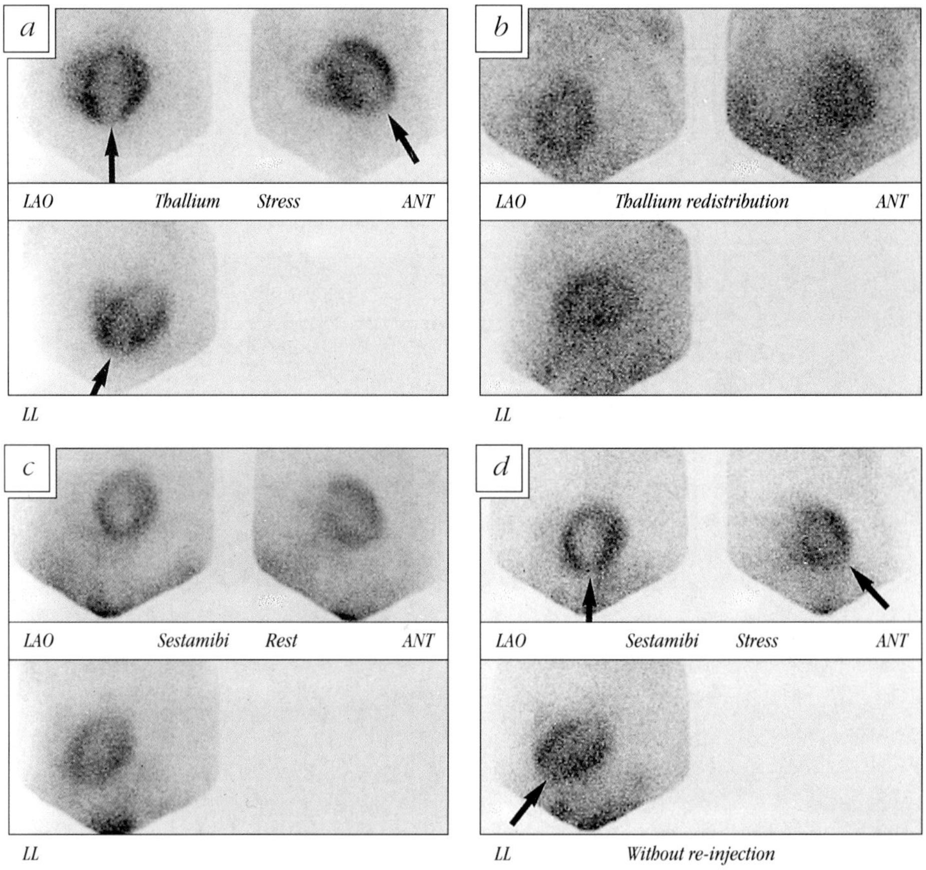

Case Study XIII.6

Gated sestamibi tomographic imaging to assess myocardial perfusion and function

These images (Fig. XIII.6a) were obtained in a patient with a previous inferolateral MI. The perfusion abnormality involving the inferior wall on the short axis view, and the posterolateral wall on the horizontal long axis (HLA) view can be appreciated on both the diastolic and systolic frames. The perfusion defect is seen with greater contrast on the diastolic frame (especially in the short axis view). However, the systolic frame concomitantly demonstrates the systolic deformation of the ventricular silhouette resulting from myocardial dysfunction (especially in the posterolateral region). Also noteworthy on these images is the presence of a zone of relative hypofixation in the apical area. This relative hypofixation is a normal finding given the smaller thickness of the apex and the partial volume effect. It disappears, however, during systole consecutive to the normal apical wall thickening, providing further evidence for normality.

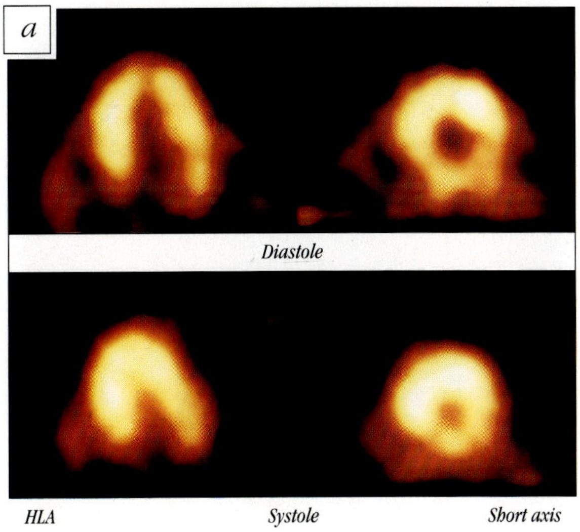

Case Study XIII.7

Myocardial dysfunction following reperfusion: myocardial stunning

Regional myocardial function may not recover for weeks after successful reperfusion in patients treated by fibrinolysis for impending MI.

The patient illustrated here has been treated by fibrinolysis for an acute lateral infarction. Perfusion images in diastole and systole (short axis view) demonstrate heterogeneous perfusion in the anterolateral wall, remaining abnormal in the superior region but partially re-established in the lateral region (Fig. XIII.7a). Functional images (systole minus diastole), however, demonstrate persistent wall motion abnormality in this area corresponding to myocardial stunning (Fig. XIII.7b, arrow), while partial re-establishment of flow attests to this region's viability.

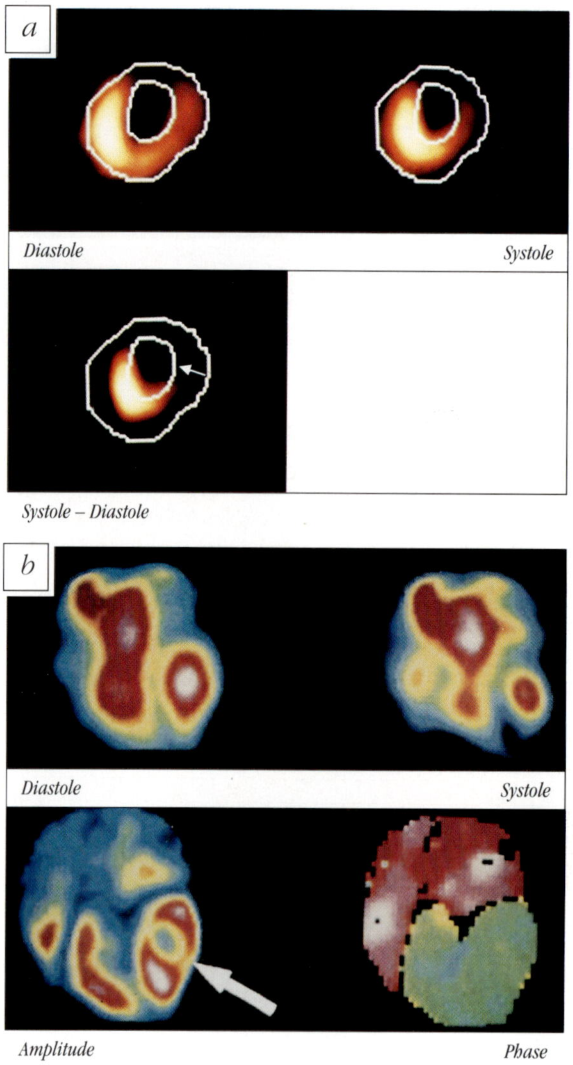

Case Study XIII.8

High FDG uptake in a patient with unstable angina and hibernating myocardium

Mrs CD is a 65-year-old female suffering from recent inferoposterior MI (1 month earlier). She was admitted for recurrent chest pain and the resting ECG showed episodes of ST–T wave abnormalities in the posterolateral region (leads DI and V6). She was treated for unstable angina. Two days later she was submitted for a positron emission tomography (PET) FDG/flow study to assess myocardial ischaemia and viability.

The PET shows an abnormal perfusion scan (Fig. XIII.8a, left, upper panel) with decreased uptake of the flow tracer in the lateral wall of the LV. However, this lateral wall concentrates glucose preferentially in this region while the anteroseptal wall has low FDG uptake (Fig. XIII.8a, right, upper panel).

This patient was submitted to revascularization and studied again later. The posterolateral wall is better perfused while regional wall motion has improved and ischaemia is no longer discernible (Fig. XIII. 8a, left, lower panel).

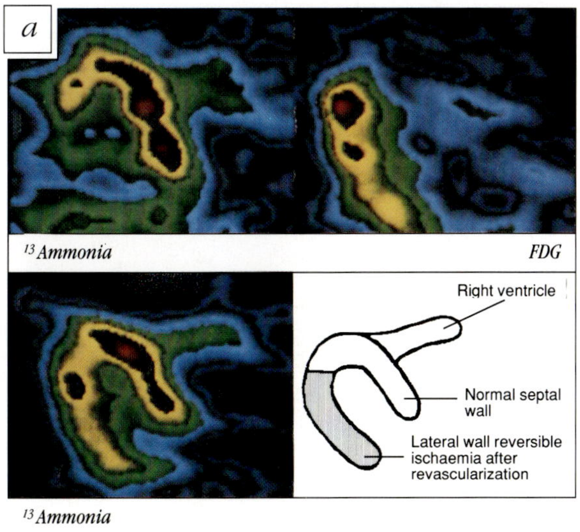

This case illustrates the potential benefits of revascularization in patients with unstable angina and ischaemic but viable (hibernating) myocardium.

At present no studies have been reported comparing ammonia and sestamibi in this setting. However, several institutions have started to use sestamibi in combination with FDG to assess myocardial viability.

INDEX

References under 'Sestamibi' and 'Perfusion' are only to the techniques and principles referring to those headings. Readers should refer themselves to the specific cardiac conditions in which sestamibi and myocardial perfusion are used.

Abbreviations used: CAD, coronary artery disease.